For Churchill Livingstone:

Senior Commissioning Editor: Ninette Premdas
Project Development Manager: Mairi McCubbin
Project Manager: Jane Dingwall
Designer: Judith Wright
Illustrations Manager: Bruce Hogarth

Coronary Heart Disease Prevention

A Handbook for the Health-Care Team

Edited by

Grace M. Lindsay BSc(Hons) PhD RGN RM

Reader in Clinical Nursing Research,
Glasgow Caledonian University, Glasgow, UK

Allan Gaw MB ChB MD PhD

Director of Clinical Trials Unit,
Glasgow Royal Infirmary, Glasgow, UK

Second Edition

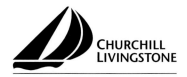

CHURCHILL
LIVINGSTONE

EDINBURGH LONDON NEW YORK OXFORD PHILADELPHIA ST LOUIS SYDNEY TORONTO 2004

CHURCHILL LIVINGSTONE
An imprint of Elsevier Science Limited

First edition 1997
Second edition 2004

ISBN 0 443 07117 9

British Library Cataloguing in Publication Data
A catalogue record for this book is available from the British Library

Library of Congress Cataloging in Publication Data
A catalog record for this book is available from the Library of Congress

Note
Medical knowledge is constantly changing. Standard safety
precautions must be followed, but as new research and clinical
experience broaden our knowledge, changes in treatment and
drug therapy may become necessary or appropriate. Readers are
advised to check the most current product information provided
by the manufacturer of each drug to be administered to verify the
recommended dose, the method and duration of administration, and
contraindications. It is the responsibility of the practitioner, relying on
experience and knowledge of the patient, to determine dosages and
the best treatment for each individual patient. Neither the Publisher
nor the editors or contributors assume any liability for any injury
and/or damage to persons or property arising from this publication.

The Publisher

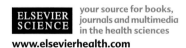

your source for books,
journals and multimedia
in the health sciences
www.elsevierhealth.com

The
publisher's
policy is to use
**paper manufactured
from sustainable forests**

Printed in China by Elsevier

Contents

Contributors

Gillian E. Armstrong BSc MCSP
Senior Physiotherapist, Cardiac Rehabilitation,
Glasgow Royal Infirmary University NHS Trust, Glasgow, UK

Kanarath P. Balachandran MBBS MD MRCP(UK)
Specialist Registrar in Cardiology, Southmead Hospital and
Bristol Royal Infirmary, Bristol, UK

Paul Bennett BA(Hons) MSc PhD
Director of Research, Bristol Doctoral Training Programme in Clinical
Psychology, University of Bristol, Bristol, UK

Douglas Carroll BSc PhD
Professor of Applied Psychology, School of Sport and Exercise Sciences,
University of Birmingham, Birmingham, UK

Joan L. Curzio PhD RGN
Project Leader, Research Initiative for Scotland, Glasgow Caledonian
University, Glasgow, UK. Formerly Nurse Researcher,
Department of Medicine and Therapeutics, University of Glasgow,
Western Infirmary, Glasgow, UK

Parijat De MD MRCP
Specialist Registrar, Diabetes and Endocrinology,
University Hospital of Wales, Cardiff, UK

Marc Evans MD MRCP
Lecturer in Medicine, Department of Medicine,
University Hospital of Wales, Cardiff, UK

Elizabeth Farish PhD FRCPath
Consultant Biochemist, Department of Biochemistry,
Stobhill NHS Trust, Glasgow, UK

Allan Gaw MB ChB MD PhD
Director of Clinical Trials Unit, Glasgow Royal Infirmary,
Glasgow, UK

Bruce A. Griffin BSC PhD RPHNutr
Reader in Nutritional Metabolism, Centre for Nutrition and Food Safety,
School of Biological and Life Sciences, University of Surrey,
Guildford, UK

Susan S. Kennedy BSc RGN DN SCM
Nurse Co-ordinator, Distance Education,
Nursing and Midwifery School, Glasgow, UK

Grace M. Lindsay BSc(Hons) PhD RGN RM
Reader in Clinical Nursing Research, Glasgow Caledonian University,
Glasgow, UK

A. Ross Lorimer MD FRCP (Glasgow, London, Edinburgh)
Honorary Professor in Medicine, Consultant Physician and Cardiologist,
Glasgow Royal Infirmary, Glasgow, UK

Gordon T. McInnes BSc PhD MD FRCP FFPM
Senior Lecturer and Honorary Consultant Physician,
Department of Medicine and Therapeutics, University of Glasgow,
Western Infirmary, Glasgow, UK

Laura McIntosh BN RGN
Heart Failure Nurse Specialist, Greater Glasgow Primary Care Trust,
Glasgow, UK

Doreen McIntyre MA(Hons) MPH PGCE
Chief Executive, No Smoking Day, London, UK

Keith G. Oldroyd MD(Hons) MRCP
Consultant Cardiologist, Hairmyres Hospital, East Kilbride, UK

Alan Rees BSc MD FRCP
Consultant Physician, University Hospital of Wales, Cardiff, UK

James Shepherd PhD FRCPath FRCP FRSE
Professor of Pathological Biochemistry and Honorary Consultant Clinical
Biochemist, Department of Pathological Biochemistry, Glasgow Royal
Infirmary, Glasgow, UK

Nicola Walker MRCP BSc(Hons)
Research Fellow, Department of Medical Cardiology,
Glasgow Royal Infirmary, Glasgow, UK

Kirsten A. Whitehead BSc(Hons) SRD DipADP MPN
Senior Dietitian, Department of Dietetics and Nutrition,
Nottingham City Hospital, Nottingham, UK

Preface

The prevention of coronary heart disease (CHD) has never been more important. Throughout the world death rates from cardiovascular causes are rising and are estimated to overtake infectious diseases as the leading global cause of death for the first time in human history. Underlying these trends are important and encouraging figures from many developed countries where CHD rates are now falling. However, in others the rates are rising, and rising fast. Currently, it is estimated that in the time it has taken you to read to the end of this first paragraph approximately 12 more people have died of CHD throughout the world.

Since the first edition of this handbook was published in 1997 there has been a remarkable number of new developments in the various fields that collectively contribute to the prevention of coronary disease. It was our aim with the first edition to capture the essential information from each of these diverse fields of practice and bring them together in a single volume for the health-care professional. With this second edition, our aim remains unchanged. However, virtually every component chapter has had to be extensively revised and rewritten to accommodate the important developments noted above. New large lipid-lowering drug trials have consolidated and extended our understanding of the importance of this treatment strategy. Similarly, therapeutic advances in the use of thrombolytic, antiplatelet and antihypertensive drugs, as well as the introduction of new drugs to manage diabetes, have altered our clinical practice. Cardiac rehabilitation has developed further and become firmly established in most centres, while antismoking therapy and the use and prescription of exercise are now regarded as key components of any preventive programme. Advances in our use of dietary advice and in particular the introduction of functional foods have also altered clinical practice.

These developments are amongst those that our co-authors have carefully incorporated into their chapters. The writing team, from across the health-care professional spectrum, has been joined by some new members in this edition. We welcome our new contributors and congratulate all our authors on focusing on the essential knowledge base required for a clear understanding of CHD prevention in practice; it is a practical approach to this subject that we have tried to promote.

This book, like the first edition, is written for those health-care professionals who are actively engaged in clinical practice: who are seeing patients on a daily basis and who need a handbook to assist them in assimilating the ever-expanding knowledge base upon which their practice is built. We hope that this second edition, updated, revised and reformatted, will prove as useful and as popular as the first.

Grace M. Lindsay
Allan Gaw
Glasgow 2004

ACKNOWLEDGEMENT

The volume editors wish to thank those authors who originated some of the chapters in the last edition and whose work has provided the foundation for the current volume: Douglas Carrol and Elizabeth Keith.

Coronary heart disease: epidemiology, pathology and diagnosis

1

Nicola Walker   A. Ross Lorimer

■ CONTENTS

EPIDEMIOLOGY

Worldwide, one third of all deaths each year are due to cardiovascular diseases, including 7 million heart attacks and 5 million strokes (WHO 2001). Coronary heart disease (CHD) is the single most important cause of death and, more importantly, the single biggest cause of premature death in modern, industrialized countries. CHD covers a spectrum of diseases including angina, acute coronary syndromes, myocardial infarction, ischaemic cardiomyopathy with chronic heart failure, and a proportion of cases of sudden cardiac death. The CHD mortality in Western countries reached a peak in the late 1960s, since when there has been a substantial decline in the mortality rates. Despite this, in 1998 in the United Kingdom 22% of all deaths were attributed to CHD – one in four men and one in five women (Heart Statistics 2001). There are no grounds for complacency as CHD is an increasing cause of death in Central and Eastern Europe and Asia (Tunstall-Pedoe et al 1999).

Since 1979, throughout the world, all registered health events have been coded using the International Statistical Classification of Diseases, Injuries and Cause of Death (ICD, 10th revision). For health events related to CHD, ICD numbers 410–414 are used. In most epidemiological studies, CHD events are defined by these ICD codes and this allows useful comparison between different populations.

The factors that impact on the epidemiology of CHD include age, gender, geography, ethnic origin and socio-economic class.

Age, gender and geography

The rates of CHD increase with increasing age. Mortality rates are generally much higher for men than women. The MONICA (WHO Monitoring Trends and Determinants in Cardiovascular Disease) project has shown that the coronary event rates in women averaged 24% of those of men (Tunstall-Pedoe et al 1999). The gender distinction is present at all ages but is less after the menopause. Coronary morbidity and mortality rates in women generally lag behind those for men by about 10 years, but beyond the seventh decade in life become similar in men and women.

The trends in CHD mortality rates over a 10-year period from the mid-1980s for men and women in 27 countries are shown in Figure 1.1. There is a wide variation in these mortality rates, the highest coronary event rate for men being found in North Karelia, Finland, and for women in Glasgow, UK.

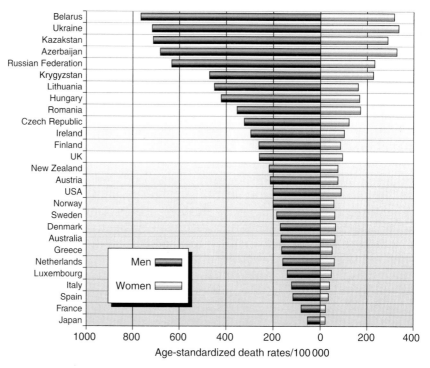

Figure 1.1 International comparison of incidence of coronary heart disease (adapted from BHF website www.heartstats.org/homepage.asp).

The lowest rates for men were found in Beijing, China, and in Catalonia, Spain, for women (Tunstall-Pedoe et al 1999).

Since 1970, worldwide trends in coronary event rates in men show a dramatic decline in countries such as the USA (Cooper et al 2000) and many Western and Northern European countries, for example by 38% in Finland between 1984 and 1994. In contrast, countries in Central and Eastern Europe and Asia have shown marked increases (41% between 1984 and 1994 in Romania) as the population risk profile worsens (Tunstall-Pedoe et al 1999). It is generally accepted that these falls have resulted from a combination of risk factor modification (e.g. improved diet and reduced smoking) and medical interventions (e.g. coronary care units, defibrillators, and thrombolysis).

In Scotland, approximately 500 000 people have CHD, with 180 000 requiring treatment for symptomatic disease. Since 1986, the proportion of deaths in Scotland caused by CHD has fallen from 29% to 23%. However, although age-adjusted mortality has declined from its peak in the early 1970s, approximately 12 500 Scots die from CHD each year, many prematurely (Lorimer 2001). These findings are similar nationwide and the National Service Framework for Coronary Heart Disease drew international comparisons, as demonstrated in Figure 1.2 (DoH 2000).

Ethnic origin

Studies of ethnic groups within the United Kingdom have demonstrated a higher than average CHD prevalence within the South Asian community (Bangladeshis and Pakistanis more than Indians (Bhopal et al 1999)) and a lower than average prevalence in those of Afro-Caribbean origin (Cappuccio 1997).

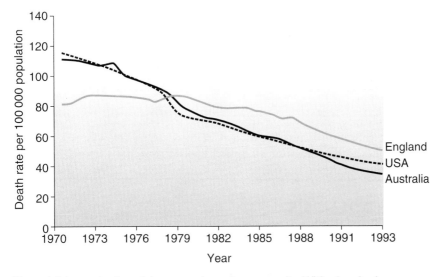

Figure 1.2 International trends in coronary heart disease mortality. Whilst there has been a reduction in mortality in all three of the countries illustrated, it is worrying that England has failed to achieve the level of reduction seen in either the USA or Australia.

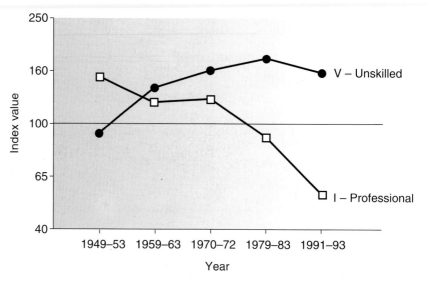

Figure 1.3 Effect of socio-economic class on the demographics of coronary heart disease mortality over time.

Social class

CHD mortality varies across different social classes. Rates in the most deprived groups are much greater than those seen in the affluent groups (Fig. 1.3) (DoH 2000). It is interesting to note that the current relationship between affluence and CHD is a reversal of the previous situation. When CHD first emerged as an important cause of death it apparently occurred predominantly in social class I. People in this group have made lifestyle modifications and diminished their risk of CHD but now, as the disease emerges in non-Westernized countries, it is once again the most affluent who are susceptible. This has important implications for both aetiology and treatment.

A search for the origins, cause and subsequent prevention of CHD has proceeded from early epidemiological studies of populations to prospective cohort studies where a population sample is identified, clinically assessed and then monitored for a number of years for signs of disease. The MONICA study has allowed international comparison. The aetiology of CHD has therefore been the subject of intense study over the last five decades and many contributory or risk factors have been identified. These are discussed in detail in Chapter 2.

ATHEROGENESIS

The spectrum of diseases encompassed by the title CHD has a common pathology – coronary artery narrowing as a consequence of atherosclerosis. Until recently, atherosclerosis was thought to be a progressive process resistant to modification and it was thought that the severity of the resultant disease reflected the degree of arterial obstruction. The observation that

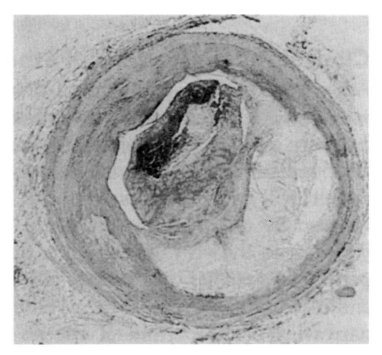

Figure 1.4 Histopathological specimen showing the consequences of acute plaque rupture with thrombus formation.

a modest stenosis, as observed at angiography, can be associated with subsequent coronary thrombosis has resulted in a re-evaluation of the underlying pathology. Atherosclerosis is now recognized to be a dynamic pathological process, which is defined as a focal, inflammatory fibroproliferative response to multiple forms of endothelial injury. The majority of fatal thromboses are due to atherosclerotic plaque rupture, when the coagulation cascade is activated by exposure to the thrombogenic contents of the plaque (Fig. 1.4).

Recent studies have tried to define what makes an atherosclerotic plaque vulnerable to rupture, and how to modify the plaque to reduce this risk. It has become clear that the composition of the plaque is of greater significance than the actual size of the lesion.

All infants have focal thickening of the coronary artery intima due to smooth muscle cell proliferation. Although this is an important hallmark of the developing atherosclerotic plaque, it is not unique to this condition as it is considered to be a simple adaptive response.

The first abnormalities to be recognized as truly atherosclerotic are fatty streaks. These are small lesions that on inspection are hardly raised and are caused by focal collections of foam cells within the intima. Foam cells are lipid-rich cells usually derived from macrophages, but smooth muscle cells can also become foam cells. Necropsy studies in children and young adults (Stary 1989) reveal the presence of atherosclerotic plaques ranging in size from the fatty streak to larger plaques. The fatty streak lesion may be the precursor of larger atherosclerotic plaques but also may be an entirely reversible phenomenon. This has been confirmed from necropsy studies of infants from societies around the world where atherosclerosis as a cause of death is relatively rare. These infants, although unlikely to have died from CHD if they had lived to maturity, have many fatty streaks in their arteries.

Progression of the fatty streak to a larger, more complex lesion is thought to occur via two key processes. First the foam cells, engorged with lipid, begin to die and break down in the centre of the fatty streak. Release of their cytoplasmic content leads to the presence of extracellular lipids and the secretion of growth factors as part of the inflammatory response.

Smooth muscle cell proliferation and migration from the media is the second process involved in the progression of the fatty streak. Smooth muscle cells push into the lipid-rich plaque where they divide and begin to synthesize a connective tissue matrix composed of elastic fibre proteins, collagen and proteoglycans. Both the increase in cell numbers and the laying down of collagenous matrix serve to increase the bulk of the plaque, which now protrudes into the artery lumen and is referred to as a raised fibrolipid or advanced plaque. The central core of the plaque is lipid rich and is surrounded by the fibrous cap – a composite of smooth muscle cells, macrophages, T lymphocytes and occasional mast cells. The presence of T cells reflects the active inflammatory nature of the plaque.

The stability of the plaque is defined by the strength of the fibrous cap. Smooth muscle cells produce collagen fibrils that add support to the plaque and these cells repair and maintain the cap. The inflammatory cells in the cap control the release of cytokines which can induce premature apoptosis (programmed cell death) of smooth muscle cells and thus destabilize the fibrous cap. These cytokines can also trigger apoptosis of endothelial cells, revealing the subendothelial matrix that is rich in tissue factor, which is a potent stimulus of the coagulation cascade (Libby 2001).

Plaque rupture and thrombosis

The features of a vulnerable plaque – one which is at risk of rupture and consequent thrombosis – include a thin fibrous cap, a large volume of inflammatory cells, a small number of smooth muscle cells and a large lipid core (Kolodgie et al 2001). Stable plaques differ mainly by their thick fibrous cap enclosing the lipid core and preventing exposure of the core to the circulating blood (Fig. 1.5).

Davies & Thomas (1985) have shown that in patients with either crescendo angina or acute myocardial infarction, thrombus formation is an important, rapidly changing and dynamic process. Post-mortem studies have shown that coronary thrombi are nearly all related to the rupture of an atheromatous plaque. The initial clot which forms is an aggregation of platelets (white thrombus), but with time the initiation of the coagulation cascade results in a fibrinous clot developing (red thrombus). The existence of these two types of clots helps explain the mechanisms by which some of the pharmacological agents act (see Chapter 9 for further detail).

The factors that determine the degree of occlusion of the artery lumen are partly local, including the size and geometry of the intimal tear, whether

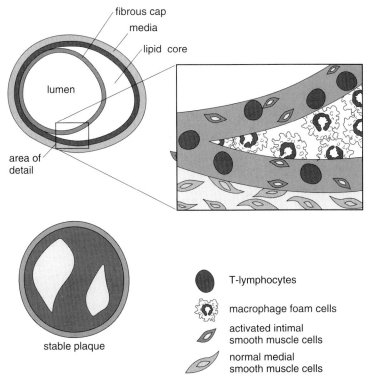

fibrous cap
media
lipid core
lumen
area of detail

T-lymphocytes

macrophage foam cells

activated intimal smooth muscle cells

normal medial smooth muscle cells

stable plaque

Figure 1.5 Illustration of the features of a vulnerable plaque compared to a stable plaque. Note the thin fibrous cap and lipid-rich core of the vulnerable plaque (adapted from Rackley 2001).

lipid is extruded into the lumen itself, the degree of stenosis and blood flow rate at the site. The systemic thrombotic or thrombolytic potential at the time also plays a part in determining the extent of obstruction. Not all plaque fissuring will result in these dire consequences. The plaque may restabilize and heal over but at a cost – the healed plaque will now be larger than before (Davies 1995).

Regression of the atherosclerotic plaque

The concept of therapeutic intervention producing reversal or regression of atherosclerotic lesions originated in the 1940s. Post-mortem examinations on individuals who had suffered great weight losses prior to their death not related to malignancy revealed that the extent of plaque development in the aorta and coronary arteries was much less than expected. Many studies have been conducted to confirm and evaluate these observations.

Lifestyle

In the Lifestyle Heart Trial (Ornish et al 1998), the objective was to determine if lifestyle changes in diet, exercise, smoking and stress could affect coronary atherosclerosis. Patients with angiographically documented CHD were assigned to an experimental group or to a usual care control group.

The experimental group patients were prescribed a regimen that included a low-fat vegetarian diet, smoking cessation, stress management training, moderate aerobic exercise and group support. After only 1 year, patients in the experimental group showed significant overall regression of coronary atherosclerosis in contrast to the control group who, having made less comprehensive lifestyle changes, showed significant overall progression of coronary atherosclerosis. After 5 years, these findings were confirmed with reduced severity of coronary artery stenoses and reduced numbers of myocardial infarctions, cardiac-related hospital admissions and cardiovascular deaths in the experimental group (Ornish et al 1998).

Lipid-lowering therapy

The lipid hypothesis has always postulated that reduction in lipid levels should result in reduced coronary atherosclerosis and fewer clinical CHD events. Various methods have been utilized, including diet and pharmacological interventions such as cholestyramine, fibrates, niacin and more recently statins. All of these have produced evidence of benefit.

In the Familial Atherosclerosis Treatment Study (Brown et al 1990), middle-aged men who had moderately elevated low density lipoprotein (LDL), a family history of CHD and angiographic evidence of CHD had reduced frequency of progression of coronary lesions and increased frequency of regression and reduced incidence of CHD events if prescribed lipid-lowering therapy.

There are now a large number of trials in both primary (e.g. WOSCOPS (Shepard & Packard 1995)) and secondary (e.g. 4S (Scandinavian Simvastatin Survival Study 1995), CARE (Sacks et al 1996) and LIPID (1998)) prevention which demonstrate that lipid lowering with statins reduces the risk of further coronary events.

Angiographic studies have shown that while statins (HMG CoA reductase inhibitors) have a potent ability to lower LDL-cholesterol and coronary events, the reduction in coronary events is greater than can be accounted for by the reduction in size of atherosclerotic plaque (Libby 2001). Thus it has been suggested that statins may have a plaque-stabilizing function, probably as a consequence of an anti-inflammatory role. This has been supported by the work of Aikawa et al (1998), who have shown that lipid lowering improved plaque stability and reduced inflammation within the atheromatous lesion. The power of statins has recently been confirmed by the Heart Protection Study (Heart Protection Study Collaborative Group, 2002), which looked at the use of statins in high-risk patients not fulfilling current indications for statin use and showed a reduction in cardiovascular events. The results of this study are likely to alter prescribing habits, extending the use of statins to all who have evidence of CHD and also all diabetics over the age of 40.

Angiotensin-converting enzyme inhibitors

Another important intervention in plaque stabilization is the use of angiotensin-converting enzyme (ACE) inhibitors. Angiotensin II is a known inflammatory mediator and there is an increasing body of evidence supporting the modulation of the renin–angiotensin system in reducing cardiovascular deaths. The most impressive (or well publicized) of these is the HOPE Study which showed little reduction in blood pressure but a reduction in cardiovascular events (HOPE Study Investigators 2000).

Surgical intervention

The medical and surgical management of the atherosclerotic lesion itself, rather than its clinical sequelae, is relatively new. Surgical intervention by means of bypass grafting of stenosed vessels provides symptomatic relief and improves survival (Davis et al 1995), but in itself does nothing to correct the underlying disease process. A careful atherosclerotic risk profile assessment and the correction of the major risk factors should always accompany such a dramatic and expensive intervention. This will only be possible with the co-operation of patients, which in turn will depend on providing them with the facts.

Non-coronary manifestations of atherosclerosis

Atherosclerosis is a pathological process that is not exclusive to the coronary arteries but can occur in widespread vessels and areas. Atherosclerosis can affect the peripheral arteries, resulting in leg muscle ischaemia presenting clinically as calf muscle pain when walking that is relieved by rest – intermittent claudication. The severity of this condition can vary from mild inconvenience to very severe limitation when there is pain even at rest. Patients with peripheral vascular disease may also complain of cold extremities, poor skin and ulceration that may progress to gangrene. These result from atherosclerotic narrowing of the peripheral arteries and reduced blood flow to the lower limbs. The abdominal aorta is frequently affected by atherosclerosis and although there is seldom complete occlusion of blood flow, there can be serious clinical consequences. The atherosclerotic lesions weaken the aortic wall and can contribute to the development of aneurysms, particularly in the abdominal aorta. Rupture of an aortic aneurysm may result in sudden death. When the cerebral arteries are affected by atherosclerosis, the patient may suffer a spectrum of disease ranging from transient ischaemic attacks (TIAs) to a fatal cerebrovascular accident. The precise clinical presentation of cerebrovascular disease depends on the area of the central nervous system deprived of blood.

The presence of peripheral vascular or cerebrovascular disease should alert the clinician to the possibility of significant CHD and appropriate risk factor modification should be instigated (see Chapter 2 for details).

CLINICAL PICTURE

There are a number of clinical presentations of CHD. The most common of these are:

- angina pectoris, which may be stable or unstable
- acute coronary syndromes including myocardial infarction (which may be recognized or silent)

- asymptomatic ischaemia
- cardiac failure
- sudden death.

Although it is convenient to consider these as different endpoints in the CHD process, it is important to remember that these conditions are inter-related and the individual patient can move from one group to another.

DIAGNOSIS OF CORONARY HEART DISEASE

In recent years there has been a major change in the nomenclature of chest pain syndromes related to CHD. Chronic stable angina describes the classic anginal symptoms that are precipitated by exertion or stress and relieved with rest. The term 'acute coronary syndromes' covers the spectrum of disease from unstable angina through to acute myocardial infarction. Acute ischaemia, as documented by ST changes on ambulatory electrocardiogram (ECG) monitoring, frequently occurs in the absence of clinical symptoms, reflecting the instability of the patient with significant CHD (Deedwania & Carbajal 1991).

The differential diagnosis of ischaemic chest pain includes:

- cardiac causes, e.g. pericarditis
- chest causes, e.g. pulmonary embolus
- oesophageal causes, e.g. oesophagitis, gastro-oesophageal reflux disease
- gastrointestinal causes, e.g. pancreatitis, cholecystitis
- musculoskeletal causes, e.g. costochondritis.

Angina pectoris

Angina pectoris is a symptom complex due to reversible myocardial ischaemia. The symptoms are those of chest pain or tightness that can radiate to one or both arms, to the teeth, throat or back. Pain is brought on by effort or emotion or may occur spontaneously at rest. Patients with angina pectoris can be divided into clinical subgroups by symptoms. Those with stable angina have a reproducible pattern in terms of intensity and duration of pain and precipitating factors. Unstable angina includes those with recent onset of symptoms (less than 6 months) or a changing pattern often involving spontaneous pain at rest or with crescendo worsening of symptoms.

It must be remembered that angina pectoris is a symptom and not a diagnosis. It is most often due to underlying atherosclerotic CHD, but can be due to other causes such as anaemia, hyperthyroidism and aortic valve stenosis. It should also be remembered that myocardial ischaemia may not cause pain or discomfort – this is particularly likely in the elderly and diabetic populations. Box 1.1 describes many of the symptoms associated with angina.

The pathogenesis of angina is usually based on an underlying stenotic lesion of one or more coronary arteries. Angina pectoris results from a transient imbalance of myocardial oxygen supply and demand. The factors that influence demand are:

- heart rate
- myocardial contractility

- myocardial wall tension – the product of left ventricular end-diastolic volume (preload) and myocardial muscle mass
- systolic blood pressure – a clinical indicator of afterload (Podrid & Rose 2001).

■ **BOX 1.1   Symptoms of angina pectoris**

- Last from 30 seconds to 20 minutes
- Are precipitated by exertion or stress
- Described by the patient as *pressing, squeezing, tightness* or *a weight*
- Sometimes radiate to left arm, neck or lower jaw
- Are relieved by rest or nitrates

Acute coronary syndromes including myocardial infarction

This is the term that covers unstable angina – ischaemic chest pain which is prolonged and not relieved by rest or sublingual nitrates – and acute myocardial infarction. Acute myocardial infarction develops when myocardial ischaemia occurs for sufficient time to cause necrosis of a localized area of the myocardium. The initial reduction in myocardial blood flow may be secondary to:

- intracoronary thrombus – often associated with plaque rupture
- haemorrhage into an atheromatous plaque
- platelet aggregation in the presence of severe atheroma leading to reduced flow and perhaps thrombus
- prolonged coronary artery spasm – more common in smokers and cocaine abusers.

Infarction may occur without total coronary artery occlusion when coronary flow falls as a result of severe hypotension. This can be associated with systemic haemorrhage or shock. The pain of myocardial infarction is similar to that of angina pectoris but results from irreversible myocardial ischaemia. The pain does not subside with rest or nitrate therapy and may last for several hours. The intensity of pain gives no indication of the severity of the infarction. Indeed, particularly in the elderly, myocardial infarction may be 'silent' and present not with pain but with the consequences of infarction such as acute left ventricular failure. Accompanying symptoms are summarized in Box 1.2. Such symptoms are largely due to associated autonomic disturbance. Up to two thirds of all deaths from MI occur within 2 hours of onset, mainly as a result of dysrhythmia. The majority of these deaths occur outside hospital (Norris 1998).

As described above, the term 'acute coronary syndrome (ACS)' covers the spectrum from unstable angina (UA) to myocardial infarction (MI). Myocardial infarctions are classified acutely as either ST elevation MI (STEMI) or non-ST elevation MI (NSTEMI), and only latterly can the terms Q-wave and non Q-wave MI be applied.

> ■ **BOX 1.2 Symptoms of acute coronary syndromes**
>
> - Severe crushing central chest pain
> - Dyspnoea
> - Syncope
> - Cold sweat
> - Pallor
> - Nausea

Q-wave MIs were previously thought to represent transmural infarction, in contrast to the subendocardial infarction thought to be associated with non Q-wave ECG changes. Autopsy evidence does not support this description (Phibbs 1983). It is now becoming clear that the terms Q-wave and non Q-wave are descriptive. The ECG presence of Q-waves is associated with increased mortality in the first 30 days after the MI, but after this time there is no difference in the clinical course of those patients with Q-wave or non Q-wave ECG changes (Abdulla et al 2001). These terms are thought to reflect the magnitude of the myocardial infarction – a non Q-wave event suggests a smaller MI (Phibbs et al 1999).

The diagnosis of ACS is based on the combination of clinical symptoms and signs, ECG changes and enzyme changes. The most important differentiation that should be made as early as possible is whether the patient has a STEMI because this is the one condition that has a specific therapy – thrombolysis (see Chapter 9 for further detail) – that benefits from expeditious use.

Cardiac failure

Cardiac failure can be defined as 'a clinical state resulting from the inability of the heart to provide sufficient blood for tissue metabolic needs'. The clinical syndrome of cardiac failure has long been recognized but its management remains a major problem and as survival from acute sequelae of CHD increases, the population affected by cardiac failure will rise. At least 25% of patients with CHD have heart failure and the long-term prognosis is determined by the extent to which cardiac performance is impaired (McMurray & Stewart 2000).

There have been recent major advances in our understanding of the pathophysiology of heart failure and its management. The role of ACE inhibitors and β-receptor antagonists has been especially important in improving symptoms and prognosis in those with impaired left ventricular function.

CHD is a major, although not the only, factor in depressing left ventricular function. Dyspnoea is the predominant feature due to increasing pulmonary vascular engorgement and decreased compliance of the left ventricle.

Sudden death

Reducing the rate of sudden death is an important challenge in cardiology. While prevention of sudden death is, of course, the ultimate aim, resources should also be available to take advantage of the considerable advances in the resuscitation of those with cardiac arrest. These improvements have been largely due to the more widespread availability of defibrillators and the training of paramedic personnel. In sudden cardiac death, 85% of subjects have evidence of CHD (Kannel & Thomas 1982); indeed, sudden cardiac death is the first cardiac event in 15% of patients with CHD (Kannel et al 1975). Other causes include structural heart disease in 10% (such as cardiomyopathy and valvular heart disease. In 5% no structural abnormality was detected (Kannel & Thomas 1982). This group of patients, with structurally normal hearts, may have had an arrhythmic cardiac arrest as a consequence of electrolyte imbalance (e.g. hypokalaemia) or ion channel disorders, such as those found in Brugada syndrome and long QT syndrome.

The mode of death is arrhythmic – usually ventricular fibrillation – and may occur in either the presence or absence of acute myocardial infarction (Cobb et al 1980). The early recognition of cardiac arrest and the initiation of prompt basic life support, while awaiting facilities for advanced life support (principally defibrillation) and transfer to hospital, increase the likelihood of successful resuscitation (Finn et al 2001). There is currently a great deal of interest in the role of public access defibrillators (Woollard 2001), but one should not lose sight of the importance of public training in the recognition and management of cardiac arrest.

Patients who have been successfully resuscitated from cardiac arrest (or aborted sudden death) require careful investigation in order to identify the optimum management strategy. Some of these patients will require the insertion of an implantable cardioverter-defibrillator (ICD) which is able to recognize and treat malignant arrhythmias (Bailey et al 2001). The MADIT II (Multicenter Automatic Defibrillator Implantation Trial II) study has recently been prematurely terminated because of efficacy in the ICD arm with a reduction of 30% in sudden cardiac death. This trial may aid the identification of patients who would benefit from this technology, although this has significant implications in terms of both cost and psychological impact.

INVESTIGATION OF CORONARY HEART DISEASE

As with all investigation strategies, the most important part of the investigation is the clinical history and examination, including the identification of clinical signs and symptoms, significant past medical and drug history, and risk factor profile. This assessment is very important in establishing the likely diagnosis and differential diagnoses prior to progressing to diagnostic tests. Initial blood tests (Box 1.3) are directed at excluding alternative causes for chest pain (e.g. anaemia or hyperthyroidism) and evaluating risk factors (e.g. renal dysfunction, diabetes and hyperlipidaemia). With these

---

■ **BOX 1.3   Blood tests in the initial assessment of CHD**

- Full blood count
- Urea and electrolytes
- Glucose
- Lipid profile
- Thyroid function tests

■ **BOX 1.4   Summary of possible investigations for CHD (see text for details)**

Non-invasive	*Invasive*
Rest ECG	Blood tests
Exercise tolerance test	• Troponin
Echocardiography	• CK and CK-MB
Stress echocardiography	• AST
SPECT	Coronary angiography and
PET	ventriculography

---

components of the initial assessment, a pretest probability can be assigned to the individual patient indicating whether CHD is likely on a scale of low, medium or high. This can then indicate investigation and aid interpretation of tests.

Since angina is a symptom complex, objective confirmatory evidence for the diagnosis is usually sought. The severity of pain is not a guide to the severity of the disease. Minor coronary artery disease can be associated with severe chest pain and major coronary artery disease can have apparently mild symptoms. Both the Scottish Intercollegiate Guidelines Network (SIGN) (2001) and the British Cardiac Society have published guidelines detailing the investigation and management of stable angina (de Bono 1999). Box 1.4 summarizes the non-invasive and invasive options for the investigation of CHD.

Electrocardiography

The main initial investigation is electrocardiography. A resting ECG should always be recorded. It may or may not be abnormal. Indeed, the resting ECG is normal in 50% of those with a history of possible angina. The resting ECG may show evidence of a previous infarction or changes representing ischaemia, such as ST segment depression or T-wave inversion (Fig. 1.6). The ECG during an acute ischaemic event may show ST elevation, ST depression or T-wave inversion or be normal.

As the initial investigation in acute chest pain it is important that the ECG is performed and reviewed quickly in order to optimize the patient's care.

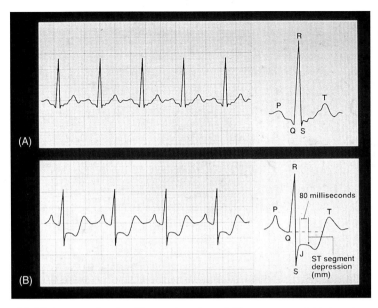

Figure 1.6 ECG tracings showing: (A) normal tracing and (B) acute myocardial ischaemia.

If the initial ECG is normal then it should be repeated after 15 minutes in case there are evolving changes. If the index of suspicion is high for ACS then continuous ST segment monitoring may be appropriate.

The ECG can identify the myocardial territory at risk and can suggest the responsible artery, e.g. anterior changes suggest the involvement of the left anterior descending artery, inferior changes are usually associated with a right coronary artery lesion, although this depends on the individual's coronary anatomy.

The resting ECG can identify an alternative cause for the chest pain, e.g. widespread ST-T elevation suggesting pericarditis or the range of changes associated with pulmonary embolus, or risk factors for CHD such as the strain pattern suggestive of left ventricular hypertrophy associated with long-standing hypertension.

The ECG may also identify consequences of CHD such as arrhythmias. Continuous ECG monitoring is advised for patients with acute coronary syndromes because of the risk of life-threatening arrhythmias.

Exercise electrocardiography

Exercise (stress) testing helps to diagnose myocardial ischaemia. Stress testing by treadmill or bicycle ergometer is important for making the diagnosis, risk stratifying the patient and establishing the degree of disability. Patients with chest pain at low risk of CHD may be reassured by a negative exercise tolerance test but there is the potential for unnecessary concern and invasive investigation due to false-positive results. It is essential to use a standard protocol. Bruce in Seattle developed the best known protocol (Bruce & Hornsten 1969). The angle and speed of the treadmill are increased at regular intervals of 3 minutes. The total workload is easily calculated and the

ECG monitored for the development of ST depression as an indicator of myocardial ischaemia.

Ischaemic changes developing within a few minutes of starting graded exercise can be an indication for more detailed investigation such as coronary angiography. Stress testing will allow the diagnosis of CHD to be made in a further 35% of patients with a normal resting ECG. Thus, 85% of patients with CHD will be diagnosed with the combination of history, resting ECG and exercise tolerance test.

The exercise stress test provides an objective non-invasive measure of a patient's cardiovascular capacity; the level of exercise achieved also has prognostic value. It is widely available, easily repeated and has a low (but not absent) mortality and morbidity: mortality 1:20 000; combined morbidity and mortality 1:1000 (Stuart & Ellestad 1980). Experience and resuscitation equipment are required for those supervising exercise testing. The uses of exercise testing are clearly described in the American College of Cardiologists/ American Heart Association (ACC/AHA) guidelines for exercise testing (Gibbons et al 1997). The most straightforward indications include:

- clinical assessment
  - chest pain of unknown cause
  - stable angina
  - after myocardial infarction
- evaluation of treatment
  - medical therapy
  - after coronary artery bypass grafting
  - after myocardial infarction.

Exercise testing is recommended following myocardial infarction to help identify those at risk of further cardiovascular events. A normal exercise test indicates a good prognosis. An exercise test limited by pain or by the development of ischaemic ECG changes or dysrhythmia can identify those at risk and requiring further investigation. Many units undertake symptom-limited exercise testing just before discharge (usually 6 days post-infarct) and again at 6 weeks. Some patients with a positive test at discharge will have a negative test at 6 weeks. This may be the consequence of resolution of thrombus and vessel recanalization or development of collateral circulation. Others may develop ischaemic changes at 6 weeks when exercise performance has improved and the underlying ischaemia can be identified. Predischarge exercise tolerance testing is indicated in all suitable patients.

Cardiac enzyme changes

Intracellular enzymes are released when ischaemia results in myocardial necrosis. Changes in cardiac enzymes after MI follow a characteristic pattern over time and are of considerable value in making a diagnosis (Fig. 1.7). The following enzymes are usually measured in the first 3 days following a suspected MI:

- troponin T or I
- total creatine kinase (CK) and creatine kinase MB isoenzyme (CK-MB)
- aspartate transaminase (AST).

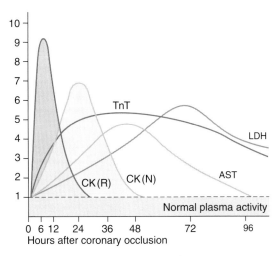

Figure 1.7 Schematic of the rise in cardiac enzymes following acute myocardial infarction. CK(R) indicates the rapid rise and fall if there is reperfusion, compared to CK(N) when there is no reperfusion.

The troponin complex consists of three subunits: TnC, TnI and TnT. TnC binds to calcium, TnI binds to actin and TnT binds to tropomyosin. Cardiac-specific forms of TnI and TnT exist (cTnI and cTnT) and this has allowed the development of specific antibodies which can be used in assays.

Because cTnI and cTnT are not normally present in the circulation, their detection can demonstrate even minor myocardial necrosis. At present, there is only one manufacturer of a cTnT assay so there is a single range of values available. By contrast, there are several cTnI assays and so each laboratory must determine its own reference range for the assay in use.

Troponin and CK levels rise rapidly after muscle damage and peak in approximately 24 hours. This allows rapid diagnosis of a suspected MI. Troponin levels rise within 6 hours of onset of chest pain and the elevation persists for at least 10 days, thus making them useful in the diagnosis of acute chest pain and late-presentation MI. However, their persistent elevation may mask reinfarction and so the other cardiac enzymes must be used in combination with the clinical picture and ECG. The FRISC Study (Lindahl et al 2001) has demonstrated that the patients with the highest cTnT results carried the highest risk of further myocardial infarction or death.

The use of the troponin assays has resulted in a redefinition of myocardial infarction (Joint ESC/ACC Committee 2000) and it has been suggested that this may lead to a 30% rise in the number of MIs documented. The important issue remains that even a small area of myocardial necrosis confers a detrimental prognosis. In order to clarify the extent of MI, it has been suggested that it should be defined in terms of size, left ventricular function and whether the infarct was spontaneous or as a result of intervention (e.g. angioplasty or coronary artery bypass grafting) (Fox 2000).

CK-MB is a specific isoenzyme found in cardiac muscle. A raised level implies cardiac damage whereas a raised total CK may follow muscle damage anywhere in the body. For example, it will be raised following an intramuscular injection.

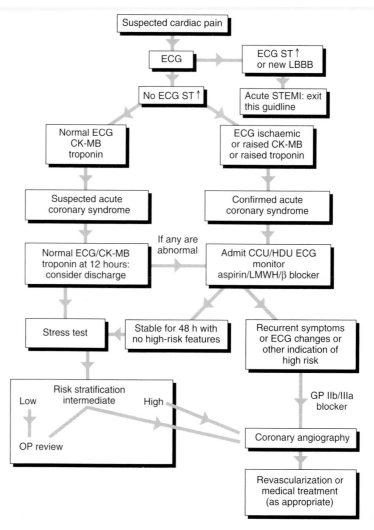

Figure 1.8 Algorithm incorporating troponin in the assessment of chest pain where ECG changes do not meet thrombolysis criteria (adapted from BCS/RCP 2001).

AST is found in heart muscle and in the liver while alanine transaminase (ALT) is predominantly found in the liver. Increased AST with a normal ALT indicates cardiac muscle damage while raised AST and ALT would point to liver damage as the cause of raised enzyme levels.

Sometimes a patient may only be seen 2–3 days after a possible infarction. The lactate dehydrogenase (LDH) enzyme will still be increased at this time when CK and AST have returned to normal. The use of LDH has been superseded by the troponin assays.

The British Cardiac Society has recommended the use of troponins in the initial assessment of suspected cardiac chest pain. A suggested management algorithm is shown in Figure 1.8 and this demonstrates the use of troponins in initial risk stratification.

Radionuclide assessment

The use of radionuclides enhances the non-invasive detection of CHD. Radionuclides are injected intravenously and a gamma camera provides an image of the distribution of radioactivity. This technique is known as single photon emission computed tomography (SPECT) and planar scans can also be imaged. Information can be obtained at rest or after exercise. Technetium-99 m labelled compound, usually in the form of sestamibi (tetrofosmin and teboroxime are two other agents), is an isotope that initially remains largely within the blood pool and can be used to estimate the dynamic performance of the heart, especially left ventricular volume and contractility. Thallium-201 is an isotope that is taken up by the myocardium itself. The uptake reflects relative myocardial blood supply. The better the blood supply, the higher the uptake of thallium.

Areas of ischaemia demonstrate poor uptake and are detected as 'cold' areas on the myocardial image. Such areas may remain 'cold' at rest and indicate scar or infarct tissue. They may also, however, reperfuse and this indicates areas of reversible ischaemia that might benefit from revascularization. Nuclear cardiology is especially useful in assessing whether or not an intervention such as coronary angioplasty has been of benefit. Impaired myocardial perfusion if present can be detected without the need for invasive angiography.

Another important role for nuclear cardiology is when conventional exercise testing is not possible because of arthritis or peripheral vascular disease. The heart can be 'stressed' by pharmacological methods such as by injecting dipyridamole or dobutamine, which enhance differences in perfusion and again demonstrate 'cold' areas of impaired blood supply. Nuclear cardiology techniques are a useful adjunct to conventional exercise testing by ECG analysis but do not replace it.

Nuclear cardiology can offer even greater information in CHD using positron emission tomography (PET). This uses technetium radioisotopes and allows correlation of myocardial perfusion with function. PET may be most useful in detecting areas of myocardial viability – regions of myocardium that may benefit from revascularization despite their appearance as poorly contractile (Wackers et al 2001).

In summary, to evaluate myocardial perfusion and wall motion the most frequently used nuclear techniques involve thallium-201. Ventricular function can be assessed with technetium-99 m and myocardial viability studies often use PET scanning.

Echocardiography

Cardiac ultrasound (echocardiography) is now established as a major non-invasive investigation. Initially used in the diagnosis of valvular abnormalities, congenital heart disease and rheumatic heart disease, echocardiography is now a mainstay in the assessment of the consequences of CHD. It does not deal with the coronary circulation but with ventricular dimensions and function. The ability of the heart muscle to contract can be observed and measured both in terms of localized areas and of global ventricular function. The terms used are:

- *dyskinesis* – expansion or dilatation instead of contraction, usually an indication of an aneurysm
- *akinesis* – absent contraction; this can be found when there is a large infarct or scar tissue
- *hypokinesis* – diminished movement, often when there is impaired coronary blood flow.

Left ventricular function can be quantified in terms of ejection fraction (EF) which can be estimated from the left ventricular end-diastolic dimension (LVEDD) and end-systolic dimension (LVESD), although this method is inaccurate in the presence of wall motion abnormalities.

$$EF = \frac{LVEDD^3 - LVESD^3}{LVEDD^3} \times 100\%$$

An EF is usually around 60–70%. Reduction in the EF to below 25% is associated with a poor prognosis following infarction. Regular echocardiograms can be a useful method of following progress and assessing effects of treatment.

The use of stress echocardiography is becoming established as the most sensitive non-invasive method of diagnosing CHD (Fleishmann et al 1998). This technique compares echocardiographic images at rest and during stress – either exercise or pharmacological. Stress-induced regional wall motion abnormalities are highly suggestive of the diagnosis of CHD, and identifies patients who should be considered for coronary angiography.

Magnetic resonance imaging

Magnetic resonance imaging (MRI) is a tool that images tissue without the use of radiation. It can visualize the function of the myocardium, assess myocardial viability and even identify atheromatous plaques in the epicardial coronary arteries.

The difficulties with this technique include its restricted access (not all centres have cardiac MRI equipment or specialist experience), the images take time to acquire and patients may find the procedure very noisy and claustrophobic.

With further technical refinements, cardiac MRI may become the technique of choice in evaluating the coronary arteries for stenoses as it avoids the risks associated with coronary angiography (de Feyter et al 2000).

Electron beam computed tomography

Electron beam computed tomography (EBCT) uses X-ray radiation in a specialized 'ultrafast' scanner to assess the coronary arteries. Contrast studies can visualize the left main coronary artery and left anterior descending arteries well, but the resolution is insufficient for other areas (de Feyter et al 2000). EBCT is also used to look at coronary calcification, which is indicative of coronary atherosclerosis (Wexler et al 1996).

EBCT is not widely used at present. A recent article suggested that it was equivalent in sensitivity and specificity to exercise testing (de Feyter et al

2000, Nallamothu et al 2001). However, the ACC/AHA did not support its use in their expert consensus document (O'Rourke et al 2002). One of the main reasons for this is the cost implication (Shaw & O'Rourke 2000) and also its limited data provision compared to other modalities.

Coronary angiography and left ventriculography

Cardiac catheterization allows radiographic visualization of the left ventricle and coronary arteries. Catheters are inserted into the femoral artery (Judkin's technique), brachial artery (Sones' technique) or radical artery and manipulated retrogradely to the left ventricle. Injection of contrast medium and recording on video, film or digitally gives information on coronary artery anatomy (Fig. 1.9) and left ventricular structure and contractility. Selective coronary angiography in multiple projections remains the principal diagnostic study in selecting patients for coronary angioplasty or coronary bypass surgery. It is still the most accurate index available for assessing prognosis in patients with angina pectoris and is probably still the final arbiter in studies of obscure chest pain.

Coronary angiography is being used increasingly for patients with acute coronary syndromes. It can determine the number of vessels affected and the site and severity of lesions, which can help direct therapy – see Chapter 9 for further detail.

Coronary angiography is not without risk and each unit performing this procedure should determine its own complication rate for use in patient consent. Published data (Davidson & Bonow 2001) suggest that for those undergoing non-urgent coronary angiography, the risks are as follows:

- death   0.14–0.75%
- myocardial infarction   0.07–0.6%
- cerebrovascular accident   0.03–0.2%

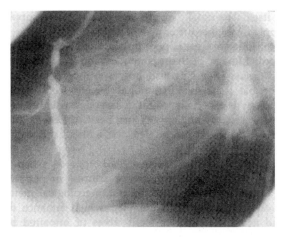

Figure 1.9 Coronary angiography. Radio-opaque dye has been injected into the coronary arteries through a fine catheter inserted into the femoral artery in the groin and passed up to the aortic root.

- arrhythmia   0.56–1.3%
- vascular complications   0.4%.

The risk of complication following coronary angiography is increased in patients who are moribund, hypotensive or shocked, have aortic or mitral valve disease, renal insufficiency or chronic heart failure or cardiomyopathy. Patients aged over 80 are considered to be at higher risk (Davidson & Bonow 2001). The risks quoted above do not apply to patients with acute coronary syndrome undergoing coronary intervention.

RISK ASSESSMENT IN ACUTE CORONARY SYNDROMES

Over the past decade there has been a radical shift in the management of patients with acute coronary syndromes (see Chapter 9). It is now important to identify the most appropriate management for each individual patient. Two timeframes need to be considered – the acute phase and the long term. The aim is to identify the patients at highest risk of death and target the most invasive therapy to them. This strategy also prevents overly aggressive management of lower risk patients.

Acute phase

The TIMI (Thrombolysis In MI) Study Group has been a driving force in the development of trials in the management of ACS. They have used their vast databases of patient data to derive risk scores for UA/NSTEMI (Antman et al 2000) (Fig. 1.10) and STEMI (Morrow et al 2000) (Fig. 1.11). These risk scores allow the categorization at presentation of an individual patient and identify those most likely to benefit from aggressive therapy.

Long term

Stress testing remains the key in identifying patients who are at risk of further ischaemic events following ACS. The first 30 days after the index event are critical, as studies have shown that greater than 60% of all major events in the first year occur in this window (Stevenson et al 1993). Therefore, most units now accept that predischarge exercise testing (symptom limited) is appropriate. Box 1.5 shows features suggesting higher risk that may indicate that coronary angiography is appropriate. A negative test should be viewed as reassuring. An assessment of left ventricular function should also be made with either echocardiography or radionuclide ventriculography.

Chest pain assessment units

Chest pain is a common presenting complaint in the emergency department. In order to optimize the management of these patients, an increasing number of centres are developing 'chest pain assessment units' which allow the early triage of patients to a specialized area (Cannon & Braunwald 2001). There, the patient can be rapidly assessed and STEMI quickly identified, thus reducing door-to-needle time (Cannon et al 1999). Protocols can be

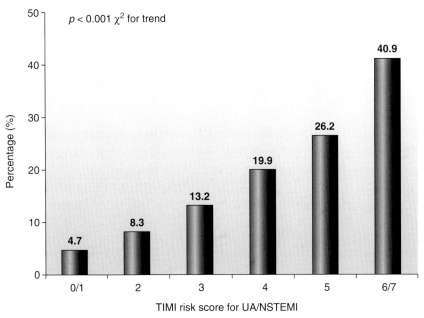

Figure 1.10 Identification of high-risk patients following UA/NSTEMI (Antman et al 2000).

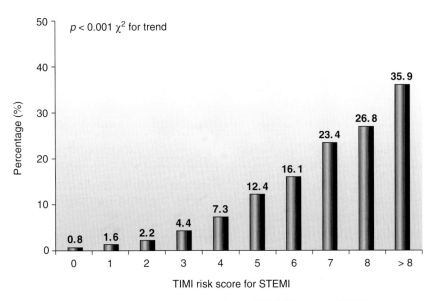

Figure 1.11 Identification of high-risk patients following STEMI (Morrow et al 2000).

instituted to identify low-risk patients (Zalenski et al 1998). The remaining patients can be optimally managed in terms of treatment and investigation.

There is evidence that chest pain assessment units can reduce hospital admissions for chest pain by 20–30% (Gibler et al 1995, Graff et al 1997). Patients who are discharged as low risk for CHD can have further investigations arranged as outpatients to identify the cause of their chest pain.

■ **BOX 1.5   High-risk features of post-MI stress test**

- ST-T depression
- Low exercise tolerance
- Failure of blood pressure to rise with exercise, or to fall
- Arrhythmias during exercise

The discharge comment 'chest pain – MI excluded' is not a diagnosis, it is an indication for further examination.

CONCLUSION

Coronary heart disease remains an important diagnosis in 20–25% of the population of industrialized countries. It is rising in incidence in developing countries. The underlying pathophysiology is becoming clearer and this is impacting on the range of strategies used to prevent the development of CHD and treat its sequelae. CHD leads to a range of clinical consequences including angina, myocardial infarction, heart failure and sudden death.

The diagnosis of CHD can be reached through non-invasive means such as clinical assessment and ECG tracings at rest and during exercise. More invasive investigations include coronary angiography and radionuclide imaging techniques. There are methods to risk stratify patients to aid management planning in both the acute phase and longer term.

A significant number of those investigated for CHD do not have the disease. These patients require further investigation to identify the cause of their chest pain in order to optimize management and prevent repeated admissions.

■ **KEY POINTS**

- CHD is the greatest single cause of death in the industrialized world, occuring in both sexes, but presenting earlier in men. Rates are improving in some groups while worsening in others.
- It may present as sudden death, myocardial infarction, or angina pectoris with chest pain being the classic symptom.
- A good history is the most important aid in the diagnosis of angina but there are many other techniques available for the full evaluation of CHD.
- Angina pectoris is a symptom complex due to reversible myocardial ischaemia.

REFERENCES

Abdulla J, Brendorp B, Torp-Pedersen C, Kober L 2001 Does the electrocardiographic presence of Q waves influence the survival of patients with acute myocardial infarction? European Heart Journal 22: 1008–1014

Aikawa M, Rabkin E, Okada Y et al 1998 Lipid lowering by diet reduces matrix metalloproteinase activity and increases collagen content of rabbit atheroma: a potential mechanism of lesion stabilisation. Circulation 97: 2433–2444

Antman EM, Cohen M, Bernink PJ et al 2000 The TIMI risk score for unstable angina/non-ST elevation MI: a method for prognostication and therapeutic decision making. Journal of the American Medical Association 284(7): 835–842

Bailey JJ, Berson AS, Handelsman H, Hodges M 2001 Utility of current risk stratification tests for predicting major arrhythmic events after myocardial infarction. Journal of the American College of Cardiology 38(7): 1912–1915

Bhopal R, Unwin N, White M et al 1999 Heterogeneity of coronary heart disease risk factors in Indian, Pakistani, Bangladeshi and European origin populations: cross-sectional study. British Medical Journal 319(7204): 215–220

British Cardiac Society and Royal College of Physicians 2001 Guideline for the management of patients with acute coronary syndromes without persistent ECG ST segment elevation. Heart 85(2): 133–142

Brown G, Albers JJ, Fisher LD et al 1990 Regression of coronary artery disease as a result of intensive lipid-lowering therapy in men with high levels of apolipoprotein B. New England Journal of Medicine 323: 946–955

Bruce RA, Hornsten TR 1969 Exercise stress testing in evaluation of patients with ischaemic heart disease. Progress in Cardiovascular Disease 11(5): 371–390

Cannon CP, Braunwald E 2001 Unstable angina. In: Braunwald E, Libby P, Zipes DP (eds) Heart disease: a textbook of cardiovascular medicine, 6th edn. WB Saunders, Philadelphia

Cannon CP, Johnson EB, Cermignani M, Scirica BM, Sagarin MJ, Walls RM 1999 Emergency department thrombolysis critical pathway reduces door-to-drug times in acute myocardial infarction. Clinical Cardiology 22(1): 17–20

Cappuccio FP 1997 Ethnicity and cardiovascular risk: variations in people of African ancestry and South Asian origin. Journal of Human Hypertension 11(9): 571–576

Cobb LA, Werner JA, Trobaugh GB 1980 Sudden cardiac death. I. A decade's experience with out-of-hospital resuscitation. Modern Concepts in Cardiovascular Disease 49(6): 31–36

Cooper RC, Cutler J, Desvigne-Nickens P et al 2000 Trends and disparities in coronary heart disease, stroke, and other cardiovascular diseases in the United States: findings of the National Conference on Cardiovascular Disease Prevention. Circulation 102: 3137–3147

Davidson CJ, Bonow RO 2001 Cardiac catheterization. In: Braunwald E, Libby P, Zipes DP (eds) Heart disease: a textbook of cardiovascular medicine, 6th edn. WB Saunders, Philadelphia

Davies MJ 1995 Acute coronary thrombosis – the role of plaque disruption and its initiation and prevention. European Heart Journal 16(suppl L): 3–7

Davies MJ, Thomas A 1985 Plaque fissuring – the cause of acute myocardial infarction, sudden ischaemic death and crescendo angina. British Heart Journal 53: 363–373

Davis KB, Chaitman B, Ryan T, Bittner V, Kennedy JW 1995 Comparison of 15-year survival for men and women after initial medical or surgical treatment for coronary artery disease: a CASS registry study. Journal of the American College of Cardiology 25(5): 1000–1009

de Bono D 1999 Investigation and management of stable angina: revised guidelines 1998. Heart 81: 546–555

de Feyter PJ, Nieman K, van Ooijen P, Oudkerk M 2000 Non-invasive coronary artery imaging with electron beam computed tomography and magnetic resonance imaging. Heart 84: 442–448

Deedwania PC, Carbajal EV 1991 Silent myocardial ischaemia – a clinical perspective. Archives of Internal Medicine 151(12): 2273–2382

Department of Health 2000 National Service Framework for Coronary Heart Disease. Department of Health, London

Finn JC, Jacobs IG, Holman CD, Oxer HF 2001 Outcomes of out-of-hospital cardiac arrest patients in Perth, Western Australia, 1996–1999. Resuscitation 51(3): 247–255

Fleischmann KE, Hunink MG, Kuntz KM, Douglas PS 1998 Exercise echocardiography or exercise SPECT imaging? A meta-analysis of diagnostic test performance. Journal of the American Medical Association 280(10): 913–920

Fox R 2000 Myocardial infarction redefined. Circulation 102: e9023

Gibbons RJ, Balady GJ, Timothy BJ et al 2002 ACC/AHA guidelines for exercise testing. Journal of the American College of Cardiology 40(8): 1531–1540

Gibler WB, Runyon JP, Levy RC et al 1995 A rapid diagnostic and treatment center for patients with chest pain in the emergency department. Annals of Emergency Medicine 25(1): 1–8

Graff LG, Dallara J, Ross MA et al 1997 Impact on the care of the emergency department chest pain patient from the Chest Pain Evaluation Registry (CHEPER) study. American Journal of Cardiology 80(5): 563–568

Heart Outcomes Prevention Evaluation Study Investigators 2000 Effects of an angiotensin converting-enzyme inhibitor, ramipril, on cardiovascular events in high-risk patients. New England Journal of Medicine 342: 145–153

Heart Protection Study Collaborative Group 2002 MRC/BHF Heart Protection Study of cholesterol lowering with simvastatin in 20,536 high-risk individuals: a randomized placebo-controlled trial. Lancet 360: 7–22

HeartStatistics 2001 www.heartstats.org

Joint European Society of Cardiology/American College of Cardiology Committee 2000 Myocardial infarction redefined – a consensus document of the Joint European Society of Cardiology/American College of Cardiology Committee for the Redefinition of Myocardial Infarction. Journal of the American College of Cardiology 36(3): 959–969

Kannel WB, Thomas HE Jr 1982 Sudden coronary death: the Framingham Study. Annals of the New York Academy of Science 382: 3–21

Kannel WB, Doyle JT, McNamara PM, Quickenton P, Gordon T 1975 Precursors of sudden coronary death. Factors related to the incidence of sudden death. Circulation 51(4): 606–613

Kolodgie FD, Burke AP, Farb A et al 2001 The thin-cap fibroatheroma: a type of vulnerable plaque: the major precursor lesion to acute coronary syndromes. Current Opinion in Cardiology 16(5): 285–292

Libby P 2001 Current concepts of the pathogenesis of the acute coronary syndromes. Circulation 104(3): 365–372

Lindahl B, Diderholm E, Lagerqvist B, Venge P, Wallentin L, the FRISC II (Fast Revascularisation during InStability in CAD) Investigators 2001 Mechanisms behind the prognostic value of troponin T in unstable coronary artery disease: a FRISC II substudy. Journal of the American College of Cardiology 38(4): 979–986

Long-Term Intervention with Pravastatin in Ischaemic Disease (LIPID) Study Group 1998 Prevention of cardiovascular events and death with pravastatin in patients with coronary heart disease and a broad base of initial cholesterol levels. New England Journal of Medicine 339: 1349–1357

Lorimer AR 2001 Coronary Heart Disease/Stroke Task Force Report. Scottish Executive, Edinburgh

McMurray JJ, Stewart S 2000 Epidemiology, aetiology and prognosis of heart failure. Heart 83: 596–602

Morrow DA, Antman EM, Charlesworth A et al 2000 TIMI risk score for ST-elevation myocardial infarction: a convenient, bedside, clinical score for risk assessment at presentation. An Intravenous nPA for Treatment of Infarcting Myocardium Early II (InTIME II) trial substudy. Circulation 102: 2031–2037

Nallamothu BK, Saint S, Bielak LF et al 2001 Electron-beam computed tomography in the diagnosis of coronary artery disease: a meta-analysis. Archives of Internal Medicine 161: 833–838

Norris RM 1998 Fatality outside hospital from acute coronary events in three British health districts, 1994–1995. British Medical Journal 316: 1065–1070

Ornish D, Schweritz LW, Billings JH et al 1998 Intensive lifestyle changes for reversal of coronary heart disease. Journal of the American Medical Association 280(23): 2001–2007

O'Rourke RA, Brundage B, Froelicher VF et al 2002 American College of Cardiology/American Heart Association Expert Consensus Document on electron beam computed tomography for the diagnosis and prognosis of coronary artery disease. Journal of the American College of Cardiology 36(1): 326–340

Phibbs B 1983 "Transmural" versus "subendocardial" myocardial infarction: an electrocardiographic myth. Journal of the American College of Cardiology 1: 561–564

Phibbs B, Marcus F, Marriot HJC, Moss A, Spodick DH 1999 Q-wave versus non-Q-wave myocardial infarction: a meaningless distinction. Journal of the American College of Cardiology 33(2): 576–582

Podrid PJ, Rose BD (eds) 2001 Pathophysiology and diagnosis of ischemic chest pain. Up To Date, Wellesley, MA

Rackley CE 2001 The role of plaque rupture in acute coronary syndromes. In Podrid PJ, Rose BD (eds) Pathophysiology and diagnosis of ischemic chest pain. Up To Date, Wellesley, MA

Sacks FM, Braunwald E, the Cholesterol and Recurrent Events Trial Investigators 1996 The effect of pravastatin on coronary events after myocardial infarction in patients with average cholesterol levels. New England Journal of Medicine 335: 1001–1009

Scandinavian Simvastatin Survival Study 1994 Randomised trial of cholesterol lowering in 4444 patients with coronary heart disease: the Scandinavian Simvastatin Survival Study. Lancet 344: 1383–1389

Scottish Intercollegiate Guidelines Network (SIGN) 2001 Management of stable angina – SIGN guideline number 51. SIGN, Edinburgh

Shaw LJ, O'Rourke RA 2000 The challenge of improving risk assessment in asymptomatic individuals: the additive prognostic value of electron beam tomography? Journal of the American College of Cardiology 36: 1261–1264

Shepherd J, Cobbe SM, Ford I et al 1995 Prevention of coronary heart disease with pravastatin in men with hypercholesterolaemia. West of Scotland Coronary Prevention Study Group. New England Journal of Medicine 333: 1301–1307

Stary HC 1989 Evolution and progression of atherosclerotic lesions in coronary arteries of children and young adults. Arteriosclerosis 9(suppl 1): 119–132

Stevenson R, Ranjadayalan K, Wilkinson P, Roberts R, Timmis AD 1993 Short and long term prognosis of acute myocardial infarction since introduction of thrombolysis. British Medical Journal 307(6900): 349–353

Stuart RJ, Ellestad MH 1980 National survey of exercise stress testing facilities. Chest 77: 94–97

Tunstall-Pedoe H, Kuulasmaa K, Mahonen M, Tolonen H, Ruokokoski E, Amouyel P 1999 Contribution of trends in survival and coronary-event rates to changes in coronary heart disease mortality: 10-year results from 37 WHO MONICA project populations. Monitoring trends and determinants in cardiovascular disease. Lancet 353(9164): 1547–1557

Wackers FJT, Soufer R, Zaret BL 2001 Nuclear cardiology. In: Braunwald E, Libby P, Zipes DP (eds) Heart disease: a textbook of cardiovascular medicine, 6th edn. WB Saunders, Philadelphia

Wexler L, Brundage B, Crouse J et al 1996 Coronary artery calcification: pathophysiology, imaging methods, and clinical implications. A statement for health professionals from the American Heart Association Writing Group. Circulation 94: 1175–1192

Woollard M 2001 Public access defibrillation: a shocking idea? Journal of Public Health Medicine 23(2): 98–102

World Health Organization 2001 Cardiovascular mortality and morbidity. www.who.int

Zalenski RJ, Rydman RJ, Ting S, Kampe L, Selker HP 1998 A national survey of emergency department chest pain centers in the United States. American Journal of Cardiology 81(11): 1305–1309

FURTHER READING

Braunwald E, Libby P, Zipes DP (eds) 2001 Heart disease: a textbook of cardiovascular medicine, 6th edn. WB Saunders, Philadelphia

Gaw A, Packard CJ, Shepherd J 1994 Lipids and atherosclerosis. In: Bloom AL, Forbes CD, Thomas DP, Tuddenham EGD (eds) Haemostasis and thrombosis, 3rd edn. Churchill Livingstone, Edinburgh, pp 1153–1168

Mills P (ed) 2001 Education in heart, volume 1. BMJ Books, London

WEBSITES

www.heartstats.org
A useful source of epidemiological facts

www.cardiosource.com
A website with brief summaries of cardiovascular trials

www.timi.tv
Link to the TIMI registry and details of the MI risk stratification

www.doh.gov.uk/nsf/coronary.htm
Link to the National Service Framework for Coronary Heart Disease

Risk factor assessment

Grace M. Lindsay

2

■ CONTENTS

INTRODUCTION

The importance of underlying risk factors in the treatment and management of coronary heart disease (CHD) can be captured in the following quotation:

> 'Coronary disease does not really begin with crushing chest pain, pulmonary edema, shock, angina or ventricular fibrillation, but rather with the more subtle signs like a poor coronary risk profile' (Kannel 1976).

The subtlety of the poor coronary risk profile alludes both to its subclinical nature and in many cases individual risk factors that are not strikingly high, so that active steps have to be taken in order to reveal their presence. Estimation of risk is an integral part of preventing CHD, particularly because there is now sound evidence that effective intervention can not only decrease risk but also halt the continued development of atherosclerosis or even reverse the process (Kunz 2002). This chapter addresses the concept of CHD risk, its assessment, interpretation and role in the prevention of CHD in practice.

RISK

The terms 'risk' or 'risk factor' are used often but sometimes without the meaning being clear. The word 'risk' originates from the French *risque* and is a fairly modern addition to the English language. Collinson & Dowie (1980) report that the word did not enter the language until the mid-17th century and then appeared in anglicized spelling in insurance transactions during the second quarter of the 18th century.

One of the immediate difficulties that arises when trying to define risk is that it has both a technical definition, e.g. risk assessment or hazard management, and a strong colloquial usage. In common use the word 'risk' is associated with the chances of loss rather than gain. The *Oxford English Dictionary* definition of risk includes 'hazard, chance of bad consequences, loss, etc.'. The consideration of risk in decision making is to recognize that the future can never be known with certainty and, at best, comes with a range of possibilities.

Risk and uncertainty are often used interchangeably. Both concepts can be defined as being basically a problem of lack of information about future events that might arise. Knight (1933) distinguishes between the two concepts by arguing that *risks* are future outcomes to which it is possible to attach probabilities, whereas *uncertainty* is a situation where a probability cannot be ascribed. CHD risk factor assessment is concerned with the nature of risk, where probabilities can be ascribed to outcome and where modification of risk can have a beneficial effect on outcome.

The term 'risk factor' is widely used to describe those characteristics found in individuals that have been shown in observational epidemiological studies, autopsy studies, metabolic studies and genetic studies to relate to the subsequent occurrence of CHD.

In global terms, risk factor categories cover personal, lifestyle, biochemical and physiological characteristics, some of which are modifiable while others are not.

Risk factor hypothesis

A search for the origins, cause and subsequent prevention of CHD has proceeded from early descriptive epidemiological studies of populations (Keys 1980) to prospective cohort studies. In the latter, a population sample was identified, clinically assessed in terms of CHD risk factors and then monitored for a number of years for signs of disease (Anderson 1987, Castelli 1984, Dawber et al 1951). One of the first major prospective studies to monitor and document incidence of CHD was started in the small community of Framingham in the United States (Dawber et al 1951). As stated by Shaper et al (1985), it has 'become synonymous with the risk factor concept and is the source of much of our knowledge about the risk of CHD in individuals'. The study started with a small number of male and female volunteers (n = 740) in 1948 and has subsequently grown into a major prospective observational study (Anderson 1987). Follow-up of the recruits and in some cases their offspring is still ongoing today and data from the study have given investigators valuable information about the relationship between various risk factors and CHD. The main risk factors for CHD were identified as smoking, hypertension, hyperlipidaemia, diabetes mellitus and family history of CHD (Castelli 1984). This study was also notable because it was one of the few large epidemiological studies of CHD that included women in its cohort.

Quantifying the risk

Statistical techniques have been used to estimate the strength of association between risk factors and the likelihood of developing CHD. There are two main approaches: univariate and multivariate analysis.

Univariate analysis

This seeks to test the effect of one variable at a time on the subsequent risk of occurrence of disease or a specified outcome without consideration of any other factors. Because many factors are related or dependent on each other, e.g. with increased obesity there is an associated increase in blood pressure, such associations should be interpreted with care. To determine if a risk factor is exerting an effect in its own right, the more complex multivariate analysis should be employed.

Multivariate analysis

This tests the effect of several risk factors at the same time and estimates the strength of the relationship. It also tests whether the relationship is independent of the effects of some other variables or dependent on them. Examination of risk factor 'dependence' is concerned with the search for aetiology. However, it is important to remember that even if a risk factor can be explained by its relationship to another factor (dependent) for an individual, such an increased risk factor still contributes to increased CHD risk.

Relative and absolute risk

A further complexity in the interpretation of CHD risk for the individual depends on whether the risk is quoted in *absolute* terms or is *relative* to other individuals or other factors.

Absolute risk defines the expected rate of CHD events for any given combination of age, gender and other risk factors. *Relative risk* is the ratio between the absolute risk in an individual and the absolute risk in someone of the same age and gender who has no other CHD risk factors.

Relative risk is therefore comparative in nature and it can be applied to grade risk within groups of individuals. For example, a young smoker will have a high relative risk compared to an age- and gender-matched non-smoker but will have a low absolute risk. By contrast, with rising age absolute risk increases and relative risk falls, because in old age CHD is more common even in the absence of major CHD risk factors.

■ **BOX 2.1   CHD risk factors**

Lifestyle

- Tobacco smoking
- Diet high in saturated fat and calories, low in fruit and vegetables, high in sugar
- Physical inactivity
- Stress
- Excess alcohol
- Obesity

Biochemical or physiological

- Elevated plasma cholesterol
- Elevated BP
- Low plasma HDL-cholesterol
- Elevated plasma triglyceride
- Diabetes mellitus
- Thrombogenic factors

Personal

- Age
- Gender
- Family history (first degree)
- Personal history

Identification of risk factors

As noted above the Framingham Study (Dawber et al 1951) began in the 1940s and was designed to generate information that would help in the early detection and prevention of CHD. Some of the risk scoring charts described later in the chapter are based on algorithms devised from analysis of the Framingham data sets.

Several other prospective population studies were initiated in the United States in the 1950s and 1960s and a summary of their results has been published in the final report of the Pooling Project (Pooling Project Research Group 1978). Along with the Seven Countries Study (Keys 1980), they indicate factors that seem to predict a major part of the subsequent CHD. These were documented as level of blood pressure, serum cholesterol, relative weight and ECG abnormalities.

The web of causation for heart disease was clearly complex and as more experience of the disease process was gained, it became apparent that more factors than had already been documented had a role to play. While a multitude of factors have been potentially associated with CHD, St George (1983) reviewed the literature and quantified the number of well-documented risk factors to be of the order of 20. However, in practice, attention focuses on the factors presented in Box 2.1. In terms of clinical practice it is useful

■ BOX 2.2   Major CHD risk factors routinely assessed in clinical practice

Modifiable

- Smoking
- Elevated plasma cholesterol
- Elevated BP
- Obesity
- Physical inactivity
- Excess alcohol
- Stress

Immodifiable

- Family history of CHD
- Personal history of CHD
- Diabetes mellitus
- Age
- Gender

to consider risk factors as either modifiable or immodifiable as detailed in Box 2.2.

RISK FACTORS FOR CORONARY HEART DISEASE

Three important, independent and modifiable risk factors have received particular attention, namely hyperlipidaemia, hypertension and smoking, with the weight of evidence suggesting a causal relationship with CHD. Because of their importance in the aetiology of CHD together with diabetes mellitus, separate chapters are devoted to each, namely Chapters 3, 4, 5 and 12, respectively. The evidence for the association of other risk factors is less strong, but clearly demonstrates a link with the development of CHD; these will now be considered in more detail.

Age and gender

Coronary heart disease increases with age in both men and women. It is rare in the first two decades of life, becoming more prevalent after the age of 30 and much more marked in males than in females below the age of 60 years. Beyond 60 years, CHD in females increases at an accelerated rate and after the seventh decade the rate approaches that in males (Fig. 2.1). It is unclear whether atherosclerosis is a result of the ageing process per se or the cumulative effect of the known risk factors exerting their effect over time.

Epidemiological studies reveal that women are relatively protected against CHD while premenopausal and that this protection is less evident in the postmenopausal years. Interpretation of risk factors in females, the

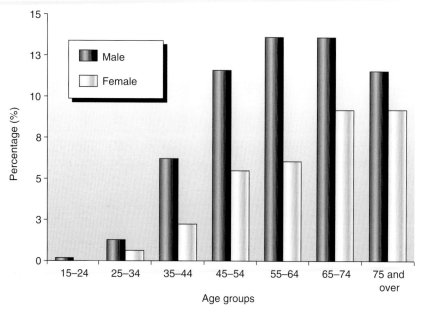

Figure 2.1 CHD death rates as a percentage of all deaths in men and women according to age bands, in England and Wales, 2000 (ONS 2001).

effects of hormonal status and the role of hormonal replacement therapy will be dealt with in more depth in Chapter 11.

Family history

A significant family history is considered to be present if CHD is diagnosed in first-degree relatives before the age of 60 years. The clustering of risk factors such as hypertension, diabetes and obesity is also common. Most of these groupings are a result of interactions between genetic factors and environmental influences so it is difficult to determine the relative effect of genetic factors, except in those with familial hypercholesterolaemia. Familial hypercholesterolaemia, in its heterozygous form, occurs in about 1 in 500 of the population, with the homozygous form being extremely rare. It is thought that the genetic component of CHD risk is likely to be the result of the influence of many genes, i.e. polygenic, rather than a single gene effect. In practice, recognizing a positive family history of CHD is important because other individuals at high risk can be identified and therefore made a priority for CHD risk factor assessment and management (Neufeld & Goldbourt 1983).

Physical activity

Long-term physical activity is known to be important in maintaining body weight and muscle tissue, in lowering blood pressure and in raising high density lipoprotein (HDL) cholesterol. Experimental studies using angiography in primates (Kramsch et al 1981) indicated that aerobic exercise reduces the severity of atherosclerosis even in the presence of an atherogenic diet.

Indirect measures of ischaemia using electrocardiograph (ECG) treadmill testing have demonstrated a favourable response to physical training. Moreover, using this same methodology, men who were less physically fit were twice as likely to suffer a myocardial infarction than their fitter counterparts (Peters et al 1993). The role of physical activity will be discussed in more detail in Chapter 7.

Obesity

Obesity has been described as one of the most important avoidable risk factors for a number of life-threatening diseases and for serious morbidity (Garrow 1992). The Department of Health statistics report that the prevalence of serious obesity doubled in Britain between the years 1980 and 1991, with the trend continuing to increase (Bennett et al 1995). The relationship between obesity and all-cause mortality has been shown to be 'J-shaped'; that is, the thinnest people show some excess risk compared to those who are 'normal' or slightly overweight. However, with increasing obesity all-cause mortality increases and this is largely due to an increase in cardiovascular mortality (Larsson 1992). Body mass index (BMI) calculated from weight/height^2 has been recommended as the best estimate of obesity in adults (Garrow 1992). Degrees of obesity are graded using the following classification: mild (BMI 25–29.9), moderate (BMI 30–40) and severe (BMI >40).

During a 15-year prospective follow-up study of a total of over 16 000 middle-aged males and females, mortality from CHD was shown to be positively and independently associated with BMI for both men and women. The BMI-associated risk was 1.03 ($p = 0.027$) after adjusting for age, hypertension, hyperlipidaemia and smoking (Jousilatiti et al 1996). Additional evidence supporting obesity as an independent CHD risk factor has been provided from the Nurses' Health Study, a US cohort study which is following more than 120 000 women (Manson et al 1995). The study demonstrated a progressive increase in CHD event rates with increasing BMI. The risk of death was 60–70% higher among women with a BMI of 29–32 than among women with a BMI of 25–27. A strong positive relationship between the degree of obesity and presence of hypertension, hypertriglyceridaemia, hyperinsulinaemia and low levels of HDL-cholesterol has been shown to exist (Kaplan 1989), supporting the rationale for multiple risk factor screening in obese individuals.

In addition to assessment of degree of obesity, additional risk has been shown to be associated with centrally distributed excess body weight. Increased waist circumference (central obesity) reflects total and abdominal fat accumulation and has been shown to relate strongly to health risk, including the risk of CHD (Han & van Leer 1995, Lean et al 1995).

Psychosocial factors

In studies that have demonstrated a role for psychological factors in the development of CHD, the following factors have been outlined. These include type A/hostility personalities, depression, anxiety, low levels of control, job demands and low levels of social support which can contribute individually or in combination to lack of coping and high levels of perceived stress (Barefoot et al 1996, Hemingway & Marmot 1999, Rubeman et al 1984). Psychosocial factors may affect health-related behaviours such as smoking, diet, alcohol consumption or physical activity.

Some consider stress to be an important risk factor, none more so than the patient who has suffered a myocardial infarction. The difficulty of assessing stress lies in defining 'stress', as an activity that may be stressful for one person may be regarded as a positive challenge by another. The possible mechanisms by which stress exerts its negative effects on CHD risk have been cited as increases in blood pressure and heart rate, increased plasma cholesterol levels and adverse effects on coagulation and fibrinolysis (Johnston 1993). In lifestyle counselling, it is important to include an assessment of the level of stress perceived by patients. Guidelines for cardiac rehabilitation have recommended that assessment for the presence of significant anxiety and depression should be made as part of routine care (SIGN 2002). They recommend the use of the Hospital Anxiety and Depression Scale (Zigmond & Snaith 1983), a short self-completed questionnaire. Individualized strategies to reduce stress can greatly improve patient well-being.

Socio-economic deprivation

There is no single definition that encompasses the complex concept of deprivation. It is considered to exist across different dimensions of life such as lack of material goods and resources, lack of membership and social contacts within society, low income, poor housing and unemployment. Deprivation scores (Carstairs & Morris 1991) have been developed as a measure of socio-economic deprivation, based on postcode, and subsequently updated using 1991 census data (McLoone 1994). It is composed of four indicators of disadvantage including overcrowding, male unemployment, no car ownership and head of household social class 4 or 5. The deprivation score is divided into seven separate categories, ranging from high (7) to very low deprivation (1).

The sensitivity of socio-economic circumstances to CHD is highlighted by the existence of large differences in incidence across socio-economic groups (BHF 2002). Socio-economic-related gradients in health have been explained in terms of their association with both social position and with different material circumstances such as bad housing, poor diets, inadequate heating, unemployment and poverty (Wilkinson 1997). Furthermore, psychosocial effects of adverse social position have been implicated in the generation of health inequalities through an increased exposure to risk of chronic mental and emotional stress together with the related coping strategies of cigarette smoking and alcohol excess.

Thrombogenic factors

Fibrinogen is an important factor in controlling blood coagulation. Elevated plasma levels of fibrinogen have been shown to be a risk factor for a CHD event (Kannel et al 1987). In addition, other haemostatic factors such as factor VII and plasminogen activator inhibitor have been associated with increased

CHD risk. However, in current clinical practice these measurements are not widely performed and are rarely used in routine CHD risk factor assessment.

Increased propensity for platelet aggregation has been found to be associated with an increased risk of CHD events (Elwood et al 1991). Unfortunately the methods used for measuring this parameter have not been fully established, so yet again this risk factor cannot be used in overall risk assessment. However, compelling evidence from clinical trials of patients with established CHD has demonstrated beneficial effects of antiplatelet drugs, particularly aspirin. Comparing the results of several trials of aspirin usage, the Antiplatelet Trialist Collaboration Group (1994) concluded that in patients with CHD the use of low-dose aspirin (75–150 mg) reduces future CHD events by one-quarter. It is important to note that these findings cannot, with present knowledge of risk and benefits, be extrapolated to advocating use of aspirin in a healthy population to reduce the risk of CHD events.

MULTIPLE RISK FACTORS

'A single risk factor … is not sufficiently sensitive to identify all individuals at high risk of coronary heart disease' (Assmann & Schulte 1990).

It has gradually become more evident that CHD mortality could not be explained solely on the basis of the effect of single risk factors. Analysis of existing data to examine the effects on CHD mortality when more than one risk factor is present revealed that the risk factors interacted synergistically, i.e. in a multiplicative rather than an additive manner, to increase markedly the risk of CHD (Grundy 1986). Observational and intervention studies in populations were conducted to examine the effect of multiple risk factors on subsequent risk of CHD.

The USA Multiple Risk Factor Intervention Trial (MRFIT 1982, Neaton et al 1984) shows that male 5-year CHD death rates per 1000 were 17.4 when the individual was a smoker, had diastolic blood pressure of greater than 90 mmHg and a cholesterol level greater than 6.5 mmol/l. In contrast, when an individual was a non-smoker, had a diastolic blood pressure less than 90 mmHg and a cholesterol level of less than 6.5 mmol/l then the rate was much lower at 2.4 per 1000.

In the British Regional Heart Study, Shaper et al (1985) collected data on middle-aged men over a period of 2 years and examined the relationship between CHD risk factors and the rate of CHD events at a 5-year follow-up. The aim of this study was to see if it was possible to identify men at high risk of CHD. The parameters used as indices of risk were smoking, mean blood pressure, previous diagnosis of CHD and diabetes, family history of CHD, ECG evidence of CHD and plasma total cholesterol. A score was developed on the basis of these risk factors and it was found that the top fifth of the score distribution identified 59% of men who subsequently had a major CHD event. It was also evident that the bulk of CHD incidence does not occur in those individuals who lie at the upper end of any single risk factor distribution but rather in those individuals who have moderate elevations in a number of risk factors.

Data from the Framingham Study, described above, also show how steeply CHD risk rises when combinations of risk factors are present (Castelli 1984). Similar trends can be seen in men and women living in the West of Scotland. Male smokers in Renfrew and Paisley with cholesterol greater than 6 mmol/l (top 40% of distribution) and diastolic pressure greater than 97 mmHg (top 20% of distribution) had a fourfold higher CHD mortality than men who did not smoke, whose cholesterol was less than 6 mmol/l and diastolic blood pressure less than 97 mmHg. The relative risk for women with multiple risk factors was even greater, although this probably reflects the fact that absolute rates for low-risk women were lower than for low-risk men (Isles et al 1989).

Evidence from trials which have sought to evaluate the impact on CHD mortality of attempts to change multiple risk factors have been mixed (McCormick & Skrabanek 1988). One of the first of these trials was carried out in Oslo (Hjermann 1983) and focused on changes in cholesterol and smoking in men aged 40–49 of whom 70% were smokers and had elevated cholesterol levels (7–9.5 mmol/l). The subjects were randomly assigned to an intervention or a control group, intervention taking the form of dietary and antismoking advice. After 5 years the results indicated a successful change of both risk factors in the intervention group compared with the control group and that the rate of fatal and non-fatal CHD events was reduced by 45%. However, as in many other intervention studies, there was no significant reduction in all-cause mortality.

The Multiple Risk Factor Intervention Trial (Cutler et al 1985) was carried out in the United States. It was most notable because of its size, having recruited more than one third of a million high-risk men (age range 35–57 years). From these men, a cohort of 12 866 was selected on the basis of their CHD risk and randomized to usual care or intervention. Intervention was in the form of lifestyle changes to lower cholesterol, stop smoking and reduce weight, and drug treatment for hypertension. Over an average 7-year follow-up period risk factor levels declined in both groups but to a greater extent in the intervention group. Mortality from CHD was reduced in both groups but, disappointingly, there was no significant difference in CHD mortality between the two groups. Explanations for this have included:

- the adverse effects of antihypertensive treatment on lipids in the intervention group
- the fact that the control group were aware of their 'high-risk' status and this influenced their own health-related behaviour in such a way as to lower their risk factor status
- the 'un-blinding' of control individuals to the intervention programme of the treatment group who in many cases came from the same occupational environment.

Other studies involving population intervention programmes have been able to show modest reductions in CHD mortality in response to reduction in levels of risk factors (Farquhar et al 1970, Kornitzer et al 1983, Puska et al 1983). Therefore multiple risk factor intervention has been advocated as the best approach to reducing the incidence of CHD.

Risk factor screening strategies

Because CHD and the related risk factors are common in the Western world and resources are limited, it is important to define priorities in screening so that those individuals likely to gain the greatest benefit from intervention are identified. Two general distinctions are employed in practice: secondary and primary prevention strategies.

Secondary prevention

The highest priority should be given to those patients with established CHD and other atherosclerotic vascular disease (Wood et al 1998). This constitutes secondary prevention and will include patients with angina and those who have suffered a myocardial infarction or have undergone percutaneous transluminal coronary angioplasty (PTCA) or coronary artery bypass grafting (CABG) and other forms of vascular disease including stroke and peripheral vascular disease. These groups should not be overlooked in the belief that because they have a positive diagnosis of vascular disease, their risk factors have already been corrected. A recent European survey has revealed ample scope for improvement in the detection, recording and intervention of the major cardiac risk factors amongst patients with established CHD (Euroaspire 1998).

Primary prevention

The next groups of individuals to tackle are those asymptomatic subjects with one or more major CHD risk factors. This includes subjects with hypercholesterolaemia, hypertension, diabetes or a family history of premature CHD, smokers and the obese. In current practice the debate continues in terms of how far primary prevention screening should extend to the general population at large.

RISK FACTOR SCORING TOOLS

In order to take into account the effect of several CHD risk factors in their assessment of an individual's global risk, scoring systems have been designed based on data from epidemiological studies. These systems are used to calculate the marginal contribution of a given risk factor to overall risk of CHD with various additive or multiplicative weights assigned to the various factors. The cumulative score does not aim to provide a precise risk indicator for a disease of such complexity but it does provide the healthcare practitioner with a better estimation of overall risk where several risk factors are present. Three different forms of scoring systems are reviewed.

Risk factor calculator

The Infarct Risk Spirit Calculator (Fig. 2.2) has been developed to assist in the provision of an objective overall risk of a myocardial infarction in an individual patient. It is based on results of the ongoing Prospective Cardiovascular Munster Study which began in 1979 (Assmann & Schulte 1989). Nine parameters are included in its estimation of risk and these are listed in Box 2.3.

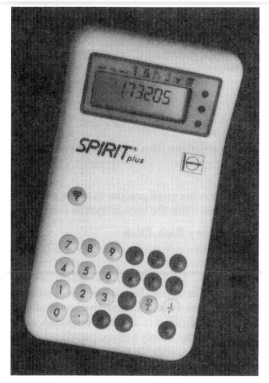

Figure 2.2 Boehringer-Mannheim Infarct Risk Spirit Calculator (reproduced by permission of Boehringer-Mannheim).

■ **BOX 2.3   CHD risk factors considered in the infarct risk calculator**

- Total plasma cholesterol
- Plasma triglycerides
- Plasma HDL-cholesterol
- Blood pressure
- Smoking (Y/N)
- Age
- Diabetes mellitus
- Angina
- Family history (myocardial infarction in relatives under 60 years old)

After entering the value of all nine parameters, the probability of suffering a myocardial infarction within 4 years is calculated and displayed as a percentage. In addition to this numerical estimation of risk, the calculator also provides a quantitative evaluation in terms of high, medium or low risk. The estimation takes into account a wide range of factors so from this perspective it is good. Providing a numerical value for risk that can be interpreted by the patient is very useful, particularly when a new score, based on the patient making changes, may be calculated so that the patient can see the improvement in risk factor status, e.g. a new score can be given that anticipates stopping smoking. One of the disadvantages is that the evaluation of smoking does not take into account number of cigarettes smoked or length of time as a smoker. In addition, all nine parameters may not be available at a routine screening clinic, e.g. triglycerides must be measured in a fasting sample. The manufacturers state that the calculator can still be used by entering 'normal' values for the missing data; however, this may interfere with the validity of the scoring system and it is not good practice to guess values of physiological measurements for patients when the tests cannot be carried out.

The Dundee Coronary Risk-Disk

This is a simple circular slide rule device (Fig. 2.3) which places patients in a rank order from 1 (high risk) to 100 (low risk) based on their relative position in the general population, from a score that integrates the three major, modifiable risk factors of smoking, blood pressure and serum cholesterol (Tunstall-Pedoe 1991). It is based on a prospective study of middle-aged men followed for a 5-year period (Rose et al 1983). It focuses on modifiable risk factors alone, excluding gender, family history, presence of CHD and diabetes mellitus. Although these immodifiable risk factors cannot be changed they must affect the interpretation of risk from any other factors and should be taken into account along with the predictive score using the Risk-Disk. The risk assessment is given in terms of relative risk, i.e. the risk compared to another individual of the same age.

Actual values of the three risk factors are used, avoiding assessment of individual risk factors by cut-off points. However, there are many factors that are not included, for instance BMI or HDL-cholesterol. Therefore other factors must be considered along with the score obtained from the disk. Again the limitation of using results based on experience gained solely in

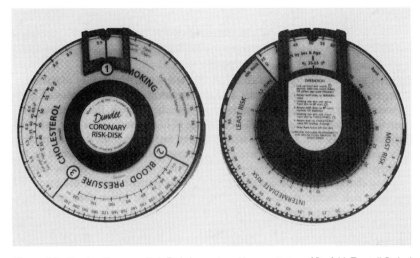

Figure 2.3 Dundee Coronary Risk-Disk (reproduced by permission of Prof. H. Tunstall-Pedoe).

men exists with this tool. The Risk-Disk has been endorsed by the Coronary Prevention Group and by the British Heart Foundation.

The British Regional Heart Study: GP score

A scoring system based on the British Regional Heart Study has been developed to identify men and postmenopausal women at high risk of myocardial infarction, for use in general practice by doctors or nurses. It is based on the belief that prediction of major CHD cases can be improved by assessing the combined effects of several risk factors and the presence of pre-existing disease. A questionnaire was administered asking people to recall any chest pain they have experienced in response to various activities. The score is calculated from the formula outlined in Box 2.4. The score is interpreted in terms of risk of CHD in a 5-year period as set out in Table 2.1.

The score does not include a cholesterol measurement but the authors suggest that the score is used as a basis for deciding who should have their cholesterol level measured. Neither does it take into account the number of cigarettes smoked, justifying this on the results from the British Regional Heart Study which found, of the indices of smoking, that 'years smoking' was the one which most strongly correlated with risk of CHD. There is a more detailed score developed from the data from the same study, taking into account age, a cholesterol measurement and an electrocardiograph. When evaluated, the top fifth of score distribution identified 59% of the men who subsequently had a CHD event during the following 5 years, compared to 53% of men using the simplified score detailed above.

■ **BOX 2.4   Scoring algorithm for the British Regional Heart Study: GP score**

$7\times$ years of smoking cigarettes
$+6.5\times$ mean blood pressure (mmHg)
$+270$ if the individual recalls a diagnosis of CHD
$+150$ if there was evidence of angina in the health questionnaire
$+85$ if either parent had died of CHD
$+150$ if diabetic

Table 2.1 Interpretation of scores obtained using the British Regional Heart Study: GP score

Score reference range	Risk of CHD event in 5 years
High risk: >1000	1 in 10
900–999	1 in 25
Average: 800–899	1 in 30
700–799	1 in 100
Low risk: <700	1 in 250

The Second Joint Task Force of European and other Societies on Coronary Prevention

These guidelines (Pyörälä et al 1994) have been produced jointly by the Task Force of the European Society of Cardiology, European Atherosclerosis Society and European Society of Hypertension. This collaboration demonstrates the growing consensus in risk factor evaluation and it is likely that these recommendations will gain wider acceptance. The guidelines endorse assessment of the total burden of CHD risk that an individual is exposed to rather than considering solely the effect of single risk factors such as smoking, hypertension or hyperlipidaemia in isolation. This approach acknowledges previously discussed concepts, i.e. aetiology is multifactorial, risk factors have a multiplicative effect and global risk factor assessment should be practised. It has also made an important step forward in providing separate assessment for men and women in recognition of the different profile of CHD in relation to gender. The aim of these recommendations is to summarize from the clinical perspective the most important issues in CHD prevention on which there is good agreement and thereby to give practitioners the best possible advice, thus facilitating their work in CHD prevention.

In assessing CHD risk status in an individual, the presence or absence and severity of each individual risk factor has to be considered. Age, gender, systolic blood pressure, smoking status and plasma total cholesterol level are included in the risk evaluation. In addition, the assessment recommends that patients with CHD, a strong family history of premature CHD, diabetes mellitus or low HDL-cholesterol levels be considered at higher risk. The guidelines are based on a risk function derived from the Framingham Study (Anderson et al 1991) and predict a person's absolute 10-year risk of a coronary event expressed as percentage chance (Fig. 2.4).

An individual's absolute risk of developing a coronary event in the following 10 years is found by entering the relevant measurement into the chart and identifying the grade of risk category. The percentage chance is given in the key. The chart can be used to predict the change in overall risk status as a result of changing any risk factor. The effect of increasing risk with age can be clearly followed using the chart. In general, even low-risk subjects should be offered healthy lifestyle advice to maintain their low-risk status. Advice should be intensified with increasing risk and a 20% chance of an event in the next 10 years should signal intensive risk modification efforts.

The risk assessment, although fairly comprehensive, does omit diastolic blood pressure, which may be a limitation, and factors such as family history, low HDL-cholesterol (<1.0 in men and <1.1 mmol/l in women) and raised triglyceride (>2.0 mmol/l) levels are given a broad 'increased risk' status without inclusion in a quantifiable way in the risk function. The impact of diabetes mellitus on risk status is estimated to approximately double in men and more than double in women.

The Joint British Societies Coronary Risk Prediction Charts

These (Wood et al 1998) are the most recent in a series of guidelines that have been published over the last decade. Compiled by the British Cardiac

Society, British Hyperlipidaemia Association and British Hypertension Society and endorsed by the British Diabetic Association, the guidelines again represent a consensus in management of CHD across expertise in the individual risk factor areas. The risk prediction algorithms are again based

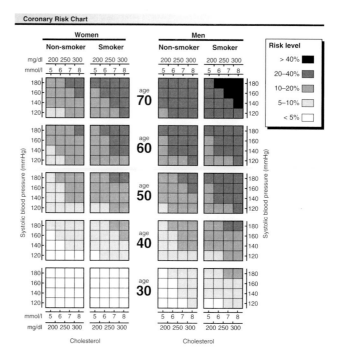

To find a person's absolute 10-year risk of a CHD event, find the table for his/her sex, age and smoking status. Inside the table, find the cell nearest to their systolic blood pressure (mmHg) and cholesterol (mmol/l or mg/dl).

To find a person's relative risk, compare his/her risk category with other people of the same age. The absolute risk shown here may not apply to all populations, especially those with a low CHD incidence. Relative risk is likely to apply to most populations.

The effect of changing cholesterol, smoking status or blood pressure can be read from the chart.

The effect of lifetime exposure to risk factors can be seen by following the table upwards. This can be used when advising younger people.

Risk is at least one category higher in people with overt cardiovascular disease. People with diabetes, familial hyperlipidaemia or a family history of premature cardiovascular disease are also at increased risk.

Risks are shown for exact ages, blood pressures and cholesterols. Risk increases as a person approaches the next category.

The tables assume HDL cholesterol to be 1.0 mmol/l in men (39 mg/dl) and 1.1 mmol/l (43 mg/dl) in women. People with lower levels of HDL cholesterol and/or with triglyceride levels above 2.3 mmol/l (200 mg/dl) are at higher risk.

Cholesterol: 1 mmol/l = 38.67 mg/dl.

Figure 2.4 Coronary risk chart derived from epidemiological data from the Framingham Study produced as part of the Joint European Guidelines of the European Society of Cardiology, European Atherosclerosis Society and the European Society of Hypertension (reproduced with permission from Pyorala et al 1994).

on the prospective database generated in the Framingham Study (Anderson et al 1991). To estimate an individual's absolute 10-year risk of developing CHD, use the table for their sex, if diabetic or not and smoking status (Fig. 2.5). Find the square matching their age, level of systolic blood pressure and the ratio of the total cholesterol to HDL-cholesterol. If there is no HDL-cholesterol result it is suggested that this is given the value of 1.00 mmol/l so in practice the lipid scale can be used for total cholesterol alone, as the European guidelines (p. 43).

CHD risk categories depend on estimated risk of CHD in a 10-year period, with those with >15% CHD risk considered high risk. Those with >30% risk should be treated now, with those in the range 15–30% being 'progressively' targeted. This results in a rather vague protocol for individuals who fall into the latter risk category and could lead to different interpretations by individual clinicians and health-care policy makers. In addition to smoking cessation, CHD risk factor targets are recommended as outlined in Table 2.2.

In addition, targets for cardioprotective drug treatment are recommended including aspirin usage, β-blockers and angiotensin-converting enzyme inhibitors.

National Cholesterol Education Program (NCEP)

As much of future clinical practice is informed by practice in the United States, a chapter devoted to CHD risk factor assessment and management would not be complete without reference to their thinking in this area. The Third Report of the National Cholesterol Education Program (NCEP) Expert Panel on Detection, Evaluation and Treatment of High Blood Cholesterol in Adults (ATP III) (NECP 2001) constitutes the NCEP's updated clinical guidelines for cholesterol testing and management. This report builds on its two predecessors, I and II, by updating the recommendations for high blood cholesterol management informed by advances in medical science in this field. ATP I outlined a strategy for primary prevention of CHD in individuals with high levels of LDL-cholesterol (≥160 mg/dl, 4.1 mmol/l) or those with borderline-high LDL-cholesterol (130–159 mg/dl, 3.4–4.0 mmol/l) and multiple risk factors (2+). ATP II affirmed the importance of this approach and added a new feature: the intensive management of LDL-cholesterol (a lower LDL-cholesterol goal of ≤100 mg/dl, 2.6 mmol/l) in persons with established

Table 2.2 CHD targets from the Joint British Societies Coronary Risk Prediction Charts

	CHD patients or 10-year CHD risk >30%	Diabetic patients
Systolic blood pressure	<140 mmHg	<130 mmHg
Diastolic blood pressure	<85 mmHg	<80 mmHg
Total cholesterol (LDL-cholesterol)	<5.0 mmol/l (3.0 mmol/l)	<5.0 mmol/l (3.0 mmol/l)
Body mass index (BMI)	<25 kg m^2	<25 kg m^2
HbA1c		<7%

DIABETES

Men

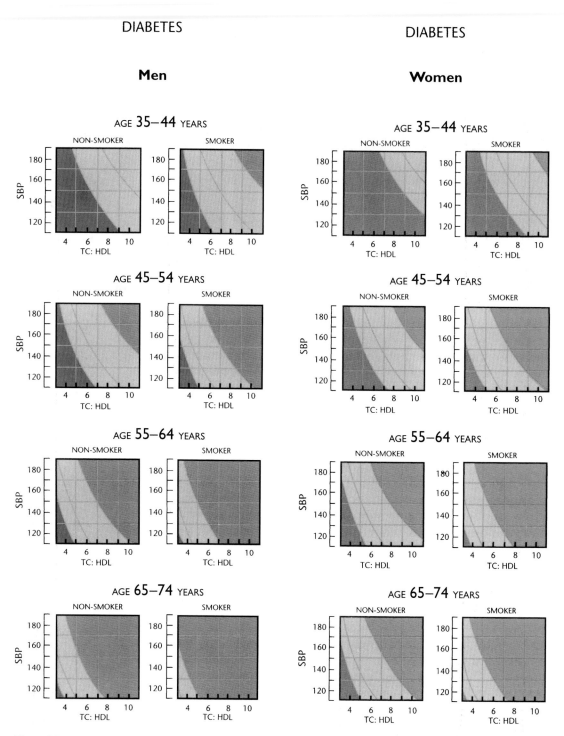

Figure 2.5 Joint British recommendations on prevention of coronary heart disease in clinical practice with permission from the University of Manchester.

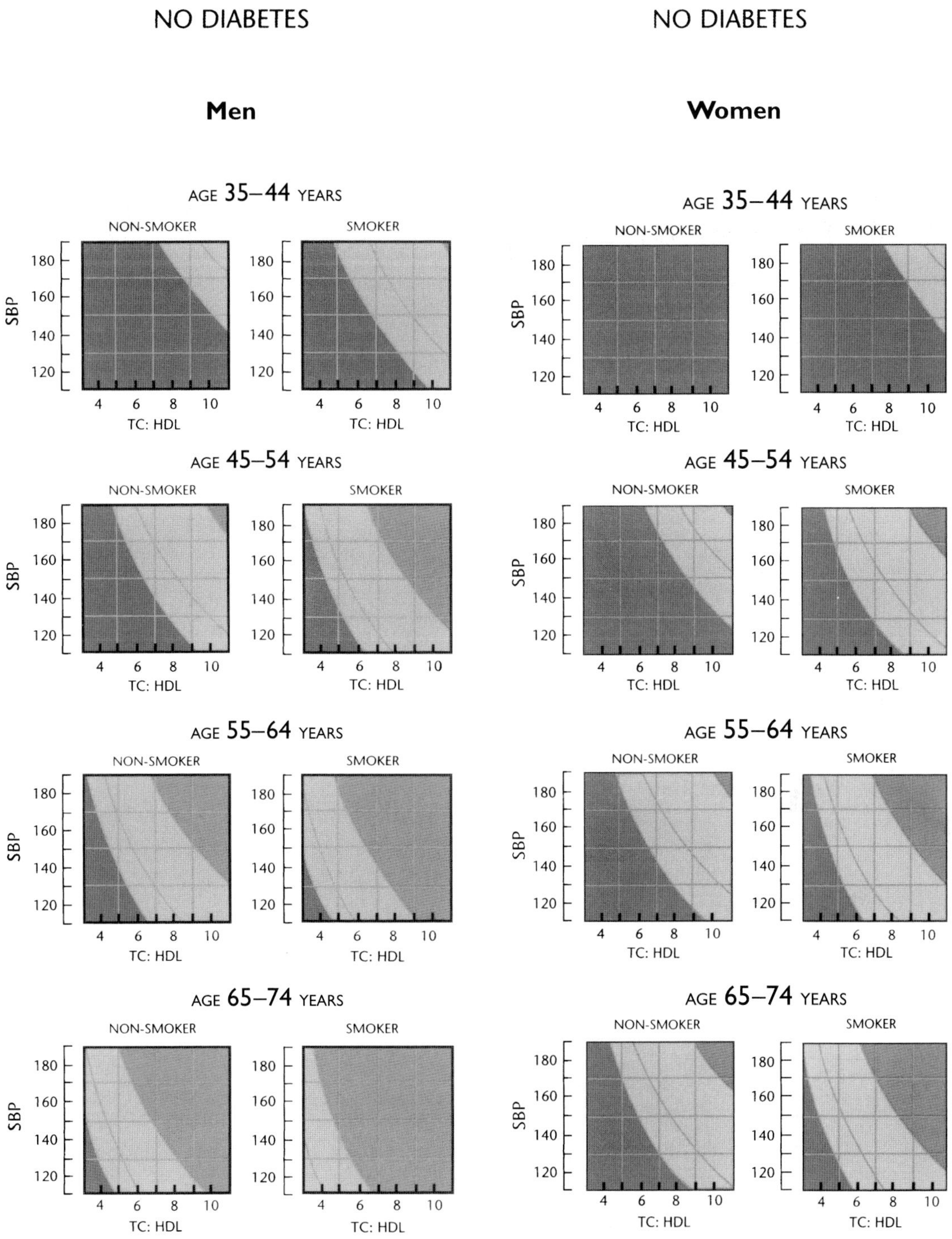

NO DIABETES

NO DIABETES

Men

Women

Figure 2.5 (Contd)

Table 2.3 Three categories of risk that modify LDL-cholesterol goals (NECP)

Risk category	LDL goal
CHD and CHD risk equivalents*	<100 mg/dl (2.6 mmol/l)
Multiple (2+) risk factors	<130 mg/dl (3.4 mmol/l)
0–1 risk factor	<160 mg/dl (4.1 mmol/l)

CHD risk equivalents: presence of CHD risk factors that confer >20% risk of developing CHD or have a recurrent event in a 10-year period. This percentage risk is estimated using the Framingham risk scoring charts.

CHD. This updateqd document adds a call for more intensive LDL lowering in primary prevention in individuals with multiple risk factors. LDL-cholesterol goals are provided for three categories of CHD risk and these are summarized in Table 2.3.

The method of risk assessment is based on a two-stage process: first, counting the number of major CHD risk factors present and second, for those with multiple risk factors, estimating 10-year CHD risk. This will allow identification of individuals whose short-term (10-year) CHD risk warrants intensive treatment.

CLINICAL RISK ASSESSMENT IN PRACTICE

CHD risk factor scoring devices are based on information gathered in populations and may require additional information in order to fully assess CHD risk at the individual level. In practice, other risk factors such as alcohol intake, stress and lack of physical exercise and obesity are also taken into account, although they do not feature in any of the scoring systems discussed above. Weight reduction in individuals who are overweight helps to control blood pressure and plasma cholesterol and aids mobility. Documentation of excess alcohol consumption and subsequent counselling should be carried out because of its possible effects on blood pressure, weight and triglyceride levels. Therefore management should be tailored to the individual factors as revealed in the screening and assessment process, including those factors known to be linked to CHD risk but not used in the score.

In summary, all risk factor scores should be viewed as merely offering guidelines and a means of identifying in a quantifiable way an individual's CHD risk. They provide a quantifiable means of monitoring improvements in risk status as a result of interventions.

Ideal goals for lifestyle behaviours and CHD risk factors can be summarized as:

- the avoidance of all forms of tobacco
- a diet low in fat and high in fruit and vegetables, compatible with ideal body weight
- plasma cholesterol levels of less than 5.0 mmol/l
- regular exercise

- blood pressure levels of 140/90 or less and 130/80 or less for diabetic patients.

In general, interventions should be aimed towards such ideals. When dealing with moderate elevations in several risk factors, because of the nature of risk interaction, modest reductions in more than one risk factor are likely to reduce risk more than aggressive reduction of a single risk factor.

■ KEY POINTS

- The aetiology of CHD is multifactorial and is described in terms of 'risk factors'.
- The term 'risk factor' is widely used to describe those characteristics found in individuals that relate to the subsequent occurrence of CHD.
- Absolute risk defines the expected rate of CHD events for any given combination of age, gender and other risk factors.
- Relative risk is the ratio between the absolute risk in an individual compared to the absolute risk in someone of the same age and gender who has no other CHD risk factors.
- Key factors that increase risk of CHD have been established.
- Risk factors interact in a multiplicative manner to greatly increase risk.
- Identifying high-risk individuals is the priority in screening strategies.
- Global risk factor assessment should be practised.
- A scoring system is a clinical tool that enables an individual to be placed in a category of risk by assessing the effect of multiple risk factors.
- Scoring systems are useful in monitoring intervention programmes to reduce risk.
- Clinical guidelines based on best practice may be integrated into patient care through risk factor scoring systems.

■ PRACTICAL EXERCISE

From your database of patient records, identify patients who are at high risk of CHD or have had a CHD event.

- What percentage of patients have had a full CHD risk factor assessment?
- Do any high-risk or CHD patients have uncorrected CHD risk factors?
- What, if any, long-term management strategies are in place?

REFERENCES

Anderson KM 1987 30-year follow-up of the Framingham Study. Journal of the American Medical Association 257: 2176–2180

Anderson KM, Wilson PWF, Odell PM et al 1991 An updated coronary risk profile: a statement for health professionals. Circulation 83: 356–362

Antiplatelet Trialist Collaboration Group 1994 Collaborative overview of randomized trials of antiplatelet therapy—I: Prevention of death, myocardial infarction, and stroke by prolonged antiplatelet therapy in various categories of patients. British Medical Journal 308: 81–106

Assmann G, Schulte H 1989 Results and conclusions of the Prospective Cardiovascular Munster (PROCAM) Study. In: Assmann G (ed) Lipid metabolism disorders and coronary heart disease. MMV Medizin Verlag, Munchen

Assmann G, Schulte H 1990 Modelling the Helsinki Heart Study by means of a risk equation obtained from the PROCAM Study and the Framingham Heart Study. Drugs 40 (suppl 1): 13–18

Barefoot JC, Helms MJ, Mark DB et al 1996 Depression and long term mortality risk in patients with coronary artery disease. American Journal of Cardiology 78: 613–617

Bennett N, Dodd T, Flatley J, Freeth S, Bolling K 1995 Health survey for England 1993. HMSO, London

British Heart Foundation 2002 Statistics. Department of Public Health, University of Oxford

Carstairs V, Morris R 1991 Deprivation and health in Scotland. Aberdeen University Press, Aberdeen

Castelli WP 1984 Epidemiology of coronary heart disease: the Framingham Study. American Journal of Medicine 76(2A): 4–12

Collinson J, Dowie D 1980 Concepts and classifications. Unit 1 of U201, Risk: a second level university course. Open University Press, Milton Keynes

Cutler JA, Neaton JD, Hulley SB, Kuller L, Paul O, Stamler J 1985 Coronary heart disease and all-cause mortality in the Multiple Risk Factor Intervention Trial: subgroup findings and comparison with other trials. Preventive Medicine 14: 293–311

Dawber TR, Meadows GF, Moore FE 1951 Epidemiological approaches to heart disease: the Framingham Study. American Journal of Public Health 41: 279–286

Elwood PC, Renaud S, Sharp DS, Beswick AD, O'Brien JR, Yarnell JW 1991 Ischaemic heart disease and platelet aggregation. The Caerphilly Collaborative Heart Disease Study. Circulation 83: 38–44

EUROASPIRE Study Group 1998 A European Society of Cardiology survey of secondary prevention of coronary heart disease: principal results. European Action on Secondary Prevention through Intervention to Reduce Events. European Heart Journal 75: 334–342

Farquhar JW, Maccoby N, Wood PD et al 1970 Community education for cardiovascular health. Lancet i: 1192–1195

Garrow JS 1992 Treatment of obesity. Lancet 340: 409–413

Grundy SM 1986 Cholesterol and heart disease: a new era. Journal of the American Medical Association 256: 2849–2858

Han TS, van Leer EM 1995 Waist circumference action levels in the identification of cardiovascular risk factors: prevalence study in a random sample. British Medical Journal 311: 1041–1045

Hemingway H, Marmot M 1999 Evidence based cardiology: psychosocial factors in the aetiology and prognosis of coronary artery disease. Systematic review of prospective cohort studies. British Medical Journal 318: 1460–1467

Hjermann I 1983 A randomised primary preventive trial in coronary heart disease: the Oslo Study. Preventive Medicine 121: 181–184

Isles CG, Hole DJ, Gillis CR, Hawthorne VM, Lever AF 1989 Plasma cholesterol, coronary heart disease and cancer in the Renfrew and Paisley survey. British Medical Journal 298: 920–924

Johnston DW 1993 The current status of the coronary prone behaviour pattern. Journal of Sociological Medicine 86: 406–409

Jousilatiti P, Tuomilehto J, Vartianinen E, Pekkanen J, Puska P 1996 Body weight, CHD risk factors and coronary mortality: 15 year follow-up of middle-aged men and women in Eastern Finland. Circulation 93(7): 1372–1379

Kannel WB 1976 Some lessons in cardiovascular epidemiology from Framingham. American Journal of Cardiology 37: 269–282

Kannel WB, Wolf PA, Castelli WP, d'Agnostino RB 1987 Fibrinogen and risk of cardiovascular disease. Journal of the American Medical Association 258: 1183–1186

Kaplan N 1989 The deadly quartet: upper body obesity, glucose intolerance, hypertriglycerides, and hypertension. Archives of Internal Medicine 149: 14

Keys A 1980 Seven Countries Study: a multivariate analysis of death and coronary heart disease. Harvard University Press, Cambridge, MA

Knight FH 1933 Risk, uncertainty and profit. Houghton Mifflin, Boston

Kornitzer M, de Backer G, Dramaix M 1983 Belgian Heart Disease Prevention Project: incidence and mortality results. Lancet i: 1066–1070

Kramsch DM, Aspen AJ, Abramowitz BM, Kreimendahl T, Hood WB Jr 1981 Reduction of coronary atherosclerosis by moderate conditioning in monkeys on an atherogenic diet. New England Journal of Medicine 305: 1483

Kunz J 2002 Can atherosclerosis regress? The role of the vascular extracellular matrix and the age-related changes of arteries. Gerontology 48(5): 267–278

Larsson B 1992 Obesity and body fat distribution as predictors of coronary heart disease. In: Marmot M, Elliot P (eds) Coronary heart disease epidemiology. From aetiology to public health. Oxford University Press, Oxford, pp 233–241

Lean MEJ, Han TS, Morrison CE 1995 Waist circumference as a measure for indicating need for weight management. British Medical Journal 311: 158–161

Manson JE, Willett WC, Stampfer MJ et al 1995 Body weight and mortality among women. New England Journal of Medicine 333: 677–685

McCormick J, Skrabanek P 1988 Coronary heart disease is not preventable by population interventions. Lancet i: 839–841

McLoone P 1994 Carstairs scores for Scottish postcode sectors from the 1991 census. Public Health Research Unit, Glasgow

Multiple Risk Factor Intervention Trial (MRFIT) Research Group 1982 Multiple Risk Factor Intervention Trial: risk factor changes and mortality results. Journal of the American Medical Association 248: 1465–1477

National Cholesterol Education Program (NECP) 2001 Third Report of the Expert Panel on Detection, Evaluation and Treatment of High Blood Cholesterol in Adults (Adult Treatment Panel III). NIH Publication No. 01-3670. National Heart, Lung and Blood Institute, National Institutes for Health, Bethesda, MD

Neaton JD, Kuller LH, Wentworth D, Borhani ND 1984 Total and cardiovascular mortality in relation to cigarette smoking, serum cholesterol concentration, and diastolic blood pressure among Black and White males followed up for five years. American Heart Journal 108: 759–769

Neufeld HN, Goldbourt U 1983 Coronary heart disease: genetic aspects. Circulation 67(5): 943–954

Office for National Statistics 2001 Mortality Statistics: cause 2000 England and Wales (DH2no. 27). Her Majesty's Stationary Office (HMSO), London

Peters PK, Cady LD, Bischoff DB 1983 Physical fitness and subsequent myocardial infarction in healthy workers. Journal of the American Medical Association 249: 3052–3056

Pooling Project Research Group 1978 Relationship of blood pressure, serum cholesterol, smoking habit, relative weight abnormalities to incidence of major coronary events. Journal of Chronic Diseases 31: 201–206

Puska P, Nissinen A, Salanen JT, Toumilchto J 1983 Ten years of the North Karelia Project: results with community-based prevention of CHD. Scandinavian Journal of Social Medicine 11: 65–68

Pyörälä K, de Backer G, Graham I, Poole-Wilson P, Wood D 1994 Prevention of coronary heart disease in clinical practice. Recommendations of the Task Force of the European Society of Cardiology, European Atherosclerosis Society and European Society of Hypertension. European Heart Journal 15: 1300–1331

Rose G, Tunstall-Pedoe H, Heller RF 1983 United Kingdom Heart Disease Prevention Project: incidence and mortality results. Lancet i: 1062–1065

Rubeman W, Weinblatt E, Goldberg JD, Chaudhary B 1984 Psychological influences on mortality after myocardial infarction. New England Journal of Medicine 311: 552–559

Scottish Intercollegiate Guidelines Network (SIGN) 2002 Cardiac rehabilitation. A national guideline. SIGN Executive, Edinburgh

Shaper AG, Pocock SJ, Walker M, Phillips AN, Whitehead TP, Macfarlane PW 1985 Risk factors for ischaemic heart disease: the prospective phase of the British Regional Heart Study. Journal of Epidemiology and Community Health 39: 197–209

St George DP 1983 Is coronary heart disease caused by environmentally induced chronic metabolic imbalance? Medical Hypotheses 12: 283–296

Tunstall-Pedoe H 1991 The Dundee Coronary Risk-Disk for management of change in risk factors. British Medical Journal 303: 744–747

Wilkinson RG 1997 Health inequalities: relative or absolute material standards? British Medical Journal 314: 591–595

Wood DA, Durrington P, McInnes G, Poulter N, Rees A, Wray R 1998 Joint British recommendations on prevention of coronary heart disease in clinical practice. Heart 80(suppl): s1–29

Zigmond AS, Snaith RP 1983 The Hospital Anxiety and Depression Scale. Acta Psychiatrica Scandinavica 67: 36

FURTHER READING

Gotto AM Jr, Farmer JA 1992 Risk factors for coronary artery disease. In: Braunwald W (ed) Heart disease: a textbook of cardiovascular medicine, 4th edn. WB Saunders, Philadelphia, pp 1125–1160

Lorimer AR, Shepherd J (eds) 1991 Preventative cardiology. Blackwell Scientific Publications, Oxford

Thompson GR, Wilson PW 1992 Coronary risk factors and their assessment. Science Press, London

Lipids and lipid-lowering drugs

Allan Gaw   James Shepherd

3

■ CONTENTS

INTRODUCTION

There are three main coronary heart disease (CHD) risk factors over which we, as individuals, have any control. These are abnormal plasma lipid concentrations, or dyslipidaemia, hypertension and smoking. This chapter will deal in detail with the first of these. The role of plasma lipids in the assessment of cardiovascular risk will be discussed, followed by a review of the trial evidence base, upon which we build our clinical use of lipid-regulating drugs. We will conclude with a brief description of the available lipid-regulating drugs, focusing particularly on the statins.

THE LINK BETWEEN LIPIDS AND CORONARY HEART DISEASE

Lipids were first implicated in the development of atherosclerosis almost 150 years ago when cholesterol was noted to be present in atheromatous lesions in arteries (Vogel 1845). However, it was not until the early years of the 20th century that the important association between dietary cholesterol and atherosclerotic lesions was confirmed experimentally (Anitschkow 1913).

This association was further confirmed epidemiologically in studies such as the Seven Countries Study (Keys 1980), where the incidence of CHD was noted to be high in countries where average cholesterol levels were high and correspondingly low in countries where cholesterol levels were low.

Using these different lines of evidence, the 'cholesterol hypothesis' was formulated. This stated that an elevated plasma level of cholesterol was a cause of CHD and by lowering the plasma cholesterol, we would reduce the CHD risk. Strong evidence to support the view that cholesterol is causally linked to the development and progression of atherosclerosis, and to CHD mortality, has come from major intervention trials that have aimed to test this cholesterol hypothesis. These studies are discussed below.

The build-up of the atherosclerotic plaque, so pivotal to the development of clinical CHD, has already been discussed in Chapter 1 and the role of lipids in this process is well established. To understand the part played by lipids in cardiovascular risk assessment, we must remind ourselves of some elementary clinical biochemistry (Gaw et al 1999).

Lipids, such as cholesteryl esters and triglyceride, are non-water soluble molecules, which must be transported around our bodies. The transport highway between our organs is the bloodstream and the immediate problem is how to carry these non-water soluble molecules through the water of our plasma. In order to circumvent this problem the lipoprotein system has evolved. Lipoproteins are multimolecular complexes that package a lipid core in a shell of water-soluble molecules. There are a number of different lipoproteins and their functions are summarized in Table 3.1. In considering cardiovascular disease we are most frequently concerned with two lipoprotein types – low-density lipoprotein (LDL) and high-density lipoprotein (HDL).

The majority of our plasma cholesterol is carried in LDL and the total cholesterol and LDL-cholesterol concentrations are closely correlated. Based on the extensive portfolio of epidemiological evidence that links cholesterol to cardiovascular risk, LDL particles are thus believed to be atherogenic and large numbers of these particles or, looked at another way, high plasma

Table 3.1 The principal plasma lipoproteins

Lipoprotein	Function
Chylomicrons	Largest lipoprotein. Synthesized by gut after fatty meal. Main carrier of dietary lipid. Rapid clearance, normally undetectable after 12-hour fast
Very low density lipoprotein (VLDL)	Similar in structure to chylomicrons but smaller. Synthesized in liver. Main carrier of endogenously produced triglyceride
Low density lipoprotein (LDL)	Generated from VLDL in the circulation. Main carrier of cholesterol, accounting for 60–70% plasma cholesterol
High density lipoprotein (HDL)	Smallest but most abundant. Protective function. Returns cholesterol to liver from peripheral tissues for excretion. Carries 20–30% of plasma cholesterol

LDL-cholesterol concentrations, are associated with an increased cardiovascular risk (Castelli 1984, Stamler et al 1986). In contrast, HDL is believed to be antiatherogenic and there is considerable evidence to support an inverse relationship between plasma HDL and CHD risk (Assmann & Schulte 1992).

Theoretically, then, a reduction in cardiovascular risk should be achieved by any strategy that lowers LDL-cholesterol and/or raises HDL-cholesterol. This was put to the test by the early intervention trials using lipid-lowering drugs in the pre-statin era. These trials aimed to test the lipid hypothesis using the best lipid-lowering drugs available at the time. Two of these studies – the Lipid Research Clinics Coronary Primary Prevention Trial (LRC-CPPT) and the Helsinki Heart Study – are discussed below. It was not, however, until the publication of the major statin trials that the clinical world really took notice of the life-saving potential of lipid-lowering therapy.

TRIAL EVIDENCE: NON-STATIN STUDIES

Lipid Research Clinics Coronary Primary Prevention Trial (LRC-CPPT)

The LRC-CPPT was one of the first major lipid-lowering trials to be conducted (Lipid Research Clinics Program 1984). This was a multicentre, randomized, double-blind study involving 3806 middle-aged men with primary hypercholesterolaemia. The participants were followed for an average of 7.4 years. Those treated with the bile acid sequestrant drug cholestyramine showed an 8.5% reduction in total cholesterol, a 12.6% reduction in LDL-cholesterol, a 3% rise in HDL-cholesterol and a 4.5% rise in triglyceride, over the placebo-treated control group. These lipid and lipoprotein changes were further enhanced in those who had adhered to the prescribed 24 g/day dosage. The drug-induced lipid changes were associated with a 19% reduction in risk of definite CHD death and/or non-fatal myocardial infarction (MI) which reflected a 24% fall in definite CHD deaths. Incidence rates of new positive exercise ECGs, angina and coronary artery bypass grafts (CABG) were significantly reduced by 25%, 20% and 21% respectively in the sequestrant resin-treated group. These findings provided the stimulus for other groups to investigate the clinical efficacy of lipid-lowering therapy and, since 1984, there has been a steady stream of larger and more powerful intervention trials.

Helsinki Heart Study (HHS)

The next major study confirmed the clinical efficacy of one of the fibrates, gemfibrozil. The HHS (Frick et al 1987), a randomized, double-blind, placebo-controlled trial designed to test the drug in reducing the risk of coronary heart disease, was conducted in Finland. A group of 4081 middle-aged men (40–55 years) with primary dyslipidaemia (non-HDL-cholesterol = 5.2 mmol/l) were recruited. Half received gemfibrozil, 600 mg twice daily, while the others received a placebo. Gemfibrozil therapy was associated with reductions in triglyceride of 35%, in LDL-cholesterol of 11% and an increase in HDL-cholesterol of 11%. The cumulative rate of cardiac endpoints (fatal and non-fatal MIs combined) at 5 years was 27.3/1000 in the gemfibrozil-treated group and 41.4/1000 in the placebo group: a reduction in CHD of 34% ($p < 0.02$).

Further analyses of the HHS data (Manninen et al 1988, 1992) have provided more detail on the relationship between the lipid changes and incidence of CHD. The success of gemfibrozil in reducing CHD events was related not only to its ability to lower LDL-cholesterol but also to its effect of raising HDL-cholesterol (Manninen et al 1988). Manninen and his colleagues (1992) went on, using subgroup analyses, to identify a high-risk group of subjects. These individuals were found to have an LDL/HDL-cholesterol ratio >5 and plasma triglyceride >2.3 mmol/l. This group profited most from gemfibrozil therapy in the HHS, with a 71% lower incidence of CHD events than the corresponding placebo subgroup. We may hypothesize that if a similar intervention trial were designed only to include this high-risk group in sufficient numbers, thereby preventing the dilutional effect seen by including all hypercholesterolaemic subjects, the clinical efficacy of a fibrate in reducing coronary morbidity might be dramatic.

Despite obvious difficulties in the interpretation of extended follow-up studies to major clinical trials, the 8.5-year follow-up of the HHS (Heinonen et al 1994) provides further supportive evidence for a beneficial effect on CHD risk attributable to fibrate therapy.

These large-scale studies with bile acid sequestrants or fibrates were viewed by many as pointing the way forward; however, others regarded their results as somewhat disappointing or at best equivocal. While significant reductions in cardiovascular endpoints were reported, these were offset to some extent by apparent increases in non-cardiovascular events (Keech 1992). Thus arose the concern among clinicians that lipid-lowering drug therapy may be a mixed blessing for their patients. This concern was founded on very thin evidence but the flames of this controversy were fanned by a series of articles written in both the lay and medical press. These articles did little to resolve the controversy and only resulted in a wholly unsupportable call for a halt to the use of all lipid-lowering drugs (Davey Smith & Pekkanen 1992). These concerns have only been put to rest by the impressive portfolio of safety data gathered across the major statin trials, where no excess of non-cardiovascular events has been observed in conjunction with the highly significant reductions in total mortality and cardiovascular morbidity. These statin trials are summarized in Table 3.2 and discussed below.

TRIAL EVIDENCE: STATIN STUDIES

Scandinavian Simvastatin Survival Study (4S)

This secondary prevention study was a double-blind, randomized, placebo-controlled trial looking at the effects of lowering cholesterol in men and women aged between 35 and 70 who had a history of angina or myocardial infarction (Scandinavian Simvastatin Survival Study Group 1994). The study recruited 4444 subjects whose cholesterol levels were between 5.5 and 8.0 mmol/l and whose triglyceride levels were less than or equal to 2.5 mmol/l. Half of the subjects were given simvastatin, 20–40 mg, while the

Table 3.2 Major CHD prevention studies with statins

Clinical trial	Drug used	Number of subjects	Relative reduction in fatal or non-fatal MI (%)
West of Scotland Coronary Prevention Study (WOSCOPS)	Pravastatin	6595	31
Cholesterol and Recurrent Events (CARE) Study	Pravastatin	4159	24
Scandinavian Simvastatin Survival Study (4S)	Simvastatin	4444	34
Long-Term Intervention with Pravastatin in Ischaemic Disease (LIPID)	Pravastatin	9014	23
Air Force/Texas Coronary Atherosclerosis Prevention Study (AF/TEXCAPS)	Lovastatin	6605	36[*]
Heart Protection Study (HPS)	Simvastatin	20 536	24[**]

[*] Expanded endpoint of combined unstable angina, fatal and non-fatal MI and sudden cardiac death.
[**] Major vascular events.

other half were given a placebo and both groups were regularly reviewed over a 5-year period.

The mean changes in lipid levels observed in the simvastatin group were as follows:

- Total cholesterol fell by 25%
- LDL-cholesterol fell by 35%
- Triglyceride fell by 10%
- HDL increased by 8%.

The primary endpoint in 4S was total mortality and Figure 3.1 demonstrates that the mortality rates of the simvastatin and placebo groups began to diverge at around 18 months into the study and continued this trend throughout the period of the trial. From these results it was calculated that there was a 30% reduction in total mortality for the patients on simvastatin.

The secondary endpoint was major coronary events and here there was also an impressive risk reduction, of 34%, for the simvastatin-treated group. The 4S also looked at two important subgroups, namely women and those over 60 years of age. The results showed that simvastatin reduced the risk of major coronary events in women to a similar extent as that seen in men and that survival rates for those over 60 years of age were significantly improved.

The study also demonstrated one important negative result: there was no increase in non-CHD mortality, such as death due to violence or cancer, observed in the simvastatin group. This puts to rest suggestions made by previous studies that lowering cholesterol may lead to increased mortality from other causes. The frequency of adverse events was similar for both the

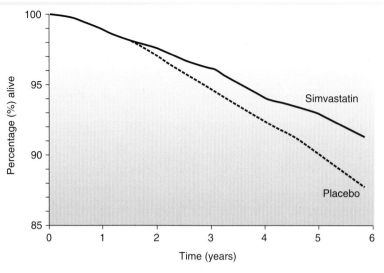

Figure 3.1 Survival curves for total mortality in 4S (adapted from Scandinavian Simvastatin Survival Study Group 1994).

simvastatin and placebo groups. Rhabdomyolysis occurred in one patient on simvastatin, but recovery followed the cessation of treatment.

Overall, the benefits of prescribing simvastatin to a group of 100 middle-aged CHD patients for 6 years were summarized as follows:

- four of the expected nine deaths would be avoided
- seven of the 21 expected MIs would be prevented
- six out of 19 revascularization procedures would be unnecessary.

A further update on the 4S was reported by the investigators (Pedersen et al 2000), where they concluded that statin treatment in patients with CHD for up to 8 years was safe and yielded continued survival benefit.

West of Scotland Coronary Prevention Study (WOSCOPS)

This study published in 1995 by Shepherd et al was of a similar design to the 4S, in that it was randomized, placebo controlled and double blind, but it differed in that it was concerned with primary prevention and only men were included. A total of 6595 men, aged between 45 and 64 years, who had no history of myocardial infarction, were recruited. Subjects were eligible for inclusion, however, if they had stable angina, provided they had not been hospitalized over the past 12 months. LDL-cholesterol levels of the participants were within the range 4.5–6.0 mmol/l. Recruits were given either placebo or pravastatin 40 mg to be taken in the evening.

The subjects were followed up over a 5-year period and those on pravastatin showed significant improvement in their lipid profile:

- Total cholesterol fell by 20%
- LDL-cholesterol fell by 26%

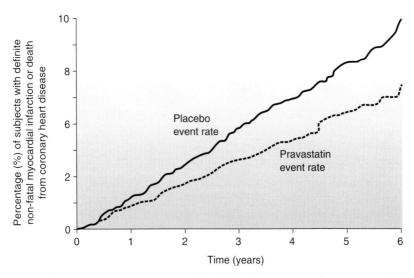

Figure 3.2 Event curve for fatal or non-fatal MI in WOSCOPS (adapted from Shepherd et al 1995).

- Triglyceride fell by 12%
- HDL-cholesterol increased by 5%.

The primary endpoint for WOSCOPS was combined CHD death and non-fatal MI and this was significantly reduced by 31% ($p < 0.001$) as shown in Figure 3.2.

Deaths from any cause were also reduced in the pravastatin group by 22% and, as with the 4S, there was no excess of non-vascular deaths. The subgroup analysis of WOSCOPS also revealed some interesting findings. In particular, it was apparent that the benefits of pravastatin therapy were not affected by age. Those aged 55 years and older obtained the same benefit as younger subjects. Similarly, smoking habits did not counter the beneficial effect of the drug. It was also noted that a significant benefit was seen in the subgroup without multiple risk factors and in those without pre-existing vascular disease.

Extrapolation of the WOSCOPS data reveals that treatment with pravastatin over 5 years of 1000 middle-aged men with hypercholesterolaemia but with no evidence of a previous MI will avoid:

- 14 coronary angiograms
- eight revascularization procedures
- 20 non-fatal MIs
- seven cardiovascular deaths
- two deaths from other causes.

Cholesterol and Recurrent Events (CARE) Study

The CARE Study was performed in multiple centres throughout the USA and Canada and was published in 1996 (Sacks et al 1996). The objective of this secondary prevention trial was to evaluate the effects of pravastatin therapy on rates of non-fatal MI and CHD death in post-MI patients without elevated total plasma cholesterol concentrations, who continue to receive standard post-MI treatments (aspirin, β-blockers, PTCA/CABG).

This was a double-blind, placebo-controlled, randomized trial of 4159 subjects aged 21–75, who were 3–20 months post-MI. The subjects in the study were randomized to receive either pravastatin (40 mg) or placebo and followed up for an average of 5 years. The primary combined endpoint was recurrent non-fatal MI or CHD death. Other endpoints of the study included coronary death, non-fatal MI, total mortality, the need for revascularization and stroke.

In the CARE Study pravastatin therapy resulted in:

- 32% reduction in LDL-cholesterol ($p < 0.001$)
- 24% reduction in fatal or non-fatal MI ($p = 0.003$)
- 31% reduction in stroke ($p = 0.03$)
- 26% reduction in CABG ($p = 0.005$)
- 22% reduction in coronary angioplasty ($p = 0.01$).

In summary, if 1000 post-MI patients with total cholesterol <6.2 mmol/l (240 mg/dl) were treated for 5 years, we would prevent 150 cardiovascular events and 51 patients would be spared from having at least one such event. For patients >60 years the corresponding figures would be 207 cardiovascular events and 71 patients. If the 1000 patients were all female the figures would be 228 cardiovascular events and 97 patients.

Air Force/Texas Coronary Atherosclerosis Prevention Study (AF/TEXCAPS)

This study randomized 6605 subjects (15% women) to either placebo or lovastatin, titrated up to 40 mg/day in order to achieve a target LDL-cholesterol goal of less than 2.84 mmol/l (110 mg/dl) (Downs et al 1998). These individuals had no clinical evidence of atherosclerotic cardiovascular disease and the interesting feature of this study was that their baseline total plasma cholesterol level was on average 5.71 mmol/l (220 mg/dl) with an LDL-cholesterol of 3.88 mmol/l (150 mg/dl). Five years of therapy changed the lipid profiles as shown below:

- Total cholesterol decreased by 18%
- LDL-cholesterol decreased by 25%
- Triglyceride decreased by 15%
- HDL-cholesterol increased by 6%.

Although these lipid changes did not result in significant reductions in CHD or total mortality, they did result in the following significant changes:

- Combined unstable angina, fatal and non-fatal MI or sudden cardiac death decreased by 37%
- Revascularizations decreased by 33%.

Long-Term Intervention with Pravastatin in Ischaemic Disease (LIPID) Study

This study revealed equally interesting data. Here, 9014 subjects (17% female), drawn from 87 centres in Australia and New Zealand and with an average total cholesterol level of 5.65 mmol/l (218 mg/dl), were randomized to pravastatin (40 mg/day) or placebo and followed for an average of 6 years (LIPID Study Group 1998). Pravastatin therapy produced the following lipid changes:

- Total cholesterol decreased by 18%
- LDL-cholesterol decreased by 25%
- Triglyceride decreased by 11%
- HDL-cholesterol increased by 5%.

and the following highly significant reductions in risk of mortality and morbidity:

- All-cause mortality decreased by 22%
- CHD deaths decreased by 24%
- Fatal CHD and non-fatal MI decreased by 24%
- Total strokes decreased by 19%.

One unique aspect of the LIPID Study arose from the decision to recruit substantial numbers of patients with unstable angina. These individuals benefited in terms of event avoidance as much as recruits with a history of myocardial infarction.

Pravastatin Pooling Project (PPP)

The PPP was designed to evaluate the consistency of the treatment effect of pravastatin on the clinical outcomes of coronary and all-cause mortality in three large, randomized, placebo-controlled studies – WOSCOPS, CARE and LIPID. These studies provided a combined patient population of approximately 20 000 followed for 5 or more years, yielding approximately 100 000 patient-years of experience. In addition to the evaluation of fatal and non-fatal cardiovascular events, a combined analysis of non-cardiovascular outcomes was pre-specified. This included evaluation of the impact of cholesterol reduction on accidental death, violence, depression, suicides or cancers. PPP evaluated the effectiveness of treatment in special populations such as the elderly, women and diabetics, and in populations with a wide range of age and lipid values.

The preliminary results of the PPP subgroup analyses (Sacks et al 2000) are shown in Figure 3.3. These data clearly demonstrate the significant clinical benefits achieved by a broad spectrum of patients using pravastatin 40 mg. In addition, the mortality data from the PPP have recently been published (Simes et al 2002). In this analysis the highly significant reductions in total mortality (-20%, $p < 0.0001$) and CHD mortality (-24%, $p < 0.001$) are confirmed. Equally important, the PPP investigators confirmed that pravastatin was not associated with an increase in non-cardiovascular mortality.

Heart Protection Study (HPS)

The HPS is a large trial designed to examine the effects of simvastatin and antioxidant vitamins (Heart Protection Study Collaborative Group 2002). Over 20 000 subjects were recruited into the HPS across a wide age range

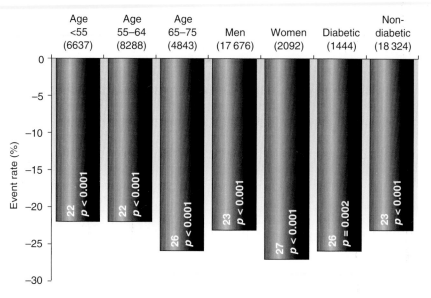

Figure 3.3 PPP subgroup data (data from Sacks et al 2000).

but all with a total cholesterol >3.5 mmol/l. In addition, all subjects were either 'secondary' prevention candidates with a history of CHD, stroke or other vascular disease or were at high risk because of a history of hypertension or diabetes. The study was designed in a two-by-two factorial format, comparing simvastatin 40 mg with antioxidants and placebo, singly or in combination. The mean follow-up was 5.5 years and the study included large cohorts of women, diabetic patients and subjects over 70 years of age.

Based on an intention-to-treat analysis, the main findings of the simvastatin arm of the HPS were as follows: total mortality fell by 12%, cardiovascular death by 17%, fatal and non-fatal stroke by 27% and all major vascular events by 24%. The corresponding figures from the intention-to-treat analysis in the PPP are 20%, 24%, 20% and 17%. Importantly, the rates of non-vascular deaths in both studies were the same in the statin-treated group and placebo-treated group.

In interpreting and comparing these data from the PPP and HPS, it is important to recognize the basic differences between the study populations. The HPS cohort was in general a high-risk group, a large number of whom entered the study with a history of stroke. In contrast, relatively few subjects in the PPP had a history of stroke. It is perhaps therefore not surprising that an apparently greater reduction in stroke risk was observed in the HPS compared to the PPP.

The HPS is an important addition to our portfolio of statin trials and strongly supports a number of key observations made previously in the large PPP study. The PPP showed a highly significant reduction in total mortality, vascular events, cardiovascular disease in women and diabetic subjects and in older adults. These have all now been further confirmed in the HPS. Importantly, the antioxidant vitamin arm of the HPS showed no benefit at all in the prevention of vascular events or all-cause mortality. The HPS did demonstrate benefits of statin therapy across a wide range of subjects with low as well as high cholesterol values. Diabetic patients without previous CHD benefited from therapy, and primary and secondary stroke prevention with statin therapy was confirmed.

LIPID-REGULATING DRUGS

There are three main classes of lipid-regulating drugs in common use: resins, fibrates and statins. In addition, a number of other drugs have been used to change the lipid profile, e.g. nicotinic acid, acipimox, probucol and fish oils. Below we describe briefly the main mechanisms of action of resins and the fibrates but devote the remainder of the chapter to the final class, for it is the statins that have now come to dominate the field of clinical lipidology.

Bile acid sequestrant resins

The bile acid sequestrant resins are able to lower LDL-cholesterol by 20–25% when given at the highest recommended dose. They are considered very safe drugs since they are not absorbed systemically and have been in clinical use for several decades. Furthermore, they are one of the few lipid-lowering compounds recommended for use in children with severe hypercholesterolaemia. The principal drawback to their more widespread prescription is the fact that they are difficult to take and patient compliance is often very poor. Approximately half of the subjects who begin resin therapy stop because of their inability to tolerate the side-effects.

Resins block the reabsorption of bile acids and thus interrupt the enterohepatic circulation. The liver compensates for this irretrievable loss of bile acids by increasing bile acid synthesis, which in turn requires increased cholesterol reserves, since cholesterol is used as the basic building block of the bile acid molecule. By increasing LDL receptor function, the liver obtains sufficient cholesterol but in so doing lowers the circulating plasma cholesterol level (Shepherd et al 1980).

Sequestrant resins have additional actions on plasma triglyceride and HDL levels. Bile acids returning to the liver in the enterohepatic circulation suppress not only cholesterol synthesis but also triglyceride production (Angelin et al 1978). The release of this inhibition by resin therapy causes an immediate rise in triglyceride synthesis and a promotion of triglyceride-rich very low density lipoprotein (VLDL) secretion so that within days of initiating therapy, VLDL triglyceride levels can increase twofold. Subsequently, the plasma triglyceride concentration usually falls back towards baseline values through an adaptation brought about by increased lipolysis. This does not occur in individuals with elevated triglyceride values prior to resin treatment. Resins are, therefore, not indicated in such individuals who have moderately or severely elevated plasma triglyceride levels.

Fibrates

Modern fibric acid derivatives, or fibrates, include bezafibrate, ciprofibrate, fenofibrate and gemfibrozil and these drugs are still prescribed worldwide, although their use has significantly declined with the introduction of the statins. These agents share a similar lipid-lowering profile, reducing plasma triglyceride levels usually by 20–50% (principally by lowering circulating VLDL levels) and plasma cholesterol by 10–25%. HDL-cholesterol is normally increased 10–30% by fibrates depending on the pretreatment level (patients with lower basal HDL respond with greater increases). The metabolic syndrome, characterized by raised plasma triglyceride and low HDL-cholesterol, is associated with high risk of CHD. Individuals with this lipid profile, i.e. plasma triglyceride >2.3 mmol/l and an LDL to HDL ratio of >5, have been shown to benefit most from fibrate therapy (Manninen et al 1992).

The mechanism of action of fibrates has been studied for many years and more recently the discovery that they act as peroxisome proliferator-activated receptor α (PPAR-α) agonists has revolutionized our understanding of their pharmacology (Staels et al 1998). The plasma concentration of VLDL is reduced up to 50% on therapy. Two main mechanisms have been proposed to explain the influence of fibrates on VLDL metabolism. The first is a fall in the return of free fatty acids to the liver secondary to suppression of their release from adipose tissue (Kissebah et al 1974), while the second is stimulation of lipoprotein lipase activity (Simpson et al 1990), the enzyme which governs triglyceride hydrolysis in plasma. Kinetic studies indicate that both mechanisms operate in vivo (Packard & Shepherd 1986, Simpson et al 1990).

The precise mechanism by which the fibrates exert their powerful HDL-cholesterol raising effect is still being studied but will almost certainly be a consequence, at least in part, of the closely interrelated metabolism of VLDL and HDL.

Statins

To understand the mechanisms by which the statins impact upon the plasma cholesterol level, we must first understand the regulation of cholesterol balance at a cellular level. The cholesterol economy of the cell is controlled by a family of recently discovered regulatory proteins, known as sterol regulatory element-binding proteins (SREBPs) (Brown & Goldstein 1997). These proteins control the transcription of the LDL receptor and at least six other key enzymatic steps in the cholesterol biosynthetic pathway (Horton & Shimomura 1999). When the cholesterol level falls within the cell, the SREBPs are activated and they interact with the cell's DNA, activating the transcription of various genes (Brown & Goldstein 1997, Edwards & Ericsson 1998).

When we give statin therapy we inhibit the key enzyme in the cell's cholesterol synthetic pathway, 3-hydroxy-3-methylglutaryl co-enzyme A (HMG CoA) reductase, and this leads to a fall in the intracellular cholesterol concentration. As described above, this sets in motion a train of events that ultimately leads to the enhanced transcription of several proteins involved in cholesterol balance including, perhaps most importantly, upregulation of the LDL receptor.

Transcription of HMG CoA reductase is also upregulated but this enzyme is not increased enough to overcome the drug effect, i.e. there is more inhibition present than enzyme produced.

The LDL receptor is a single transmembrane protein (Brown & Goldstein 1987), which binds apoB and apoE (Mahley & Innerarity 1983). The receptor therefore recognizes and interacts with particles containing these proteins but with different affinities, since apoE binds approximately 10 times more effectively than the B. In theory, then, a whole spectrum of lipoprotein particles found within the VLDL–LDL interval, which contains one or both of these proteins, could interact with, and be degraded by, the LDL receptor. Indeed, metabolic studies have now shown that statin therapy is not simply associated with an increased clearance of LDL (Shepherd et al 1980) but also of VLDL (Vega et al 1988) and intermediate-density lipoprotein (IDL) (Gaw et al 1993).

Effects on plasma LDL cholesterol

Plasma LDL-cholesterol reductions achieved with statin therapy appear to be independent of the baseline lipid phenotype. That said, it must also be appreciated that between statins there are marked differences in cholesterol-lowering effectiveness and wide interindividual variation in response to the same dose on one statin. For example, a recent study of simvastatin at 40 mg/day for 3 months produced anything from a decrement in LDL-cholesterol of over 60% to an increment of almost 10% (Dujovne 1997).

There are many small studies defining the biochemical effectiveness of the statins either individually or in comparison with each other. However, any tabular comparison of the cholesterol-lowering effects of the statins inevitably raises more questions than it answers, as small studies are often included alongside large-scale studies, results achieved in normal practice are compared with the results achieved in a controlled clinical trial setting and different doses are compared. What is obvious from studies with all the statins is that the dose–response is not a simple linear one. Doubling the dose of any statin does not double the percentage cholesterol lowering. Indeed, as a rule of thumb, each time the dose is doubled an approximately 6% further LDL-cholesterol reduction is achieved.

While there are clear pharmacological differences between the statins in terms of the cholesterol reductions seen with equivalent doses, it is probably true to say that by adjusting the doses accordingly, all statins are capable of producing equivalent reductions in LDL-cholesterol. What is not clear from studies completed so far is whether such dose adjustments will be equally free from side-effects for each statin or whether therapy with all statins, irrespective of their potency in lowering LDL-cholesterol, will have the same effect on clinical events.

Effects on plasma triglyceride and HDL

Considering their basic mechanism of action, it was assumed that statins would have no effect on triglyceride levels but this was not the case. Two studies looking at the effects of statins in patients with hypertriglyceridaemia revealed that simvastatin and atorvastatin both reduced plasma triglyceride levels in these subjects in proportion to their effects on LDL-cholesterol (Bakker-Arkema et al 1996, Stein et al 1996). This prompted a more detailed analysis of the question looking at data from different statins, at different doses. Thus, a fixed, non-dose related, triglyceride/LDL-cholesterol ratio in subjects on statin therapy, with or without baseline hypertriglyceridaemia, was discovered (Stein et al 1998). At lower plasma triglyceride levels (1.7 mmol/l, <150 mg/dl) the percentage reduction in triglyceride with statin therapy is modest in comparison to the effects of the drug on LDL. When baseline triglyceride concentration exceeded 2.8 mmol/l (250 mg/dl), the percentage triglyceride reduction achieved with any of the statins tested at any dose equalled the corresponding percentage reduction in LDL-cholesterol. All statins are therefore effective in lowering plasma triglyceride levels, in addition to their effects on plasma LDL-cholesterol, but only in baseline hypertriglyceridaemic subjects is this effect comparable to the effects on plasma cholesterol.

Two possible mechanisms have been postulated to explain the influence of the statins on triglyceride and, more specifically, VLDL metabolism. In the first, it is proposed that statins inhibit VLDL secretion by limiting the availability of free cholesterol or cholesteryl esters for lipoprotein assembly. There are in vitro and animal model studies to support this concept (Burnett et al 1997, Qin et al 1992) and recently, atorvastatin has been reported to promote apoB intracellular degradation, possibly by so lowering the cholesterol content of newly forming lipoprotein particles that they become unstable (Mohammadi et al 1998). The second mechanism suggests that drug-induced stimulation of LDL receptors promotes the direct catabolism of VLDL, particularly the cholesterol-rich remnants (Gaw et al 1993). If the latter mechanism is important, then the observation that VLDL from hypertriglyceridaemic subjects, by virtue of its surface apoE content, binds to the LDL receptor whereas VLDL from normotriglyceridaemic subjects fails to do so (Gianturco et al 1982) provides a possible explanation for the phenotype dependency of plasma triglyceride lowering by statins described above.

Collectively, what has emerged from these studies is that the initial phenotype of our patients has little bearing on the LDL-cholesterol lowering with statin therapy but when the effects on triglyceride are examined, the initial phenotype is paramount.

Accompanying the changes in triglyceride, there are small increases in HDL-cholesterol on statins, usually of the order of 5–10%. The significance of these is not clear, nor is the mechanism for the increase. In WOSCOPS, for example, the small rise in HDL could not be linked to any change in the risk of coronary events (WOSCOPS 1998).

Mechanisms of action beyond lipid modification

Close scrutiny of the statin clinical trial results has prompted some to question whether the unexpectedly rapid onset of the striking clinical benefits can be attributed to cholesterol reduction alone (Vaughan et al 1997). Laboratory and clinical evidence is certainly accumulating to the effect that individual statins may possess benefits beyond their cholesterol-lowering capability, particularly with regard to:

- plaque stabilization (Crisby et al 2001)
- endothelial function (Stahl et al 1989)

- platelet function (Rosensen & Tangney 1998)
- anti-inflammation (Ridker et al 1999)
- lipoprotein oxidation (Kleinveld et al 1993)
- rheology and blood coagulation (Lowe et al 2000, Schrör 1990)
- glucose intolerance (Freeman et al 2001).

These potential mechanisms are reviewed in detail elsewhere (Shepherd 2000) and support the premise that cholesterol lowering provides cardiovascular gain beyond the traditional notion of atherosclerotic lesion regression. Thus, these mechanisms provide a plausible explanation for the unexpectedly early benefit that these agents seem capable of producing (Andrews et al 1997, Shepherd et al 1995).

LIPID-LOWERING DRUGS IN PRACTICE

Lipid-lowering or, more correctly, lipid-regulating drugs have an important place in the management of the lipid-related risk of CHD. In secondary prevention they occupy a first-line role in this management. However, in primary prevention, and depending on the baseline global risk level and the baseline lipid values, they may occupy a second-line place after lifestyle changes have been tried and found inadequate. All patients who are found to be dyslipidaemic should receive detailed and tailored dietary advice as outlined in Chapter 6. This should be given in conjunction with safe and practicable exercise advice and, if appropriate, advice on how to stop smoking. Lipids, like all of the cardiovascular risk factors, should never be managed in isolation. If lipid-regulating drugs are used, it is important to note that drug therapy is prescribed as an adjunct to dietary therapy and not as an alternative. The patients' lifestyle changes in terms of diet should be continued and patients must be made to realize that the initiation of drug therapy does not mean that their efforts, which are sometimes considerable, have been in vain.

Another important point to be considered by both patient and prescriber is that lipid-lowering drug therapy is lifelong and requires understanding and co-operation from the patient if it is to be effective and worthwhile. Like the management of hypertension, the drug treatment of dyslipidaemia does not carry any immediate and obvious benefit or 'feel-good factor'. The concept of CHD risk should be explained to the patient along with the rationale for prevention. In the secondary prevention situation, where the patient has already suffered a coronary event, this is much easier and the patient is often well focused on the issue. However, in primary prevention more time may be needed to explain the reasons for commencing drug therapy and the long-term benefits that are expected.

The choice of lipid-regulating drug should be dictated by the evidence, for we are constantly encouraged to practise evidence-based medicine. The clinical trials have been discussed above and they immediately suggest specific drugs at specific doses for the prevention of cardiovascular events. The use of alternative therapeutic strategies may be equally effective but they do not, as yet, carry the same weight of clinical trial evidence.

CONCLUSION

The correction of raised plasma lipid levels is a problem that faces the health-care team on a daily basis. There is now abundant evidence that a wide range of individuals with high CHD risk factor scores require intervention to lower their plasma lipid levels. A range of lipid-lowering drugs is now available and the mechanisms of action of most of these are now well understood, but it is the statins that have dominated this field in the last 5 years and they are likely to do so for the foreseeable future. Some of these drugs have been proven not only to impact upon the plasma lipid profile but, much more importantly, to reduce cardiovascular risk and extend life. The even more widespread use of these drugs is curtailed not by any lack of evidence that they are clinically effective but rather by concerns over cost containment. Against these often high costs must be placed the overwhelming costs of the diseases that we are trying to prevent. Cardiovascular disease is the leading cause of death and disability in many countries and any attempt to change this will, of course, carry a significant price tag. However, our current concerns over the economics of lipid-regulating drug use may abate as the first statins lose their patent protection and prices fall. This, coupled with our developing appreciation that statins possibly provide us with even greater clinical benefits than we had anticipated, will mean that we must recalculate our current cost-effectiveness equations. Perhaps then we will be ready to offer more of our patients the cardiovascular protection afforded by these therapies.

■ KEY POINTS

- Lipoproteins are complexes of lipids and proteins, which facilitate lipid transport around the body.
- Elevated plasma LDL-cholesterol and decreased plasma HDL-cholesterol are associated with increased risk of CHD.
- Interpretation of lipid-related risk should always be part of a global CHD risk factor assessment.
- By lowering plasma cholesterol we can reduce a patient's risk of CHD and this has been proven conclusively in a wide spectrum of patient groups.
- Resins bind and remove bile acids from the body, thus forcing the liver to resort to plasma LDL-cholesterol for its needs. This in turn lowers plasma LDL-cholesterol.
- Fibrates are PPAR-α agonists and primarily lower triglyceride and raise HDL-cholesterol.
- The statins inhibit HMG CoA reductase, the rate-limiting enzyme in the cell's cholesterol production, thereby forcing the liver to resort to plasma LDL-cholesterol for its needs.
- The major lipid-lowering drug trials, 4S, WOSCOPS, CARE, LIPID, AF/TEXCAPS and HPS, have clearly demonstrated the clinical efficacy of the statins in both primary and secondary prevention of CHD.
- Lipid-lowering drug therapy is lifelong and will only be successful with the full co-operation and understanding of the patient.

■ CASE STUDY 3.1

A 48-year-old man arrives at the hospital emergency department complaining of chest tightness and numbness in his left arm. His initial ECG was equivocal but a suspected MI was later confirmed by serum cardiac enzyme changes. After an uneventful 24 hours in the CCU he was transferred to the general medical ward prior to discharge 5 days later. He was prescribed aspirin 75 mg daily and enrolled in the hospital's cardiac rehabilitation programme. He comes to your clinic 6 weeks later. His notes provide the following information.

BP:	150/105 mmHg
Smoking status:	Ex-smoker
BMI:	29.7
Lipids:	Never checked
Exercise:	None formally, but has heavy manual job

Checked on this visit
  Fasting glucose: 5.0 mmol/l (90 mg/dl)
  Fasting lipids: Total cholesterol 6.3 mmol/l (244 mg/dl), triglyceride 2.1 mmol/l (186 mg/dl), HDL-cholesterol 0.85 mmol/l (33 mg/dl)

Questions

1. What further information do you require to assess the overall coronary risk?
2. What further lifestyle advice would you offer?
3. What further drug management would you have considered as an inpatient?
4. Is there clinical trial evidence to support the acute use of a statin in this man?

Answers

1. This man has suffered a classic myocardial infarction and is now a candidate for secondary prevention. Most guidelines or risk calculators that allow the overall coronary risk to be calculated do so in primary prevention candidates. When an individual has clinical evidence of coronary disease it is unnecessary to calculate his risk score as it is, by definition, high. There is good evidence that all patients with coronary disease should receive statin therapy as all secondary prevention trials have shown unequivocal benefit in these patients.
2. This man is noted to be an ex-smoker but many patients, once they have recovered from their acute coronary event, will resume smoking. It is crucial to make this man understand that smoking is a major risk factor for coronary disease and that the single most important thing he can do to help himself is to keep off his cigarettes. His blood pressure is high and untreated and he is overweight. He should be advised to follow a sensible weight reduction diet and in view of his dyslipidaemia, should also receive detailed advice about a lipid-lowering diet. In addition, an appropriate exercise regimen should be suggested and if possible, this may be co-ordinated through the cardiac rehabilitation programme.

3. This patient is inadequately managed at present. His current dose of aspirin would be considered too low by many physicians and the use of β-blockers and ACE inhibitors should be considered. Statin therapy is also indicated in a man such as this.

4. This patient could have been in either the 4S (simvastatin) or the LIPID Study (pravastatin). Both these secondary prevention studies recruited patients with pre-existing coronary disease. The other major secondary prevention study that tested a statin (pravastatin) was the CARE Study. Although this man fits the study's main criterion of being an MI survivor, his total cholesterol level is too high to have been included in CARE.

■ PRACTICAL EXERCISE

If we are truly to practise evidence-based medicine, we should ideally prescribe those drugs and doses tested in large-scale clinical trials. Many patients are currently receiving lipid-lowering therapies or doses that have been untested. In your regular reviews of patients who are receiving risk factor management in the form of lipid-lowering drugs, consider in each case if the treatment they are receiving is backed up by the kind of robust clinical trial evidence described in detail above.

REFERENCES

Andrews TA, Raby K, Barry J et al 1997 Effect of cholesterol reduction on myocardial ischemia in patients with coronary disease. Circulation 95: 324–328

Angelin B, Einarsson K, Hellström K, Leijd B 1978 Effects of cholestyramine and chenodeoxycholic acid on the metabolism of endogenous triglyceride in hyperlipoproteinemia. Journal of Lipid Research 19: 1017–1024

Anitschkow N 1913 Uber die Veranderungen der Kaninchenaorta bei experimenteller Cholesterinsteatose. Beitrage zur pathologisten Anatomie und zur allgemeinen Pathologie 56: 379–404

Assmann G, Schulte H 1992 Relation of high density lipoprotein cholesterol and triglyceride to incidence of atherosclerosis coronary artery disease (the PROCAM experience). American Journal of Cardiology 70: 733–737

Bakker-Arkema RG, Davidson MH, Goldstein RJ et al 1996 Efficacy and safety of a new 17 HMG-CoA reductase inhibitor, atorvastatin, in patients with hypertriglyceridemia. Journal of the American Medical Association 275: 128–133

Brown MS, Goldstein JL 1997 The SREBP pathway: regulation of cholesterol metabolism by proteolysis of a membrane-bound transcription factor. Cell 89: 331–340

Burnett JR, Wilcox LJ, Telford DE et al 1997 Inhibition of HMG-CoA reductase by atorvastatin decreases both VLDL and LDL apolipoprotein B production in miniature pigs. Arteriosclerosis Thrombosis and Vascular Biology 17: 2589–2600

Castelli WP 1984 Epidemiology of coronary heart disease: the Framingham study. American Journal of Medicine 76: 4–12

Collins R 2001 The MRC/BHF Heart Protection Study. American Heart Association Scientific Sessions, Anaheim, USA

Crisby M, Nordin-Fredriksson G, Shah PK, Yano J, Zhu J, Nilsson J 2001 Pravastatin treatment increases collagen content and decreases lipid content, inflammation, metalloproteinases, and cell death in human carotid plaques: implications for plaque stabilization. Circulation 103: 926–933

Davey Smith G, Pekkanen J 1992 Should there be a moratorium on the use of cholesterol lowering drugs? British Medical Journal 304: 431–434

Downs JR, Clearfield M, Weis S et al 1998 Primary prevention of acute coronary events with lovastatin in men and women with average cholesterol levels: results of AFCAPS/TEXCAPS Research Group. Journal of the American Medical Association 279: 1615–1622

Dujovne CA 1997 New lipid lowering drugs and new effects of old drugs. Current Opinion in Lipidology 8: 362–368

Edwards PA, Ericsson J 1998 Signaling molecules derived from the cholesterol biosynthetic pathway: mechanisms of action and possible roles in human disease. Current Opinion in Lipidology 9: 433–440

Freeman DJ, Norrie J, Sattar N et al 2001 Pravastatin and the development of diabetes mellitus. Circulation 103: 357–362

Frick MH, Elo O, Haapa K et al 1987 Helsinki Heart Study: primary-prevention trial with gemfibrozil in middle-aged men with dyslipidemia. New England Journal of Medicine 317: 1237–1245

Gaw A, Packard CJ, Murray EF et al 1993 Effects of simvastatin on apoB metabolism and LDL subfraction distribution. Arteriosclerosis and Thrombosis 13: 170–189

Gaw A, Cowan RA, O'Reilly D St J, Stewart MJ, Shepherd J 1999 Clinical biochemistry: an illustrated colour text, 2nd edn. Churchill Livingstone, Edinburgh

Gianturco SH, Brown FB, Gotto AM, Bradley WA 1982 Receptor mediated uptake of hypertriglyceridemic very low density lipoproteins by normal human fibroblasts. Journal of Lipid Research 23: 984–993

Heart Protection Study Collaborative Group 2002 MRC/BHF Heart Protection Study of cholesterol lowering with simvastatin in 20,536 high-risk individuals: a randomized placebo-controlled trial. Lancet 360: 7–22

Heinonen OP, Huttunen JK, Manninen V et al 1994 The Helsinki Heart Study: coronary heart disease incidence during an extended follow-up. Journal of Internal Medicine 235: 41–49

Horton JD, Shimomura I 1999 Sterol regulatory element-binding proteins: activators of cholesterol and fatty acid biosynthesis. Current Opinion in Lipidology 10: 143–150

Keech AC 1992 Does cholesterol lowering reduce total mortality? Postgraduate Medical Journal 68: 870–871

Keys A 1980 Seven Countries Study: a multivariate analysis of death and coronary heart disease. Harvard University Press, Cambridge, MA

Kissebah AH, Adams PW, Harrigan WV 1974 The mechanism of action of clofibrate and tetranicotinylfructose on the kinetics of plasma free fatty acid and triglyceride transport in Type IV and Type V hypertriglyceridemia. European Journal of Clinical Investigation 4: 163–174

Kleinveld HA, Demacker PNM, de Haan AFJ, Stalenhoef AFH 1993 Decreased in vitro oxidisability of LDL in hypercholesterolemic patients treated with HMG CoA reductase inhibitors. European Journal of Clinical Investigation 23: 289–295

Lipid Research Clinics Program 1984 The Lipid Research Clinics Coronary Primary Prevention Trial results. I. Reduction in incidence of coronary heart disease. Journal of the American Medical Association 251: 351–364

Long-Term Intervention with Pravastatin in Ischaemic Disease (LIPID) Study Group 1998 Prevention of cardiovascular events and death with pravastatin in patients with coronary heart disease and a broad range of initial cholesterol levels. New England Journal of Medicine 339: 1349–1357

Lowe G, Rumley A, Norrie J et al 2000 Blood rheology, cardiovascular risk factors, and cardiovascular disease: the West of Scotland Coronary Prevention Study. Thrombosis and Haemostasis 84: 553–558

Mahley RW, Innerarity TL 1983 Lipoprotein receptors and cholesterol homeostasis. Biochimica et Biophysica Acta 737: 197–222

Manninen V, Elo O, Frick MH et al 1988 Lipid alterations and decline in the incidence of coronary heart disease in the Helsinki Heart Study. Journal of the American Medical Association 260: 641–651

Manninen V, Tenkanen L, Koskinen P et al 1992 Joint effects of serum triglyceride and LDL cholesterol and HDL cholesterol concentrations on coronary heart disease risk in the Helsinki Heart Study. Implications for treatment. Circulation 85: 37–45

Mohammadi AJ, Macri J, Newton R, Romain T, Dulay D, Adeli K 1998 Effects of atorvastatin on the intracellular stability and secretion of apolipoprotein B in HepG2 cells. Arteriosclerosis Thrombosis and Vascular Biology 18: 783–793

Packard CJ, Shepherd J 1986 Cholesterol 7 α hydroxylase: involvement in hepatobiliary axis and regulation of plasma lipoprotein levels. In: Fears R, Sabine JR (eds) Cholesterol 7α hydroxylase. CRC Press, Boca Raton, FL, pp 147–165

Pedersen TR, Wilhelmsen L, Faergeman O et al 2000 Follow-up study of patients randomized in the Scandinavian Simvastatin Survival Study (4S) of cholesterol lowering. American Journal of Cardiology 86: 257–262

Qin W, Infante J, Wang S, Infante R 1992 Regulation of HMG-CoA reductase, apoprotein B and LDL receptor gene expression by the hypocholesterolemic drugs simvastatin and ciprofibrate in HepG2 human and rat hepatocytes. Biochimica et Biophysica Acta 1127: 57–66

Ridker PM, Rifai N, Pfeffer MA, Sacks F, Braunwald E 1999 Long-term effects of pravastatin on plasma concentration of C-reactive protein. The Cholesterol and Recurrent Events (CARE) Investigators. Circulation 100: 230–235

Rosensen RS, Tangney CC 1998 Antiatherothrombotic properties of statins. Journal of the American Medical Association 279: 1643–1650

Sacks FM, Pfeffer MA, Moye LA et al 1996 The effect of pravastatin on coronary events after myocardial infarction in patients with average cholesterol levels. New England Journal of Medicine 335: 1001–1009

Sacks FM, Tonkin AM, Shepherd J 2000 Effect of pravastatin on coronary disease events in subgroups defined by coronary risk factors: the Prospective Pravastatin Pooling Project. Circulation 102: 1893–1900

Scandinavian Simvastatin Survival Study Group 1994 Randomised trial of cholesterol lowering in 4444 patients with coronary heart disease: The Scandinavian Simvastatin Survival Study (4S). Lancet 344: 1383–1389

Schrör K 1990 Platelet reactivity and arachidonic acid metabolism in Type II hyper-lipoproteinaemia and its modification by cholesterol lowering agents. Eicosanoids 3: 67–73

Shepherd J 2000 Ancillary benefits of the statins. In: Gaw A, Packard CJ, Shepherd J (eds) Statins: The HMG CoA reductase inhibitors in perspective. Martin Dunitz, London

Shepherd J, Packard CJ, Bicker S, Lawrie TDV, Morgan HG 1980 Cholestyramine promotes receptor mediated low density lipoprotein catabolism. New England Journal of Medicine 302: 1219–1222

Shepherd J, Cobbe SM, Ford I et al 1995 Prevention of coronary heart disease with pravastatin in men with hypercholesterolaemia. New England Journal of Medicine 333: 1301–1307

Simes J, Furberg CD, Braunwald E et al 2002 Effects of pravastatin on mortality in patients with and without coronary heart disease across a broad range of cholesterol levels. The Prospective Pravastatin Pooling Project. European Heart Journal 23: 207–215

Simpson HS, Williamson CM, Olivecrona T et al 1990 Postprandial lipemia, fenofibrate and coronary artery disease. Atherosclerosis 85: 193–202

Staels B, Dallongeville J, Auwerx J, Schoonjans K, Leitersdorf E, Fruchart JC 1998 Mechanism of action of fibrates on lipid and lipoprotein metabolism. Circulation 98: 2088–2093

Stahl GL, Fusman B, Lefer AM 1989 Cardiovascular effects of acute hypercholesterolaemia in rabbits. Journal of Clinical Investigation 83: 465–477

Stamler J, Wentworth D, Neaton JD 1986 Is the relationship between serum cholesterol and risk of premature death from coronary heart disease continuous and graded? Findings in 356,222 primary screenees of the Multiple Risk Factor Intervention Trial (MRFIT). Journal of the American Medical Association 256: 2823–2828

Stein EA, Davidson MH, Dujovne CA et al 1996 Efficacy and tolerability of low-dose simvastatin and niacin, alone and in combination, in patients with combined hyperlipidemia: a prospective trial. Journal of Cardiovascular Pharmacology and Therapeutics 1: 107–116

Stein EA, Lane M, Laskarzewski P 1998 Comparison of statins in hypertriglyceridemia. American Journal of Cardiology 81(4A): 66B–69B

Vaughan CJ, Murphy MB, Buckley BM 1997 Statins do more than just lower cholesterol. Lancet 348: 1079–1082

Vega GL, East C, Grundy SM 1988 Lovastatin therapy in familial dysbetalipoproteinemia: effects on kinetics of apolipoprotein B. Atherosclerosis 70: 131–143

Vogel J 1845 Patholog. Anat. Des meschlischen Korpers (The pathological anatomy of the human body). H Baillière, London

West of Scotland Coronary Prevention Study Group 1998 Influence of pravastatin and plasma lipids on clinical events in the West of Scotland Coronary Prevention Study (WOSCOPS). Circulation 97: 1440–1445

FURTHER READING

British national formulary 2001 British Medical Association & the Royal Pharmaceutical Society of Great Britain, London

Gaw A 2003 Statins in general practice, 2nd edn. Martin Dunitz, London

Gaw A, Cowan RA, O'Reilly D St J, Stewart MJ, Shepherd J 1999 Clinical biochemistry: an illustrated colour text, 2nd edn. Churchill Livingstone, Edinburgh

Gaw A, Packard CJ, Shepherd J 2000 Statins: the HMG CoA reductase inhibitors in perspective. Martin Dunitz, London

National Cholesterol Education Program (NCEP) Expert Panel on Detection, Evaluation and Treatment of High Blood Cholesterol in Adults (Adults Treatment Panel III) 2001 Executive summary of the Third Report. Journal of the American Medical Association 285: 2486–2497

Hypertension and antihypertensive therapy

4

Gordon T. McInnes   Joan L. Curzio
Susan S. Kennedy

■ CONTENTS

INTRODUCTION

Hypertension (high blood pressure) is defined traditionally as the blood pressure above which intervention has been shown to reduce risk (Pickering 1968). However, the relationship between blood pressure and risk is continuous with no lower threshold. Therefore, the definition of the blood pressure level which can be considered as hypertension is somewhat arbitrary.

This chapter outlines the physiological definition, epidemiology, measurement, assessment, diagnosis, management and follow-up care of hypertension. Hypertension is just one of the factors that increases risk of cardiovascular disease (MacMahon et al 1990). Therefore, hypertension care needs to be part of an integrated multiple risk factor reduction programme.

WHAT IS BLOOD PRESSURE?

Blood pressure is the pressure in the arterial system. It waxes and wanes as the heart beats. It also varies from beat to beat. The maximum pressure, i.e. systolic blood pressure, occurs as the left ventricle empties into the aorta and the resting pressure, i.e. diastolic blood pressure, occurs as the ventricle fills. The major determinants of blood pressure are cardiac output, i.e. the amount of blood expelled by the left ventricle in 1 minute of pumping, and peripheral resistance, which is determined by the tone or tension of the vascular musculature and the diameter of the vessels in the periphery.

This pressurized system is dynamic, reacting with increases and decreases in pressure to a number of stimuli, each of which affects either the cardiac output or peripheral resistance or both. These stimuli include the release or inhibition of adrenaline, noradrenaline, renin, angiotensin, aldosterone, endothelin, etc.

Blood pressure exhibits considerable variability over a 24-hour period. Levels during the day are usually higher than those at night. Blood pressure increases sharply when an individual rises in the morning and falls abruptly on retiring to bed (and sleep) at night. This fluctuation is not a circadian rhythm. The major determinant is activity (mediated by the hormonal influences outlined above) and the usual day–night pattern is lost during prolonged bedrest or reversed in nightshift workers. Superimposed on the basic blood pressure pattern are shorter term changes induced by physical and mental stress.

WHAT IS HYPERTENSION?

During assessment and even before the diagnosis of hypertension is made, it is helpful to explain that high blood pressure is not a disease. Blood pressure has an approximately normal distribution in the population and those with hypertension are merely at the upper end of the distribution. Although high blood pressure is not an illness, without treatment it increases the risk of heart attack, stroke and other vascular diseases.

Patients are often confused by the terminology – high blood *pressure* and hyper*tension*. They assume that the condition is related to stress and that feelings of tension indicate that blood pressure is elevated. Some feel completely well and have difficulty in accepting that they are at risk. It is important to explain that hypertension is an asymptomatic condition. Symptoms, such as epistaxis or headache, are only likely if hypertension is severe or if complications develop. This emphasizes the importance of early diagnosis and long-term treatment.

EPIDEMIOLOGY

Hypertension is one of the most common medical conditions in this country. Up to 20% of the entire population has high blood pressure. However, the frequency of hypertension varies in different populations. In Western societies, high blood pressure levels are more frequent in lower social classes and in the elderly (Wolf-Meier et al 2003). The rise in blood pressure with age is not seen in individuals sheltered from the influences of modern life (e.g. Italian nuns) or in rural societies (e.g Kalahari bushmen). Black Africans who move to cities have blood pressure higher than that in their contemporaries who continue to live in a rural setting. Indeed, black Africans who live in Westernized societies have blood pressure higher than native Caucasians.

The underlying mechanism for these blood pressure differences is unclear but is probably multifactorial. Dietary changes (such as increased salt intake) are likely to be of major significance. However, within populations, nature as well as nurture is important. A genetic component is suggested by the recognition of families with high incidence of hypertension.

In the vast majority of people with high blood pressure, no cause is found; this is essential (primary) hypertension. A few people with high blood pressure have an underlying cause, mostly due to kidney or glandular (hormonal) problems; this is secondary hypertension. The usual form of hypertension (essential) often runs in families. Lifestyle factors can make blood pressure higher – overeating, lack of exercise, excessive alcohol consumption, too much salt in the diet.

At least 90% of individuals with chronically raised blood pressure have essential hypertension and such individuals should be the focus of attention. However, when assessing anyone with elevated blood pressure, it must be recognized that a few patients will have a diagnosable and treatable cause for hypertension (Box 4.1). All assessment protocols need to include screening for these conditions with referral to a specialist centre for diagnosis and treatment.

In epidemiological studies, there is a close relationship between blood pressure (systolic and diastolic) and risk of stroke, coronary heart disease and other cardiovascular events (He & Whelton 1999, MacMahon et al 1990). The higher the blood pressure, the greater is the risk. This relationship is consistent in different populations, in younger and older subjects, in men and women, and is independent of other cardiovascular risk factors. The relationship is continuous across the range of blood pressure, indicating that there is no lower threshold or safe level of blood pressure. The slope of the relationship between blood pressure and stroke is about 50% steeper

---

■ **BOX 4.1 Causes of secondary hypertension**

- Renal disease:
  - glomerulonephritis
  - pyelonephritis
  - polycystic kidneys
  - renal infarction
- Renal artery stenosis
- Phaeochromocytoma
- Primary aldosteronism
- Adrenal adenoma
- Cushing's syndrome
- Coarctation of aorta
- Late polio or encephalitis
- Drug induced:
  - oral contraceptives
  - steroids
  - carbenoxalone
  - monoamine oxidase inhibitors

than that between blood pressure and coronary heart disease. However, many more coronary events are experienced in Western populations, although strokes are the predominant events in individuals from South East Asia.

Individuals with more than one cardiovascular risk factor (e.g. hypertension, hyperlipidaemia, cigarette smoking) are at greater risk from the combination of factors, increasing the risk well above that which is attributed to the factors singly (Kannel et al 1986, Primatesta et al 2001). In Westernized populations an individual with one cardiovascular risk factor is more likely to have other risk factors co-existing and therefore be at higher risk (Criqui et al 1986, Kannel 2000, MacMahon et al 1985). Other independent risk factors of particular relevance to a community health-care team include history of coronary heart disease (angina or myocardial infarction), electrocardiographic (ECG) evidence of myocardial ischaemia, prior infarction or left ventricular hypertrophy (LVH) and history of premature cardiovascular disease in a first-degree relative (e.g. parent or sibling at age <55 years in males and <65 years in females).

Finally and critically, there is now abundant evidence that reducing blood pressure reduces cardiovascular risk. Over the past four decades, numerous studies have examined the influence of drug treatment of hypertension on risk of cardiovascular events (Collins & MacMahon 1994). The usual aim was to achieve diastolic blood pressure less than 90 mmHg. The average reduction in diastolic blood pressure of 5–6 mmHg in these trials conferred a reduction of about 38% in stroke incidence, a 16% reduction in coronary heart disease events, a 21% reduction in all vascular events and a 12% reduction in all-cause mortality, all highly significant. Effects on fatal and non-fatal events were similar. The proportional reductions were the same in high- and low-risk individuals, in the young and the elderly, and in mild, moderate and severe hypertension. At least equivalent benefits are associated with treatment of systolic hypertension, even in the absence of raised diastolic pressure.

This section is only a brief summary of the epidemiological evidence; more information on risk factors for coronary heart disease can be found in Chapter 2. For readers wishing further study, a comprehensive review of epidemiological issues in hypertension can be found in the *Handbook of Hypertension* series, Volume 20: *Epidemiology of Hypertension*, edited by Professor Chris Bulpitt (Bulpitt 2000).

PATHOGENESIS OF CORONARY HEART DISEASE

The mechanisms whereby hypertension contributes to coronary heart disease pathogenesis are complex and unclear. However, much work is ongoing and evidence is accumulating for multifactorial defects.

In hypertension the structure and function of the vasculature are modified. In many hypertensives, the vascular wall is thickened with a decreased internal diameter, thus increasing peripheral resistance (Swales 1994). In these narrowed vessels, cholesterol-rich deposits have a greater chance of causing blockade and constriction is more likely to lead to vasospasm.

There are functional changes in the endothelial lining of the arteries, possibly increasing the likelihood of vasospasm. Decreased production and/or availability of vasorelaxing substances and an increase in vasoconstrictor substances have also been reported in hypertension. The vasodilator nitric oxide has received much attention in this regard (Loscalzo 1995), as has the reactive oxygen species superoxide which scavenges nitric oxide, reducing its availability, and has adverse effects on cell growth (Berry et al 2001). Platelet adhesion, platelet activation and platelet aggregation may also be increased in hypertension (Luscher 1990). Such increases can promote thrombus formation.

MEASUREMENT OF BLOOD PRESSURE

The importance of accurate blood pressure measurement cannot be over-emphasized. The level of blood pressure will determine diagnosis, if treatment is required, whether treatment is controlling blood pressure adequately and if additional or different treatment is necessary. Measurement needs to be standardized as measurements over time must be consistent to allow reliable and meaningful comparison.

The observer needs to start with a review of the equipment to be used for measurement and the effects of physical and environmental factors (Box 4.2),

---

■ **BOX 4.2   Factors that affect blood pressure measurement (compiled from O'Brien & O'Malley 1991)**

Global factors

- Digit preference
- Observer bias
- Defence reaction
- Beat-to-beat variability
- Auscultatory gap

Factors causing overestimation of BP

- Cuff bladder too narrow
- Cuff applied loosely
- Bladder not centred over artery
- Mercury column slopes away from vertical (usually due to damaged hinges)
- Too rapid deflation of mercury column during measurement – overestimates diastolic BP
- Hearing impaired or eartips not forward – overestimates systolic BP
- Arm held below heart level

Factors increasing BP

- Talking
- Standing – slight increase in diastolic BP

- Arm unsupported, causing isometric exercise of limb
- 'White coat hypertension'

Factors causing underestimation of BP

- Cuff bladder too wide (less of a problem)
- Leaks in tubing
- Heavy pressure on stethoscope over artery – underestimates diastolic BP
- Too rapid deflation of mercury column during measurement – underestimates systolic BP
- Hearing impaired or eartips not forward – underestimates systolic BP
- Arm held above heart level

Factors decreasing BP

- Rest
- Standing – slight decrease in systolic BP, marked decrease in some elderly people and those taking α-blocking drugs

before progressing to the actual measurement. The mercury sphygmo-manometer, as first designed by Rivi Rocci in 1888, is simple and elegant. Due to environmental concerns, however, mercury sphygmomanometers will be phased out of use in the near future (Feathers 2001). The robustness of this device is outstanding with its basic functioning easy to assess. The portability of aneroid sphygmomanometers makes such devices useful and popular with community staff. Unfortunately a tendency to lose accuracy due to a leaking diaphragm or stretched spring necessitates recalibration at 6-monthly intervals.

Further specific information on mercury and aneroid sphygmomano-meters can be found in Box 4.3. There is an accompanying exercise to provide

■ **BOX 4.3   Blood pressure equipment maintenance (compiled from O'Brien & O'Malley 1991)**

Briefly check equipment each time you use it. It is more likely that you will notice when it needs repair or maintenance.

Mercury sphygmomanometer

1. Hinges – they should be tight, allowing the mercury column to be straight in an upright position.
2. Mercury column – is the column clean, are the markings clear and does the mercury rest at zero?
3. Tubing and connectors – cracks and loose/leaky connections.
4. Cuff – is it clean? When was the last time the cover was washed? Is the Velcro full of lint? (This can be cleared with a suede brush.) Is it the right size for the arm?
5. Bulb – cracks, air leaks.
6. Inflation valve – can it be shut completely and opened slowly to allow for controlled deflation? Can you inflate it to above 200 mmHg in 3–5 seconds and deflate at a rate of 2–3 mmHg per second? (The control release valve is the most common source of error in the system.)
7. Service – when last serviced, note next date of service. Mercury sphygmomanometers should be checked once a year by a trained technician. It is not recommended for health professionals to handle mercury; it is a poison. (Some drug companies provide sphygmomanometer calibration and service free of charge. Alternatively, medical supply firms do it for a small fee.)

Aneroid sphygmomanometer

1. Tubing and connectors – cracks and loose/leaky connections.
2. Cuff – is it clean? When was the last time the cover was washed? Is the Velcro full of lint? (This can be cleared with a suede brush.) Is it the right size for the arm?
3. Bulb – cracks, air leaks.
4. Inflation valve – can it be shut completely and opened slowly to allow for controlled deflation? Can you inflate it to above 200 mmHg in 3–5 seconds and deflate at a rate of 2–3 mmHg per second?
5. Dial – does it zero? Do not use one with a stop pin at zero. If gauge is outwith the zero range, **do not use**. Have it serviced even if a service is not due.
6. Service – when last serviced, note next date of service. Aneroid sphygmomanometers should be checked 6 monthly by a trained technician. Their calibration should be regularly compared

against a mercury column using a Y-connector. (Some drug companies provide sphygmomanometer calibration and service free of charge. Alternatively, medical supply firms do it for a small fee.)

7. Other problems with aneroids: vacuum between diaphragms is hard to maintain and the mechanical moving parts require regular lubrication.

Automated sphygmomanometer and 24-hour blood pressure monitoring devices

1. Tubing and connectors – cracks and loose/leaky connections.
2. Cuff – is it clean? When was the last time the cover was washed? Is there lint in the valve? (This can be cleaned with a suede brush). Is it the correct size for the arm?
3. Is readout legible?
4. Service according to manufacturer's recommendation using a Y-connection to a mercury sphygmomanometer, if available. The clinical physics department in many local hospitals takes responsibility for monitoring electronic devices.

Stethoscope

1. Tubing – keep as short as possible.
2. Ear pieces – are they clean and are they tilted forward when you use them? Do they fit you properly?
3. Head – use good-quality diaphragm.

readers with an opportunity to assess their own equipment (Box 4.4). An example of an appropriate set-up for blood pressure measurement is shown in Figure 4.1.

Automated blood pressure measuring devices should in theory resolve the difficulties in manual blood pressure measurement. Many models from several manufacturers have been found wanting over the years. Standards of validation for such devices have become much more rigorous in recent years (O'Brien et al 1993). Although several newer models meet these validation standards, this is no guarantee that the manufacturer will not change a model or produce newer models with different specifications. As mercury is withdrawn from medical use under EU regulations, the need for accurate and reliable devices of this type is becoming urgent. Information on validated devices can be found on the British Hypertension Society (BHS) website (www.hyp.ac.uk/bhsinfo/index.html).

Blood pressure measurements obtained outside the clinical setting, by the use of either a home sphygmomanometer or a 24-hour ambulatory blood pressure monitor, can provide additional information about blood pressure variability. In addition to the problems with equipment validation and calibration, home blood pressure monitoring requires careful patient education. Regular review of equipment and technique is also required.

Ambulatory blood pressure monitoring can help to identify 'white coat hypertension', i.e. the occurrence of raised blood pressure only in the presence of health-care personnel. This syndrome is uncommon if clinical readings are performed carefully over time and standardized. The long-term

■ **BOX 4.4 Exercise: assessment of manual sphygmomanometer**

Please assess the equipment you have available to use.

1. Sphygmomanometer

Please specify type:

Mercury . . . . Aneroid . . . . Other (please specify) . . . .

Please describe condition and circle response where appropriate:

Cuff tubing: . . . . Cracks? Y/N

Machine tubing: . . . . Cracks? Y/N

Bulb: . . . . Cracks? Y/N

Cuff sizes available (mm × mm): . . . .

. . . .

Cuff covering type: Velcro or wrap around? . . . .

If mercury sphygmomanometer, condition of column (please circle):

Is oxidation present? Y/N Markings legible? Y/N

Does it rest at zero? Y/N If not, what is resting level? . . . . . . mmHg

If box type, is lid held at 90° when open? Y/N

Date last calibrated: . . . . Maintenance cycle: . . . . . .

Testing

Can the release valve be opened and shut smoothly? Y/N

Can you control deflation smoothly? Y/N

Does the system maintain pressure and not deflate prior to releasing value? Y/N

Can it be inflated to 200 mmHg within 3–5 seconds? Y/N (please do twice to confirm)

Can it be deflated at 2–3 mmHg per second? Y/N (please do twice to confirm)

Does the mercury return to zero after deflation? Y/N If no, does it after flick of lid? Y/N

2. Stethoscope

Type: diaphragm or bell tubing: . . . . Cracks? Y/N

Length: . . . . Ear piece condition: . . . .

3. Scales

Type: . . . .

Date last calibrated: . . . . Maintenance cycle: . . . .

epidemiological significance of ambulatory blood pressure measurement has yet to be established. The cost of ambulatory blood pressure monitoring equipment puts it out of reach of most general practices, particularly when compared with lower cost options such as home measurements.

Recommendations for the manual measurement of blood pressure have evolved over the years. A brief summary of the BHS recommended technique is given in Box 4.5. Unfortunately, the knowledge and skills of many

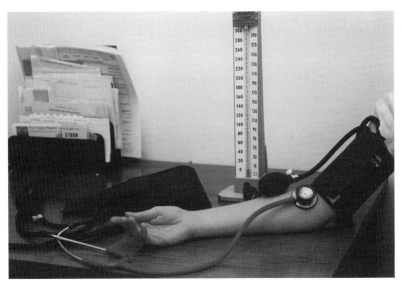

Figure 4.1 Accurate blood pressure measurement requires well-maintained equipment with the patient and equipment positioned correctly.

■ **BOX 4.5   Method recommended by the BHS for the manual measurement of blood pressure by mercury sphygmomanometer (O'Brien et al 1997)**

Positioning of patient and equipment

1. Explain procedure to patient.
2. Have patient in comfortable position with arm supported, in a warm environment with tight or restrictive clothing removed.
3. Apply cuff of appropriate size (to encompass approximately 80% of upper arm), with tubing superiorly, with the centre of the bladder over the brachial artery and the lower edge 2–3 cm above the antecubital fossa.
4. Ensure that the manometer is at eye level and within 3 feet of you.

Estimation of systolic blood pressure

1. Palpate brachial or radial pulse.
2. Inflate cuff until pulsation vanishes (systolic pressure).
3. Deflate cuff and record reading.

Measurement of systolic and diastolic pressure

1. Place stethoscope gently over maximal pulsation of brachial artery.
2. Inflate cuff to 30 mmHg above estimated systolic pressure.
3. Reduce pressure at rate of 2–3 mmHg per second or per heart beat.
4. Systolic blood pressure is noted when repetitive, clear tapping sounds appear for two consecutive beats.
5. Diastolic blood pressure is noted when repetitive sounds disappear.
6. Record reading.

health-care professionals regarding the measurement of blood pressure are inadequate (Feher et al 1992, McKay et al 1990, Wingfield et al 1996). In response, the BHS produced a video and accompanying pamphlet (Petrie et al 1990) and training programmes have been set up and evaluated (O'Brien et al 1991). This material has been updated and is available on the BHS website; it can be purchased in CD-ROM format. Ultimately, the responsibility for understanding the correct technique for the measurement of blood pressure lies with the individual practitioner.

DIAGNOSIS OF HYPERTENSION

As essential hypertension is symptomless, screening for high blood pressure is necessary. Over 75% of adults attend their general practitioner at least once every 3 years and this type of opportunistic screening has been shown to be successful (Barber et al 1979). Screening should embrace patients aged up to 80 years and even older if life expectancy is otherwise good. Opportunities for checking blood pressure present frequently and such opportunities should be taken, using the recommended method for taking blood pressure as described. Furthermore, recording the level in a standard, prominent place within each patient's notes aids future assessment. Blood pressure measurement needs to be repeated over time and a suggested guideline to follow for such a programme is given in Table 4.1.

Hypertension is usually identified by opportunistic screening. To avoid alarming the individual, it should be explained that blood pressure should be measured on several occasions to establish the sustained (usual) level. Preferably, monitoring should be carried out by a nurse who is less likely than the general practitioner to provoke an alarm reaction. The subject can be advised that blood pressure is often raised at the first contact with a health

Table 4.1 Follow-up as determined by level blood pressure

Blood pressure level	Follow-up timescale
Systolic <135 mmHg and diastolic <85 mmHg	Reassess in 5 years
Systolic 135–139 mmHg and diastolic 85–89 mmHg	Reassess annually
Systolic 140–159 mmHg and/or diastolic 90–99 mmHg	Reassess every 4 weeks for 3–6 months*
Systolic 160–199 mmHg and/or diastolic 100–109 mmHg	Reassess every week for 4 weeks and every 4 weeks for further 3 months*
Systolic ≥200 mmHg and/or diastolic ≥110 mmHg	Ask doctor to check fundi for malignant hypertension. If not malignant hypertension, reassess four more times over 2 weeks

*Shorter period in high-risk individuals, i.e. prior cardiovascular disease, target organ damage, diabetes mellitus or 10-year coronary heart disease risk ≥15% (140–159/90–99 mmHg).

professional and that it is likely to settle with familiarization. It should be emphasized that the sustained level is the one that matters in determining whether treatment is necessary, but even if this is below the threshold for treatment, annual readings are advisable since blood pressure tends to increase with age and treatment may eventually be necessary (Ramsay et al 1999).

ASSESSMENT

The period of blood pressure monitoring can be used to assess patients for other cardiovascular risk factors and evidence of blood pressure-induced damage to organs. Target organs include the brain (cerebrovascular accidents (strokes) and transient ischaemic attacks), the heart (left ventricular hypertrophy (LVH), myocardial infarction, myocardial ischaemia or heart failure), peripheral blood vessels (formation of atheroma leading to claudication, rarely aneurysms which may lead to dissection) and the eyes (retinopathy).

The baseline examination and investigations (Box 4.6) should be conducted at a return appointment in individuals with borderline, mild or moderate hypertension. The appointment is best made when both the general practitioner and nurse are available and when a venous blood sample can be sent promptly to a laboratory for analysis. The patient should be asked to bring a fresh (voided in the previous 4 hours) sample of urine.

Physical examination undertaken by the doctor will most frequently be normal. Nevertheless, rare signs of secondary causes may be present. Also, by looking in the eye for fundal changes (funduscopy), evidence of target organ changes may be detected. Serious fundal changes – bilateral exudates, flame haemorrhages or oedema of the optic discs (papilloedema) – indicate malignant hypertension. This condition is serious and requires referral to and treatment in hospital.

Urinalysis using reagent strips is easy to perform and it is worth asking the patient to give a specimen of urine at the surgery if one is not brought to the appointment. This is because proteinuria and haematuria suggest underlying renal disease, requiring further investigation. If a reagent strip shows glucose in the urine, diabetes should be considered. Hypertension with diabetes potentiates the risk of renal impairment; in such individuals, good control of both diabetes and hypertension is important.

Biochemical testing of blood is helpful to exclude several secondary causes of hypertension and identify other cardiovascular risks such as raised cholesterol and glucose. Also, serum creatinine level is an indicator of kidney function.

An electrocardiogram (ECG) provides information on the state of the heart and acts as a baseline for future comparison and assessment. In the patient with hypertension, an abnormal ECG tracing is a guide to the presence of LVH, strain and prior (sometimes silent) myocardial infarction (MI). LVH is a powerful indicator of cardiovascular risk, independent of blood pressure. Rigorous blood pressure control is vital if LVH is detected. The results of this initial physical examination and accompanying investigations as outlined above will help to determine the management of patients with hypertension.

■ BOX 4.6   Baseline procedures and investigations to be recorded

- History of cardiovascular risk factors:
  - smoking status
  - alcohol intake
  - level of exercise
  - type of diet
- Family history:
  - cardiovascular disease (including MI, stroke)
  - renal disease
- Past medical and drug history
- Height and weight. Calculate body mass index:

$$\frac{\text{Weight (kilograms)}}{\text{Height (metres)}^2}$$

- Blood pressure and pulse rate
- Physical examination including:
  - funduscopy
  - radiofemoral delay
  - carotid and abdominal bruits
  - peripheral pulses
- Test urine for:
  - protein
  - glucose
  - blood
  (Send midstream urine for culture and sensitivity testing if blood and/or protein show up on reagent strips; if negative, recheck urine and arrange follow-up as necessary)
- Blood sample for:
  - urea and electrolytes
  - creatinine
  - γ-GT
  - urate
  - random cholesterol and HDL-cholesterol
  - glucose
- Arrange for 12-lead electrocardiograph and have it reported

It is helpful to explain the purpose of clinical evaluation: identification of secondary forms of hypertension, other cardiovascular risk factors and target organ damage secondary to hypertension. Patients, not unnaturally, imagine that there must be a cause for hypertension. Careful explanation that correctable causes of high blood pressure are extremely rare and that the condition is often hereditary helps patients to come to terms with their predicament. A close relative may have hypertension and family members may have experienced cardiovascular events or complications. The patient can be reassured that family history is relevant to an individual's risk only when it affects a first-degree relative (parent or sibling) and occurs prematurely.

Hypertension is only one risk factor for cardiovascular disease and the patient should understand that the clinical evaluation includes assessment of other risks. Risk predictors include older age, male sex (and women 10 years post menopause), family history of premature cardiovascular diseases, nicotine use, excess alcohol, high blood fats (cholesterol), diabetes, obesity, sedentary lifestyle and renal impairment. Evidence of target organ damage, history of ischaemic heart disease (angina or prior MI), stroke or transient ischaemic attack, or peripheral vascular disease; clinical evidence of vascular disease (e.g. reduced or absent peripheral pulses, cardiomegaly or fundal changes on ophthalmology), and ECG evidence of LVH or MI are powerful indicators of risk. Thus, in addition to careful history and clinical examination, simple blood and urine tests and a resting ECG are necessary. Full evaluation is required to determine the need for and urgency of intervention.

MANAGEMENT OF HYPERTENSION

Aims of treatment

The objectives of antihypertensive therapy are to prevent the end-organ damage which complicates uncontrolled chronic high blood pressure (MI, cerebrovascular incidents, renal failure and heart failure) and to postpone death. There is now conclusive evidence that drug treatment of hypertension, including isolated systolic hypertension, significantly reduces the risk of such events (Collins & MacMahon 1994).

In the vast majority of individuals, hypertension is an asymptomatic condition and the aims of treatment are to prevent future damage. In effect, when we initiate antihypertensive management, we act as insurance salesmen: if the patient accepts the lifetime management plan, an event, which may not occur in any case, will be prevented in the distant future and no harm will result from the treatment prescribed. Unfortunately, with our present knowledge, we are unable to determine accurately which hypertensive subject will subsequently suffer an event or experience intolerable adverse effects of treatment. The worst scenario is the patient who is incapacitated by drug side-effects but still dies from a heart attack or stroke. All these considerations dictate that drugs used to treat hypertension should be convenient and well tolerated.

It is important to ensure that the patient is aware of the available support team – doctor, practice nurse and others. Effective treatment involves regular contacts with members of the team and follow-up is essential. Initially, there may be several visits over weeks or months but later, as treatment is established, 3-monthly appointments may be all that is needed.

Lifestyle modification

Hypertension should not be considered in isolation. Its management should form part of a primary prevention package which also addresses other correctable risk factors such as smoking, hyperlipidaemia, diabetes mellitus and obesity.

The first step in antihypertensive therapy is non-pharmacological therapy. Weight reduction in obese subjects, moderation of alcohol and salt intake and increased aerobic exercise have all been shown to reduce blood pressure to an extent similar to that of drug monotherapy (Berchthold et al 1982, MacMahon & Norton 1986, Treatment of Mild Hypertension Research Group 1991, Wassertheil-Smoller et al 1992). Discontinuation of cigarette smoking has little long-term effect on resting blood pressure but has an influence on cardiovascular (and non-cardiovascular) morbidity and mortality greater than that of blood pressure reduction (MRFIT Research Group 1986).

Non-pharmacological treatment to lower blood pressure includes achieving ideal body weight (a realistic initial target is at least 10 kg weight reduction in obese individuals), avoidance of excessive alcohol intake, improving overall level of fitness and reducing added salt to food (Table 4.2). The level of salt reduction required to have significant effects on blood pressure is difficult to achieve and maintain (Wood 1986), but there is value in reduction of excessive salt intake (Stein & Black 1993). Other lifestyle modifications which help to reduce the risk of cardiovascular disease are not to smoke and to improve the diet by reducing saturated fat intake and increasing consumption of fruit and vegetables which have a high antioxidant content.

As hypertensive individuals have no symptoms, time should be taken to explain why it is that they are being asked to make, in some cases, major changes to their lifestyles for no obvious short-term benefit. The chapters on lifestyle changes discuss the different approaches to encouraging behaviour change. Ideally the health professional should provide information to patients in response to their needs and expectations. It is not unusual for patients to be presented with a package of changes to their lifestyle to consider.

Mullen et al (1997), in a meta-analysis of trials evaluating patient education and counselling, found that both these techniques were effective for increasing preventive behaviours in people who were healthy. In particular, it was

Table 4.2 Effect of non-pharmacological intervention

Non-drug therapy	Effect on BP	Effect on risk
Normalizing glucose	No effect	Reduces risk
Normalizing cholesterol	No effect	Reduces risk
Stopping smoking	No effect	Reduces risk++
Losing weight	Lowers BP*	Unknown
Decreasing alcohol intake	Lowers BP†	Unknown
Decreasing salt intake	Lowers BP‡	Unknown
Increasing exercise	Lowers BP	Reduces risk

*Weight reduction of 1 kg can reduce BP by 2 mmHg.
†Reducing alcohol consumption to within the recommended units/week.
‡Reducing salt to 5 g/day has less pronounced effect in mild hypertension and therefore remains controversial. Patients should be advised not to add salt at the table and avoid very salty foods.

shown that health-care personnel should focus on behavioural techniques such as:

- teaching self-monitoring, e.g. home blood pressure monitoring
- use of personal communication and target setting, e.g. shared care cards
- written or other audiovisual materials, e.g. patient information leaflets.

Information materials used simply to provide knowledge are not particularly helpful but are effective if used alongside exchange of information between doctors/nurses and patients. Asking open questions allows patients to tell the health-care provider what they need to know and then they can be supported or motivated to consider beneficial changes to their behaviour. The benefits of successful lifestyle changes should be explained to patients. Their risk of vascular disease will be greatly reduced, the need for medication may be lessened and there will be other health benefits. Patients should be told that the time which can be spent on non-pharmacological measures before drugs are introduced depends on the level of the blood pressure and other cardiovascular risks (Ramsay et al 1999).

Pharmacological treatment

Long-term trials have demonstrated conclusively the benefit of antihypertensive drug therapy in reducing the risk of cerebrovascular events (Collins & MacMahon 1994); a 38% reduction in stroke is exactly that predicted from prospective epidemiological studies, given the average blood pressure change seen. The reduction in coronary heart disease events in these studies was 16% or about three-quarters of that predicted. However, this deficit is not statistically significant.

The apparent shortfall in protection against heart attack has been emphasized widely and has many hypothetical explanations although there is no direct support for any of these. It seems likely that the extent of blood pressure reduction (mean change in diastolic blood pressure of 5 mmHg), the sample size of the study population and the duration of treatment (only 3 years on average) were insufficient to demonstrate benefit. It is important to note that these trials were discontinued on ethical grounds when significant benefit in stroke prevention was demonstrated. There is certainly no valid support for the notion that drugs used in these trials (thiazides and β-blockers) had cardiotoxic influences that offset their beneficial effect on blood pressure reduction (McInnes et al 1992).

Most hypertensive patients require drug therapy. The patient should be informed that more than one drug taken in combination is usually necessary to control blood pressure and that a significant minority require three or more drugs. Different drugs act in different ways and therefore using drugs together leads to greater reduction in blood pressure. Also, not all drugs suit all patients. A prolonged period of trial and error, usually lasting several months, is necessary before the most appropriate drug(s) is identified in terms of efficacy and tolerability.

In an era of package inserts, the potential for antihypertensive agents to cause side-effects is all too apparent. This is of particular concern to individuals without symptoms. It is useful to explain that, because of this, drugs for hypertension have to be very well tolerated. The long list of potential side-effects on the package insert reflects experience in many thousands of patients and includes effects not related causally to the drug. Only a small minority of patients will experience a significant adverse event. If this occurs, the treatment will be changed. At each consultation, possible side-effects should be discussed and treatment adjusted as necessary.

Clinical trials in nearly 50 000 people with high blood pressure have shown beyond doubt that antihypertensive drug treatment saves lives and prevents heart attacks, strokes and other vascular events. The expected benefits of effective blood pressure control and attention to other risk factors merit emphasis. To help inform the patient, it can be useful to provide an estimate of 10-year risk of a major event and the reduction that can be expected from treatment (e.g. 30% to 20%). Such calculations are facilitated by the use of the British Hypertension Society risk assessment computer disk or chart (Ramsay et al 1999). The latter has the advantage of allowing easy explanation to the patient.

Risk assessment charts also assist in explaining the need for attention to all risks and not just blood pressure. Blood pressure reduction itself may have a modest effect on absolute risk but in combination with other interventions (e.g. stopping smoking and lipid-lowering drugs) the effect can be dramatic.

Antihypertensive treatment is for life, although drugs and dosages may be adjusted (sometimes downwards) over time. This message is important because patients (and doctors) expect a course of treatment to be given until a condition resolves.

Choice of antihypertensive drugs

In individuals who do not respond adequately to a reasonable trial of non-pharmacological measures, drug therapy is indicated. Several classes of drugs are effective in reducing blood pressure (Box 4.7).

Six main classes of antihypertensive drugs are available. Those with the largest and most robust body of evidence of benefit are thiazide diuretics and β-blockers. Drugs from these classes are recommended for first-line therapy unless there are specific contraindications (Ramsay et al 1999).

■ **BOX 4.7   Antihypertensive drugs**

- Diuretics
- β-Blockers
- Calcium antagonists
- ACE inhibitors
- Angiotensin II receptor antagonists
- α-Blockers
- Others

Diuretics

Diuretics were introduced in the 1950s and are still among the most widely used antihypertensive agents. Three classes of diuretics are available:

- Benzothiadiazine (thiazide) diuretics, such as bendroflumethiazide (bendrofluazide), cyclopenthiazide or hydrochlorothiazide, act at the cortical diluting segment of the distal convoluted tubule in the kidney.
- Loop (high ceiling) diuretics, such as bumetanide, furosemide (frusemide) and torasemide, act on the thick ascending limb of the loop of henle and the proximal tubule.
- Potassium-sparing diuretics, amiloride, triamterene and spironolactone, act at sodium:potassium exchange sites in the distal convoluted tubule and collecting duct.

Thiazide diuretics Thiazide diuretics are the most useful and by far the most widely used in hypertension. These drugs are fairly weak natriuretic agents with potential to eliminate 5–10% of filtered sodium (potency). However, thiazides have a gradual onset (hours) and prolonged (12 to over 24 hours) duration of action. These properties allow once-daily administration. The dose–response relation is shallow, i.e. there is little increase in sodium excretion at high doses.

In the UK, bendroflumethiazide (bendrofluazide) is the least expensive thiazide available; more expensive agents offer no advantage. Bendroflumethiazide (bendrofluazide) is completely absorbed and fairly extensively metabolized; only 30% is excreted unchanged in the urine. It has a plasma half-life of 3–4 hours but a much longer biological half-life. Diuresis starts around 2 hours after drug administration and continues for 12–18 hours. The recommended dose is 2.5 mg daily; larger doses cause more adverse effects without any improvement in blood pressure control.

Loop diuretics Loop diuretics act more abruptly (30–60 minutes) and tend to have a diuretic effect which persists for only a few (4–6) hours at usual doses. Thus these agents have to be taken at least twice daily to provide 24-hour control of blood pressure. An exception is torasemide which can be used once daily. Loop diuretics have high potency (15–25% of filtered sodium) and steep dose–response curves (high ceiling).

Loop diuretics have a very limited role in hypertension. These drugs are sometimes useful in treatment of resistant hypertension and high doses can be effective in renal failure, where thiazides are ineffective. Thiazide diuretics become progressively less effective as renal function deteriorates and are not usually useful if serum creatinine exceeds 150 μmol/l (creatinine clearance less than 50 ml/min). Loop diuretics in high doses (e.g. furosemide (frusemide) 80 mg twice daily) remain effective in renal impairment.

Potassium-sparing diuretics Potassium-sparing diuretics have weak natriuretic actions (5% filtered sodium) and although duration of action is prolonged (12–24 hours), these drugs have a minor role in antihypertension therapy. Their main use is in combination with other diuretics to limit disturbances in potassium balance. Spironolactone acts as a specific competitive aldosterone antagonist and this action is utilized in the treatment of rare patients with primary hyperaldosteronism (Conn's syndrome). However, this drug is no longer licensed in the UK for the treatment of essential hypertension because of concerns about the carcinogenic potential of a closely related analogue (canrenoate potassium).

Mechanism of action All diuretics act on the kidneys at renal tubular sites to enhance salt (sodium and chloride ion) and water loss. This results in acute reduction in plasma volume, cardiac output and extracellular fluid volume. However, enhanced sodium excretion persists only for the first few days of chronic administration. In the longer term, homeostatic mechanisms lead to recovery of plasma volume and cardiac output. Lowered blood pressure is sustained by reduction in total peripheral resistance (reverse autoregulation). Although the eventual result is reduced peripheral resistance, probably due to reduction in sodium content in vascular smooth muscle, the prime mover is renal salt and water loss.

Adverse effects Symptomatic adverse effects of diuretics are rare although frequency, nocturia and prostatism can cause problems particularly in the elderly. Thiazide diuretics cause reversible erectile impotence in about 5% of middle-aged men; accurate assessment of the frequency of this side-effect is difficult since the complaint is common in that population. Other uncommon reactions to thiazides include nausea, vomiting, diarrhoea, skin rashes, pancreatitis, agranulocytosis, aplastic anaemia and thrombocytopenia. Thiazides inhibit renal lithium clearance and may precipitate toxicity in patients treated with lithium carbonate.

High doses of loop diuretics can cause ototoxicity particularly in patients with renal impairment. The antiandrogenic action of spironolactone is associated with gynaecomastia in men and mastalgia or menstrual irregularities in women.

The major complications of diuretic therapy are metabolic disturbances. The concern is that these changes may predispose to cardiovascular disease and limit their preventive benefit.

As a direct result of their renal action, thiazide and loop diuretics promote urine potassium loss and a tendency to reduced serum potassium concentration. Urine potassium excretion follows that of sodium and returns to baseline within about 1 week but fractional renal clearance of potassium remains increased indefinitely. As a result, serum potassium concentration reaches a new plateau after about 7–10 days and thereafter is unchanged unless clinical conditions alter, e.g. increase in dose. Thereafter there is little need for continued monitoring of serum potassium. The average reduction in serum potassium with previously recommended doses of thiazides (e.g. bendroflumethiazide (bendrofluazide) 10 mg daily) is 0.6 mmol/l. Some 50% of patients become hypokalaemic at this dose but only about 2% have serum potassium levels less than 3.0 mmol/l on long-term therapy.

Although it has been suggested that diuretic-induced hypokalaemia predisposes to serious cardiac arrhythmias, there is little good evidence for this except in patients at particular risk (Box 4.8). There is no justification for

■ **BOX 4.8** **Subjects at risk of or from hypokalaemia**

Factors increasing risk of *hypokalemia*

- High doses of diuretics
- Long-acting agents (thiazides more than loops)
- Divided doses
- Women
- Young (more than old)

Factors increasing risk from *hypokalaemia*

- Concomitant digoxin
- Concomitant drugs which prolong QT interval, e.g. amiodarone, disopyramide, flecainide, sotalol
- Chronic liver disease
- Arrhythmias or antiarrhythmic therapy
- Severe or unstable angina
- Post myocardial infarction
- Primary hyperaldosteronism
- Serum potassium less than 3.0 mmol/l

routine use of potassium supplements or potassium-sparing agents although hypokalaemia (serum potassium <3.5 mmol/l) should be avoided.

If required, potassium replacement is best achieved by the use of potassium-sparing diuretics. Dietary sources of potassium (citrus fruit, bananas, dried fruit, tomatoes) are inadequate except when taken in huge amounts. Slow-release potassium chloride or combined thiazide-potassium formulation similarly contains relatively small amounts of potassium. These preparations are ineffectual since the underlying cause of hypokalaemia (increased fractional renal clearance) is not influenced and much of the absorbed potassium is merely lost in the urine.

As well as being ineffective, potassium supplements can cause serious side-effects, including oesophageal injury or ulceration. Slow-release formulations simply transfer the damage further down the gastrointestinal tract with risk of small bowel stenosis, ulceration and perforation. Hyperkalaemia is occasionally seen in patients with renal impairment or those prescribed concomitant potassium-sparing agents.

Potassium-sparing diuretics can also precipitate hyperkalaemia in patients with renal impairment or where angiotensin-converting enzyme inhibitors are prescribed simultaneously. Hyperkalaemia carries a risk for serious cardiac arrhythmias and sudden death much greater than that due to hypokalaemia.

Combined preparations of thiazide or loop diuretics and potassium-sparing agents are difficult to justify since the risk of severe hypokalaemia is generally low. Also such combinations carry a risk of severe hyponatraemia which may cause symptomatic neurological consequences, including fits and coma.

Profound hyponatraemia can arise after only a few doses and is more likely in elderly females. It seems to be particularly associated with the use of Moduretic (hydrochlorothiazide and amiloride).

Subjects at risk of or at risk from hypokalaemia are listed in Box 4.8. In such individuals, monitoring of serum potassium and use of potassium-sparing agents as necessary are indicated.

Patients receiving thiazide diuretics have a tendency to develop hyperglycaemia, perhaps as a consequence of increased insulin resistance. However, only about 1% of thiazide-treated subjects will develop diabetes mellitus during long-term exposure. There is little evidence that alteration in carbohydrate metabolism, short of diabetes, is a risk factor for cardiovascular disease.

All diuretics, other than potassium-sparing agents, may cause hyperuricaemia. Only about 2% of men and many fewer women go on to develop gout. This is most likely in obese, heavy-drinking males treated with loop diuretics. Increase in serum uric acid does not appear to be an independent risk factor for coronary artery disease.

Short-term (months) treatment with high doses of thiazides causes marked changes in serum lipoproteins (increased total cholesterol and low density lipoprotein cholesterol and reduced high density lipoprotein cholesterol). However, alterations are markedly attenuated in the long term. After 1 year's treatment, the small increase in total cholesterol (1%) is unlikely to be of clinical significance.

Dose All the metabolic effects of thiazides are dose related, while the antihypertensive effect is not dose related. Blood pressure reduction is maximal at low doses, e.g. bendroflumethiazide (bendrofluazide) 2.5 mg daily. At such doses, metabolic changes are trivial. Small reductions in serum potassium are frequent but hypokalaemia is rare.

Outcome studies A series of long-term outcome trials has demonstrated beyond reasonable doubt that thiazide-based treatment regimens reduce the chances of premature stroke and myocardial infarction in hypertension (Collins & MacMahon 1994, He & Whelton 1999).

■ KEY POINTS

- Diuretics should be used in low doses.
- Diuretics need little dose titration.
- Thiazides can be used once daily.
- Diuretics are useful in pseudotolerance: resistance to other antihypertensive agents (particularly vasodilators) due to fluid retention.
- All diuretics (particularly thiazides) are inexpensive.
- Loop diuretics are useful in renal failure.

β-Blockers

β-Adrenoceptor antagonists were accidentally discovered to be antihypertensive agents in the early 1970s and since then have entered widespread use. Like thiazide diuretics, these agents have been used widely in the trials which have demonstrated the benefits of drug treatment of hypertension (Collins & MacMahon 1994).

Mechanisms of action β-Blockers are competitive inhibitors of catecholamines at β-adrenergic receptors. These drugs decrease cardiac activity by inhibiting both the rate and force of cardiac contraction, and also decrease the normal cardiac responses to stress and exercise.

Despite lengthy experience with β-blockers in hypertension, there remains uncertainty about their mechanism of action. Candidate actions include:

- cardiac – reduced myocardial contractility, heart rate and cardiac output
- central – reduced sympathetic outflow from the brain
- renal – reduced renin release from the juxtaglomerular apparatus and hence inhibition of angiotensin II and aldosterone action; angiotensin II is a potent vasoconstrictor and aldosterone promotes renal salt and water retention.

Ancillary properties All β-blockers inhibit both β_1-receptors, found largely in the heart and peripheral vasculature, and β_2-receptors, found principally in the bronchi but also in the peripheral vasculature. Some β-blockers exhibit cardioselectivity and/or partial agonist activity.

Cardioselective drugs have preferential activity at β_1-adrenoceptors located in the heart. Cardioselectivity is relative rather than absolute. Therefore, at high doses, such drugs lose their selectivity. Cardioselective β-blockers such as atenolol and metoprolol have fewer unwanted effects due to inhibition of β_2-adrenoceptors, including less influence on airways resistance.

All β-blockers act by occupying the β-receptor and denying access to the natural stimulant (agonist). Drugs with partial agonist activity (PAA), also known as intrinsic sympathomimetic activity (ISA), act as weak agonists in resting conditions. During exercise or arousal, antagonist activity becomes dominant. β-Blockers with PAA have little demonstrable activity at rest and more marked effects on activity, e.g. little bradycardia at rest but attenuation of tachycardia on activity. In some subjects, such drugs are better tolerated (less bradycardia and coldness of extremities) than other β-blockers, but they generally have less marked antihypertensive activity.

Classification A pharmacological classification of some commonly used β-blockers is shown in Table 4.3. In addition to ancillary properties, β-blockers differ in their route of elimination and duration of action. Lipid-soluble β-blockers, e.g. metoprolol, undergo rapid extensive hepatic metabolism and tend to have relatively short half-lives and durations of action. Water-soluble β-blockers are slowly eliminated unchanged by the kidney and tend to have longer half-lives and duration of action. Plasma half-life underestimates biological half-life. Atenolol and bisoprolol are suitable for once-daily administration.

In renal impairment, dosage adjustment may be necessary with drugs which are cleared predominantly by the kidney. β-blockers which undergo extensive hepatic metabolism should be avoided in severe liver failure and

Table 4.3 Properties of β-blockers

Drug name	β₁-Selective	PAA	Water soluble	Plasma half-life (h)	Duration of action (h)	Elimination
Acebutolol	+	+/−	+/−	3	12	Renal/hepatic
Atenolol	+	−	+	6	16	Renal
Bisoprolol	++	−	+/−	10–12	>24	Renal/hepatic
Metoprolol	+	−	−	3–4	8	Hepatic
Nadolol	−	−	+	6–24	24	Renal
Oxprenolol	−	+	−	1–2	8	Hepatic
Pindolol	−	++	+/−	3–4	12	Renal/hepatic
Propranolol	−	−	−	3–6	12	Hepatic

may theoretically be involved in pharmacokinetic interactions with other drugs which undergo similar biotransformation.

Labetalol differs from other β-blockers in that it also has α-receptor blocking properties. As a result, labetalol tends to lower peripheral resistance.

Adverse effects β-Blockers are usually well tolerated. Adverse effects are generally due to unwanted blockade of β-receptors. Thus side-effects can be predicted from pharmacological actions.

• Bronchoconstriction (bronchospasm) is due to blockade of β₂-receptors in bronchial smooth muscle – these receptors modulate bronchodilatation.

• Impaired peripheral circulation and Raynaud's phenomenon are due to blockade of vasodilatory β₂-receptors and/or unopposed α-adrenergic stimulation.

• Cardiac failure or cardiac conduction defects (heart block) can arise from excessive β₁-receptor blockade.

• Symptoms of hypoglycaemia (tachycardia, sweating) may be masked since these responses depend on activation of the β-adrenergic system. β₂-Receptors also mediate the gluconeogenic and glycogenolytic responses to hypoglycaemia. Therefore, non-selective β-blockers delay the recovery following insulin-induced hypoglycaemia.

• Tiredness and fatigue during β-blocker therapy probably reflect reduced cardiac output.

• Impairment of quality of life and central nervous system effects (such as nightmares) may represent central effects of β-blockers and seem more prominent with lipid-soluble agents which more readily cross the blood–brain barrier. Atenolol, among the most water-soluble β-blockers, seems to cause little sleep disturbance.

• β-Blockers should be avoided in asthma, bradycardia and heart block. Non-selective β-blockers such as propranolol may have effects on carbohydrate metabolism at least as great as those of thiazides, but recent evidence supports the use of selective β-blockers in diabetes. Use of cardioselective β-blockers in peripheral vascular disease has been shown to be without ill effects unless drugs which decrease peripheral resistance (e.g. nifedipine) are also prescribed.

New β-blockers In recent years, highly cardioselective β-blockers such as betaxolol and bisoprolol have been introduced. Carvedilol, celiprolol and nebivolol are β-blockers with vasodilator properties. Carvedilol (like labetalol) has weak α-blocking properties. Celiprolol is said to be a cardioselective (β_1-) blocker and β_2-agonist with vasodilating activity. Nebivolol appears to stimulate nitric oxide production in the vascular endothelium. The clinical advantage of these agents compared with conventional β-blockers is yet to be established, although carvedilol, in common with other β-blockers, has overall beneficial effects in patients with stable heart failure.

■ KEY POINTS

- β-Blockers should be used in low doses to avoid side-effects. Antihypertensive efficacy is well maintained at low doses.
- β-Blockers need little dose titration.
- β-Blockers can be administered once or twice daily.
- Cardioselective β-blockers are preferred since some adverse effects are less marked.
- Other pharmacological differences between β-blockers have marginal clinical significance.
- All β-blockers are contraindicated in patients with asthma (or severe irreversible airways disease).

Calcium antagonists

The calcium antagonist class embraces three groups of drugs with distinct actions:

- dihydropyridines, e.g. amlodipine, felodipine, lacidipine, nifedipine
- phenylalkylamines, e.g. verapamil
- benzothiazepines, e.g. diltiazem.

Mechanism of action Calcium antagonists inhibit transmembrane calcium influx through slow calcium channels during membrane depolarization. Therefore, these drugs lower intracellular free calcium, the final common mediator of all vasoconstrictor mechanisms. Although all calcium antagonists reduce blood pressure, such agents have variable affinities for calcium channels at different sites in the cardiovascular system (Table 4.4).

Table 4.4 Sites of activity and pharmacokinetics of first-generation calcium antagonists

Drug name	Classification	Site of activity			Pharmacokinetics		
		Vascular smooth muscle	Myocardium	Conducting tissue	Bio-availability (%)	Elimination	Half-life (h)
Nifedipine	Dihydropyridine	+++	+/−	−	30–60	Hepatic	2–6
Diltiazem	Benzothiazepine	++	+	++	30–60	Hepatic	2–5
Verapamil	Phenylalkylamine	++	+	+++	1–20	Hepatic	3–7

Table 4.5 Adverse effects of calcium antagonists

Drug name	Vasodilatation (flushing, headache, dizziness)	Palpitation	Ankle oedema	Constipation	Heart block	Heart failure
Dihydropyridines	+++	++	++	+	−	+/−
Diltiazem	+	+	+	+	++	+
Verapamil	+	+	+	+++	++	++

Dihydropyridines have the most potent action at vascular smooth muscle sites, while only verapamil and diltiazem have measurable direct cardiac effects in humans. These two drugs suppress electrical conduction in cardiac conductive tissue and hence have a role in the management of tachyarrhythmias.

All three types of calcium antagonist tend to depress myocardial contractility. However, the direct cardiac effects are offset by reflex cardiac stimulation secondary to vasodilatation. Thus, with dihydropyridines, because of their particularly potent vasodilatory effect, the net result is a tendency to increase heart rate while verapamil and diltiazem tend to reduce heart rate (rate-limiting calcium antagonists).

Adverse effects The adverse effects of calcium antagonists are predictable from the sites and mechanisms of action (Table 4.5). Side-effects due to vasodilatation (e.g. flushing, headache and dizziness) and reflex cardiac stimulation (palpitation) are more likely with dihydropyridines. Cardiac conduction delays (heart block and bradyarrhythmias) are seen only with verapamil and diltiazem. Heart failure is also slightly more common with rate-limiting calcium antagonists but all calcium antagonists are best avoided in patients with heart failure. Ankle oedema, which appears to be due to local small vessel leakiness and is not a reflection of fluid retention, appears to be more frequent with dihydropyridines, particularly longer-acting agents. Calcium antagonist-induced ankle swelling does not respond to diuretic treatment. Verapamil causes constipation in a relatively high proportion of patients because of its direct action on gastrointestinal smooth muscle, although this symptom is not usually particularly troublesome.

The incidence of symptomatic side-effects with calcium antagonists is high relative to earlier agents. Original formulations of nifedipine (capsules) were associated with a withdrawal rate due to intolerable side-effects of 20%. Newer long-acting drugs (e.g. amlodipine) or long-acting formulations of older agents (e.g. Adalat LA) are better tolerated, with the exception of ankle oedema. Patients should be advised that ankle swelling can arise even several months after starting therapy but that it is reversible with dose reduction or discontinuation.

Pharmacokinetics The first-generation calcium antagonists (nifedipine, verapamil and diltiazem) are well absorbed but undergo extensive first-pass hepatic elimination and are readily eliminated from the body (see Table 4.4).

Table 4.6 Critical pharmacokinetics of second-generation dihydropyridines (compared with nifedipine)

Drug name	Bio-availability (%)	Time to max serum conc (h)	Half-life (h)
Nifedipine	30–60	1–2	2–6
Amlodipine	52–88	6–12	34–50
Felodipine	12–16	1–2	10–25
Isradipine	16–18	1	5–9
Lacidipine	2–52	1–2	2–10
Nicardipine	15–45	<1	1–7

As a consequence, oral bio-availability is low and plasma levels show considerable interindividual variability; elimination half-lives are short. In the original formulations, these drugs have to be administered in divided daily doses to provide 24-hour control of blood pressure.

Thus, there was a requirement for longer-acting calcium antagonists. Two approaches were adopted: naturally occurring long-acting agents and sustained-release preparations of earlier drugs.

Several new dihydropyridines have appeared in recent years (Table 4.6). The second-generation dihydropyridine, amlodipine, does not undergo significant first-pass metabolism. Therefore it has consistently high oral bio-availability and a prolonged elimination half-life. Once-daily amlodipine appears to provide smooth blood pressure control throughout the dosage interval. Other new agents in this class, such as lacidipine, probably should be administered twice daily to ensure 24-hour control.

Sustained-release formulations of otherwise short-acting drugs have inconsistent durations of action. The more reliable of these preparations include Adalat LA (nifedipine), Plendil (felodipine), Securon SR (verapamil) and Tildiem LA (diltiazem). Because of the variability between different sustained-release formulations of the same drug, these should be prescribed by proprietary rather than generic name and substitution should be avoided.

Drug interactions Because of complex bio-availability and high degree of hepatic metabolism, there is potential for interaction with drugs which undergo similar biotransformation. Pharmacokinetic interactions between calcium antagonists and carbamazepine, cimetidine, ciclosporin, quinidine and theophylline have been demonstrated but are of uncertain clinical significance. Co-administration of verapamil increases steady-state serum digoxin levels by about 100%. This can cause problems in susceptible individuals.

The most clinically relevant drug interaction with calcium antagonists is that between rate-limiting agents (verapamil and diltiazem) and other drugs with direct cardiac actions, notably β-blockers. Combined cardiodepressant effects can result in life-threatening bradyarrhythmias and heart failure.

Outcome trials Despite being the most widely used class of antihypertensive drugs in the world, evidence of benefit equivalent to that of diuretics and β-blockers in preventing cardiovascular complications has been documented only in the last few years (Blood-Pressure Lowering Treatment Trialists'

Collaboration 2000, Psaty et al 1995). Short-acting dihydropyridines may increase mortality and should be avoided (Psaty et al 1995).

■ **KEY POINTS**

- Calcium antagonists should be started at low doses to minimize the risk of side-effects.
- Some dose titration is usually necessary.
- Once- or twice-daily dosing depends on drug or formulation.
- Relatively poor tolerability.
- Major differences between drugs.
- Adverse drug interactions may cause complications. Verapamil and diltiazem should not be administered with β-blockers except under close hospital supervision.

ACE inhibitors

Theoretical considerations suggest that the renin–angiotensin system may be involved in the pathogenesis of hypertension and its complications (McInnes 1995). Drugs which inhibit this axis, such as angiotensin-converting enzyme (ACE) inhibitors, may have an important role in the management of hypertension.

Mechanism of action Renin produced by the juxtaglomerular apparatus in the kidney acts on angiotensinogen produced by the liver to generate angiotensin I. The primary action of ACE inhibitors is inhibition of ACE which converts the inactive decapeptide, angiotensin I, to the active octapeptide, angiotensin II, one of the most potent endogenous vasoconstrictors. Angiotensin II also stimulates the synthesis and release of aldosterone in the adrenal cortex; aldosterone acts on the kidneys to promote salt and water retention. Thus ACE inhibitors have dual effects to reduce blood pressure: inhibition of angiotensin II-induced vasoconstriction and aldosterone-mediated homeostasis.

Other non-specific actions may also contribute to the antihypertensive effect of ACE inhibitors. ACE modulates the breakdown of vasodilator peptides such as bradykinin; thus ACE inhibitors potentiate the kallikrein–kinin system. Indirect stimulation of vasodilator prostaglandins and inhibition of the sympathetic nervous system are other potential mechanisms.

The conversion of angiotensin I to angiotensin II occurs in the circulation but also within many tissues. Such local systems may have a critical role in the development of hypertension or its complications. ACE inhibitors do not block all of the pathways of angiotensin II production within tissues.

Classification ACE inhibitors can be classified according to their chemical structure and pharmacokinetic properties (Table 4.7).

The main structural difference between the available ACE inhibitors is the presence or absence of a sulphur-containing moiety in the molecule. Only captopril has such a grouping. It has been claimed that this may be responsible for some of the drug's adverse effects and beneficial properties.

Table 4.7 Properties of ACE inhibitors

Drug name	Sulphydryl group	Prodrug	Onset of action (h)	Peak action (h)	Duration of action (h)	Elimination
Captopril	+	−	0.5	1–4	3–12	Renal
Cilazapril	−	+	1–2	4–6	≤24	Renal
Enalapril	−	+	1–4	4–8	12–30	Renal
Fosinopril	−	+	1–2	3–4	≤24	Renal/hepatic
Lisinopril	−	−	1–2	2–8	18–30	Renal
Perindopril	−	+	1–2	4–8	≤24	Renal
Quninapril	−	+	1–2	2–6	≤24	Renal
Ramipril	−	+	0.5–2	3–8	24	Renal
Trandolapril	−	+	1–2	2–4	>24	Renal/hepatic

However, there is little evidence that the presence of sulphur in the molecule has a clinically significant influence on the action of ACE inhibitors.

Most ACE inhibitors are prodrugs, i.e. the drug is administered as a relatively inactive molecule which is metabolized during or after absorption to the active diacid, e.g. enalapril to enalaprilat. Initially, there was concern that the dependence on hepatic or prehepatic metabolism would expose these drugs to interference from other drugs similarly metabolized and reduce efficacy in patients with impaired liver function. These concerns have proved unfounded. The main consequence of using the prodrug is delay in onset of action. Prodrug ACE inhibitors take longer to demonstrate activity after administration compared with non-prodrug ACE inhibitors.

ACE inhibitors are mainly eliminated by the kidneys and the rate of elimination determines half-lives and durations of action. Thus captopril must be administered twice or three times daily to provide 24-hour control of blood pressure. In contrast, lisinopril has 24-hour duration of action at most doses and trandolapril at all doses. Most other ACE inhibitors have intermediate half-lives and durations of action.

Duration of action of ACE inhibitors is highly dependent on dose. For instance, at low doses enalapril should be administered twice daily and is a once-daily preparation only at the highest dose.

Some drugs have dual routes of elimination (fosinopril and trandolapril). This offers theoretical advantages in renal and hepatic impairment but there is little evidence that this property is of clinical significance.

Adverse effects ACE inhibitors are well tolerated but growing clinical experience indicates that significant side-effects do occur.

A dry irritating cough or other upper respiratory tract symptoms are seen in 15% of patients (10% of men and 20% of women). This adverse effect tends to accumulate with time; it may be seen after only a few days of treatment but may take several months to develop. Cough is independent of dose and is class specific rather than drug specific. Therefore changing ACE inhibitor is not helpful. However, the symptom is unpredictable; only about two thirds of patients with well-established ACE inhibitor-induced cough will experience cough on rechallenge.

An abrupt fall in blood pressure after introduction of ACE inhibitors (first-dose hypotension) is only likely if blood pressure is highly dependent on activation of the renin–angiotensin system, e.g. subjects who are sodium depleted as a result of high-dose diuretic therapy or patients with bilateral renal artery stenosis (or obstruction of the renal artery to a single functioning kidney). Such circumstances are uncommon in hypertension but, if suspected, a low test dose of ACE inhibitor should be prescribed under hospital supervision. Otherwise, ACE inhibition can safely be introduced in outpatients at usual doses. The time to onset of first-dose hypotension depends on the ACE inhibitor administered (early with captopril, late with prodrugs) but the magnitude of the fall is similar.

ACE inhibitors can cause renal impairment by two mechanisms. During first-dose hypotension, perfusion of vital organs including the kidneys may be impaired. With short-acting agents, the duration of hypotension is brief and renal ischaemia is less likely. This complication is uncommon in essential hypertension.

In bilateral renal artery stenosis (or renal artery stenosis in a single functioning kidney), glomerular perfusion is highly dependent on angiotensin II. ACE inhibition can result in sudden renal impairment reflected by a rapid rise in serum creatinine. Thus, renal function should be monitored 1–2 weeks after the introduction of an ACE inhibitor since renal artery stenosis may be unsuspected. A marked fall in blood pressure after introduction of an ACE inhibitor may be an indication that renal artery stenosis is present. Particular caution is necessary in patients with clinical evidence of peripheral vascular disease, which is a useful marker for atheromatous renal artery stenosis. Renal impairment may be severe but is usually reversible on stopping treatment.

Theoretically, elderly patients and those with renal impairment may be at particular risk of such adverse events but there is little sound evidence for this. In these patient groups, the duration of effect rather than the magnitude of the effect is likely to increase. ACE is inhibited almost completely at low doses and increasing plasma drug concentrations merely prolongs the action.

Normal renal elimination of potassium is highly dependent on aldosterone. Therefore, inhibition of the renin–angiotensin–aldosterone axis is associated with a tendency to increased serum potassium. The effect of ACE inhibitors is usually trivial but may attenuate diuretic-induced hypokalaemia. However, in patients with pre-existing renal impairment or who are receiving concomitant potassium-sparing diuretics or potassium supplements, dangerous hyperkalaemia can arise. Ciclosporin, indomethacin and probably other non-steroidal anti-inflammatory drugs also increase the risk of hyperkalaemia with ACE inhibitors. ACE inhibitors should not be administered with such drugs.

Uncommon side-effects of ACE inhibitors include rash, angio-oedema, neutropenia and dysgeuesia (disturbance of taste).

Some side-effects of ACE inhibitors (cough, angio-oedema) are likely to reflect the non-specific action of these drugs. In particular, accumulation of tissue bradykinin or other peptides is implicated.

Although ACE inhibitors are widely promoted for their favourable influence on quality of life, there is little evidence that these drugs have an advantage over currently used agents in this respect (Fletcher et al 1993, Hjendahl & Wikland 1992).

Outcome trials ACE inhibitors have been used for 20 years but evidence of benefit equivalent to that of diuretics and β-blockers has accumulated only recently (Blood Pressure Lowering Treatment Trialists' Collaboration 2000).

■ KEY POINTS

- A low starting dose is usually recommended to avoid rare dose-dependent side-effects.
- Dose titration is needed to ensure duration of action throughout the dose interval.
- ACE inhibitors can be used once or twice daily.
- ACE inhibitors are generally well tolerated.
- ACE inhibitors have beneficial effects on surrogate markers of risk and recent outcome trials indicate benefits equivalent to those with diuretics and β-blockers.
- ACE inhibitors are expensive compared with diuretics and β-blockers.

Angiotensin II receptor antagonists

Because of the presumed importance of the renin–angiotensin–aldosterone system in the pathogenesis of hypertension and the lack of specificity of the action of ACE inhibitors, recent attention has focused on drugs which inhibit the axis at other sites. This has resulted in the introduction of specific angiotensin II receptor antagonists or angiotensin receptor blockers.

Mechanism of action Angiotensin II receptors exist in two forms (AT1 and AT2). The AT1 receptor modulates all the cardiovascular effects of angiotensin II derived from all sources, including local renin–angiotensin systems. The physiological function of the AT2 receptor is unclear but stimulation of this receptor may oppose the actions mediated at the AT1 receptor. Angiotensin receptor blockers deny access of angiotensin II to the AT1 receptor. These drugs have high affinity for the AT1 receptor and exhibit little or no action at the AT2 receptor. Thus, angiotensin receptor blockers are potent, specific angiotensin II antagonists with selectivity for the AT1 receptor (McInnes 1998).

Several angiotensin receptor blockers are available – candesartan, eprosartan, irbesartan, losartan, telmisartan and valsartan. Differences between individual drugs are slight.

Angiotensin receptor blockers have antihypertensive efficacy similar to that of other drugs from the main therapeutic classes. Duration of action is at least 24 hours even at low doses. Higher doses have little additional peak antihypertensive effect but prolong duration of action even further.

Adverse reactions Angiotensin receptor blockers are very well tolerated. In contrast to ACE inhibitors, those drugs do not cause the side-effects due to non-specific actions.

Dry cough during ACE inhibition is probably due to potentiation of a peptide substrate of ACE, such as bradykinin or neurokinin. ACE is identical to kinase II, the enzyme responsible for the degradation of bradykinin and other vasoactive peptides, accumulation of which is associated with the development of cough. Angiotensin receptor blockers do not cause cough.

Since angiotensin II receptor antagonists lack the bradykinin potentiation of ACE inhibitors, these drugs should also be devoid of other rare side-effects of ACE inhibition, such as urticaria and angio-oedema, which are mediated by this mechanism.

No detrimental biochemical disturbances have been noted. Losartan has a significant uricosuric action which may be a useful adjunctive effect when used in combination with a diuretic.

Angiotensin receptor blockers induce changes in renal haemodynamics similar to those of ACE inhibitors. Thus, these drugs carry the same risk in patients with renal artery stenosis.

Outcome trials Whether these drugs will have an advantage over other agents, including ACE inhibitors, in relation to end-organ damage, such as reversal of the long-term effects of angiotensin II on cardiac hypertrophy, remains to be tested in adequate clinical trials. Several outcome studies are in progress.

■ KEY POINTS

- Specific inhibition of the renin–angiotensin axis.
- Little need for dose titration.
- Once-daily dosing.
- Well tolerated.
- Putative beneficial cardiovascular effects as with ACE inhibitors.
- Expensive.

α-Blockers

Stimulation of the α-adrenergic system causes vasoconstriction and increased arterial pressure. Thus, inhibition of vascular α-receptors is a logical approach to lowering blood pressure.

Classification Non-selective α-adrenoceptor antagonists (inhibition of α_1- and α_2-receptors) have been available for many years. However, a high incidence of side-effects and the rapid development of tolerance make these drugs unsuitable for general use. Oral phenoxybenzamine and intravenous phentolamine are now obsolete except in the management of phaeochromocytoma, where there is dramatic excess of circulating catecholamines.

More recently, selective postjunctional α_1-adrenoceptor antagonists have become available – doxazosin, indoramin, prazosin and terazosin. Indoramin is the least selective of these agents and is associated with the least favourable side-effect profile.

Mechanism of action The selective postjunctional α_1-adrenoceptor blockers reduce blood pressure by vasodilatation. Prazosin has relatively abrupt onset and short duration of action, necessitating multiple daily dosing. Doxazosin and terazosin have more gradual and prolonged actions and are suitable for once-daily dosing.

Adverse effects Postural hypotension, particularly after the initial dose, is a commonly experienced problem. The α-adrenergic system is activated with adoption of the upright posture. Thus, α-blockers are most effective with the patient erect. Indeed, these drugs have relatively little activity in the supine posture.

Other major side-effects – headache and palpitation (due to reflex tachycardia) – are predictable from the vasodilator properties of α-blockers. Fatigue, sedation and sexual dysfunction have also been reported. With doxazosin and prazosin, problems with sexual dysfunction are probably no more common than in the general population.

Avoidance of orthostatic hypotension Because of the frequency of postural hypotension, precautions are required during the initiation of α-blockade. A low starting dose before the patient retires to bed at night is recommended; an abrupt fall in blood pressure is then unlikely. Diuretics should be withheld for 24–48 hours before dosing since the magnitude of postural blood pressure reduction is greater if the patient is sodium depleted. If tolerated, the dose of α-blocker is then gradually increased over several weeks.

Doxazosin and terazosin are absorbed slowly and therefore have a gradual onset of action, making postural hypotension less likely. Even with newer drugs, however, postural symptoms are still troublesome.

The inconvenience of the dosing schedule greatly reduces the attraction of α-blockers. These drugs are not popular as first-line agents in the UK.

Outcome trials α-Blockers have beneficial effects on serum lipid profiles. About 5% reduction in total cholesterol and low density lipoprotein cholesterol and a similar increase in high density lipoprotein cholesterol can be expected during long-term therapy.

Recent evidence (ALLHAT 2000) suggests that, as first-line therapy, the most widely used α-blocker (doxazosin) is similar to a diuretic in preventing coronary heart disease and all-cause mortality. However, doxazosin was associated with an increased risk of stroke and heart failure. It is uncertain whether the same problems pertain when doxazosin is used in addition to diuretics, but the prescriber may wish to discuss this with the patient before initiating therapy. α-Blockers should be used as monotherapy only if all other main-line drugs are not tolerated.

■ KEY POINTS

- Low starting dose recommended.
- Lengthy period of dose titration necessary.
- Once- or twice-daily dosing.
- Poorly tolerated compared with other first-line agents.
- Reduce atherogenic lipid fractions.
- Expensive.

Other antihypertensive drugs

Drugs occasionally used in the management of hypertension include:

- direct vasodilators, e.g. hydralazine, minoxidil, diazoxide and sodium nitroprusside, are sometimes used in hypertensive emergencies
- centrally acting agents, e.g. clonidine, methyldopa, reserpine, are now very rarely used in the UK; moxonidine is a selective imidazoline-receptor agonist better tolerated than earlier agents
- adrenergic neurone blockers, e.g. bethanidine, debrisoquine, guanethidine, are largely of historical interest
- ganglion blockers, e.g. trimetaphan, may be used in hypertensive crises
- tyrosine hydroxylase inhibitors, e.g. metirosine, may be useful in patients with severe hypertension due to phaeochromocytoma.

Adverse effects

Direct vasodilators These are powerful antihypertensive agents but cause predictable side-effects. The most common are tachycardia and fluid retention. Therefore, these drugs are best used in combination with β-blockers and diuretics. In addition, drug-specific side-effects are seen.

Hydralazine The principal drawback with use of hydralazine is a systemic lupus erythematosus (SLE)-like syndrome which arises more commonly in females and is dose dependent. Hydralazine undergoes onward metabolism by acetylation in the liver. The extent of acetylation is under genetic control; the SLE-like syndrome is more common in slow acetylators where hydralazine levels are higher. The daily dose of hydralazine should be limited to 50 mg in women and 100 mg in men. The development of malaise, weight loss or arthritis should raise suspicion of the SLE-like syndrome.

Minoxidil This potent vasodilator causes particularly marked fluid retention. A loop diuretic is usually required to compensate for this. Minoxidil frequently causes unsightly hair growth (hypertrichosis). As a result, this drug is not popular with women and, even in men, the site of hair growth can cause cosmetic problems. Hair growth across the forehead is common in patients taking minoxidil.

Centrally acting antihypertensive drugs These cause predictable unwanted actions, e.g. somnolence and lethargy. Such drugs also commonly cause dry mouth and nasal stuffiness. Side-effects are less common with moxonidine.

Clonidine The main complication of clonidine use is the rapid offset of its action if a dose is missed. Blood pressure returns quickly to pretreatment levels but rarely to higher levels. Therefore the usual appellation of 'rebound hypertension' is not entirely accurate.

Methyldopa Long-term treatment with methyldopa may be associated with increases in hepatic enzyme activity as assessed in serum samples. In affected patients, methyldopa induces a mild hepatitis. Since this may go on to cirrhosis in a few patients, liver enzymes should be monitored during methyldopa therapy and the drug discontinued if abnormalities appear.

■ **KEY POINTS**

- These drugs are potent antihypertensive agents with steep dose–response curves, i.e. increasing doses lead to marked increases in efficacy.
- Treatment is complicated by many subjective side-effects which also tend to be dose related.
- These drugs are reserved for refractory patients, i.e. failure to respond adequately to first-line drugs in combination, or patients with particular problems, for example hypertensive crises (diazoxide, sodium nitroprusside or trimetaphan) or phaeochromocytoma (metirosine).
- There is little need to institute these drugs in general practice.

General comments

Efficacy The major antihypertensive agents (thiazides, β-blockers, calcium antagonists, ACE inhibitors, angiotensin II receptor antagonists and α-blockers) have similar efficacy (McInnes 1998, Treatment of Mild Hypertension Research Group 1991). Between 30% and 40% of patients with mild hypertension are likely to respond adequately to monotherapy. The response rate depends on the initial level of blood pressure and the level accepted as adequate control (usually diastolic blood pressure less than 85 mmHg and systolic blood pressure less than 140 mmHg).

Much higher response rates (80–90%) are often quoted in promotional literature. These rates refer to patients with very mild hypertension observed without adequate controls. Thus, such response rates include placebo responders (usually about 30%) and are hugely optimistic.

Dose Dose–response curves are relatively shallow. By employing low doses, side-effects are much less likely but it must be remembered that duration of action is dependent on dose. Therefore, at low starting doses, efficacy should be assessed at the end of the dosage interval to avoid undertreatment.

Factors influencing responsiveness Response rate is not influenced importantly by patient characteristics. Age, sex and plasma renin concentrations have been used to predict responses to particular drugs but results have usually been unconvincing. Elderly hypertensives appear to respond better to thiazide diuretics than to β-blockers but few other differences have been noted. Black patients of Afro-Caribbean origin respond well to diuretics and calcium antagonists and less well to β-blockers and ACE inhibitors. This response pattern may reflect the usual low renin status of such patients.

Drug choice in co-existent disease There are marked differences between drugs in side-effect profiles. Drug tolerability may be influenced by patient characteristics. The presence of co-existent diseases may determine the appropriate choice of drug (Table 4.8).

Thus, in a patient with asthma or severe airways disease, a β-blocker is contraindicated because of the risk of provoking bronchospasm. Even cardioselective agents should be avoided.

Table 4.8 Antihypertensive drugs in co-existent diseases

	Thiazide	β-Blocker	Calcium antagonist	ACE inhibitor	All antagonist	α-Blocker
Airways disease	+	−	+	+	+	+
Angina	+	++	++	+	+	+
Heart failure	++	(+)/++	−	++	++	+
Diabetes	+	+	+	+	+	(+)
Claudication	+	(+)	+	(+)	(+)	+
Renal failure	−	+	+	(+)/++	(+)/++	+

++, Positive indication; (+), Caution; +, No contraindication; −, Contraindication.

In angina, a β-blocker or a calcium antagonist would be a good choice because these drugs have antianginal properties. A combination of β-blocker plus dihydropyridine calcium antagonist may be particularly useful. Post myocardial infarction, a β-blocker is preferred.

Patients with overt heart failure should be given a diuretic and ACE inhibitor (or angiotensin receptor blocker if cough) regardless of whether there is hypertension. Recent evidence indicates that β-blockade improves outcome in patients with heart failure stabilized on diuretic and ACE inhibitor. Treatment should be started at low doses with careful monitoring. This is best undertaken under hospital supervision. Although theoretically advantageous due to their vasodilatory action (cardiac offloading), calcium antagonists generally cause a deterioration in ventricular function.

Intermittent claudication may be worsened by treatment with β-blockers which reduce cardiac output. However, controlled studies suggest that cardioselective agents have little adverse effect, unless combined with dihydropyridine calcium antagonists which may divert blood flow to non-ischaemic tissue. ACE inhibitors should be used with caution in patients with clinically overt peripheral vascular disease because of the high risk of bilateral renal artery stenosis.

In significant renal impairment, thiazides have little effect. A loop diuretic is preferable. It is usually recommended that ACE inhibitors should be used in low doses but there is little evidence that this is necessary.

It is particularly important to emphasize to high-risk patients the need to achieve rigorous blood pressure control and this usually means multiple drugs. In diabetes mellitus, all main-line antihypertensive drugs can be used alone or in combination. Low-dose diuretics are not harmful and are usually essential; there is as yet no convincing evidence of superiority for ACE inhibitors. Tight control of blood pressure is more important than specific drugs (UKPDS Group 1998a).

High-risk patients need to be reminded that very small additional reductions in blood pressure can achieve marked benefits in cardiovascular risk reduction (Hansson et al 1998, UKPDS Group 1998b). Such individuals must also understand the need to treat all risk factors, e.g. lipid-lowering therapy for hyperlipidaemia if 10-year coronary heart disease risk ⩾30% (Ramsay et al 1999). Many patients take aspirin in the belief that it protects against cardiovascular disease. However, aspirin, although cheap, is not cheerful; high-risk patients gain benefit but low-risk patients may be harmed (Ramsay et al 1999).

Drug interactions

Antihypertensive drugs are often used in combination or along with drugs prescribed for other conditions. Therefore, it is important that significant drug interactions are not encountered.

With other antihypertensives The antihypertensive effects of most agents are additive. This means that low doses of more than one drug can be combined to improve blood pressure control without necessarily imposing a greater burden of adverse effects.

β-Blockers and ACE inhibitors have less than additive effects since both drug types interfere with the renin–angiotensin system. Part of the antihypertensive effect of calcium antagonists appears to be mediated by renal sodium loss; dihydropyridine calcium antagonists and thiazide diuretics have a less than additive antihypertensive effect. However, such combinations are useful in many patients.

There is little evidence that any antihypertensive drug combination has a greater than additive effect. However, thiazides and ACE inhibitors appear to be particularly effective in combination. ACE inhibitors block the activation of the renin–angiotensin system secondary to diuretics; stimulation of this system may offset the blood pressure-lowering effect of thiazides.

Adverse interactions between antihypertensive agents are uncommon. However, concomitant use of β-blockers with verapamil or diltiazem may cause profound bradycardia and heart block, and precipitate heart failure. This combination should be avoided. ACE inhibitors (or angiotensin receptor blocker) and potassium-sparing diuretics both increase serum potassium concentrations and combined use is associated with the risk of life-threatening hyperkalaemia. Potassium-sparing diuretics should be discontinued if an ACE inhibitor (or angiotensin receptor blocker) is prescribed.

With other drugs Some drugs can attenuate the effect of antihypertensive drugs and lead to loss of blood pressure control. Non-steroidal anti-inflammatory drugs (NSAIDs) cause sodium retention and are often implicated in such interactions. These agents are often used in elderly patients and blood pressure should be carefully monitored when NSAIDs are introduced to older patients with hypertension.

NSAIDs can also cause hyperkalaemia and renal impairment when used with ACE inhibitors and potassium-sparing agents. Again this is a particular problem in the elderly and in those with pre-existing renal impairment.

Diuretic-induced hypokalaemia rarely leads to problems but even mild hypokalaemia can be dangerous in patients receiving drugs which prolong the QT interval (see Box 4.8). The major risk is the dimorphic ventricular arrhythmia, torsade de pointes, which can result in sudden death.

With foods When prescribing blood pressure-lowering therapy to hypertensive patients, their concurrent diet should be considered in one or two exceptional circumstances. Patients taking ACE inhibitors should not take potassium supplementation in the form of medication, salt substitutes or two or more servings of a potassium-rich food daily as this can result in hyperkalaemia (serum potassium greater than 5.5 mmol/l) (Ray et al 1999). Patients drinking grapefruit juice while taking calcium antagonists are at risk of hypotension and increased heart rate. Other citrus fruit juice can be taken safely (Bailey et al 1991). Liquorice can increase blood pressure if doses of 50 g daily are ingested for 2 weeks or more (Sigurjonsdottir et al 2001).

Factors influencing choice of drugs

Drugs used to treat hypertension should satisfy certain criteria:

- efficacy in reducing blood pressure
- convenience for the patient (i.e. once- or twice-daily administration) and the prescribing physician (no need for prolonged dose titration)
- tolerability
- safety
- compatibility with other drugs
- modification of outcome (reduction of morbid events).

Most first-line antihypertensive agents satisfy most of these criteria. However, thiazides and β-blockers have the enormous advantage of good safety records during long-term, widespread experience. The full potential of the more expensive newer agents remains to be established.

If all other factors are equal, consideration should be given to cost. Thiazides are by far the least expensive agents. Bendroflumethiazide (bendrofluazide) 2.5 mg daily costs less than £10 per year (2003 prices). Newer agents (calcium antagonists, ACE inhibitors, angiotensin II receptor antagonists and α-blockers) are much more expensive at equivalent doses.

Use of antihypertensive drugs

Most patients with sustained hypertension require more than one drug in combination to achieve adequate control. The conventional approach is stepped care.

Stepped care The principles of stepped care are:

- drugs have additive antihypertensive effects
- use of drugs at submaximal doses results in side-effects which are less than additive
- addition of some drugs attenuates the side-effects of others, e.g. ACE inhibitors lessen diuretic-induced hypokalaemia.

In this approach, drugs are added in a stepwise manner until control is achieved. If side-effects supervene, other drugs can be tried. Although usually described as restrictive, the policy is infinitely flexible.

An example of stepped care:

- Step 1: bendroflumethiazide (bendrofluazide) or β-blocker
- Step 2: bendroflumethiazide (bendrofluazide) plus β-blocker
- Step 3: add ACE inhibitor or dihydropyridine calcium antagonist or α-blocker.

There is little to choose between thiazides and β-blockers in the absence of specific contraindications. Thiazides are less expensive and appear to be better tolerated in women. β-Blockers may have a marginal advantage in tolerability in men.

Other options can be employed:

- Step 1: ACE inhibitor
- Step 2: add calcium antagonist
- Step 3: add α-blocker.

Very rarely, a fourth drug from another therapeutic class may have to be added. In such patients it is advisable to include a diuretic even in patients in whom such drugs are normally contraindicated, e.g. a history of gout; the risk from diuretic-induced hyperuricaemia can be avoided by co-administration of allopurinol.

Popular combinations are available in fixed-dose formulations. These are convenient, may improve compliance and can prove economical for patients who pay prescription charges.

Limitations of stepped care Compliance may deteriorate with multiple drugs. Although compliance is mainly influenced by the frequency with which drugs have to be taken, many patients find multiple drugs inconvenient, particularly if dosing times differ.

When patients are taking multiple drugs, it is often difficult to be certain of the contribution to blood pressure control made by individual drugs. Therefore, a patient may be taking a drug which is having little beneficial effect but nonetheless be exposed to the risk of side-effects from that drug.

Even if all drugs are contributing to blood pressure control, side-effects may accumulate. Side-effects from submaximal doses of drugs are usually less than additive but the frequency is generally greater than that attributable to one drug alone.

The costs of multiple drugs are additive. To ensure economic prescribing, it is imperative that individual drugs are contributing to control.

Stepped care is subject to the law of diminishing returns. About 40% of truly hypertensive patients will respond to step 1: 65% to step 2 (i.e. 40% responding to step 1 and 40% of remaining 60% to step 2) and 75–80% to step 3. Thus, fewer and fewer patients (in absolute numbers) respond to each additional drug.

New approaches Because of the perceived shortcomings of stepped care, other approaches have been advocated. These treatment plans are termed individualization and substitution.

Individualization In individualization, drugs are matched to the requirements of individual patients. The attempt is to gain specific benefit and/or to avoid adverse effects. Unfortunately, other than in the examples listed in Table 4.8, our ability to achieve this is limited.

Substitution The aim of substitution is to control blood pressure with the minimum number of drugs. Drugs are administered in series to identify the most suitable agent(s) in terms of efficacy and tolerability. If there is an inadequate response or an adverse reaction to a particular drug, that agent is withdrawn and replaced with another. Substitution depends on the untested assumption that patients who fail to respond to one drug will eventually respond to another. This policy is time consuming, unpopular with the patient and usually unsuccessful.

Limitations of individualization and substitution It is difficult and may be impossible to identify patients who will respond particularly well to a given drug. Despite popular misconceptions, factors such as age, sex and plasma renin activity are poor predictors of responsiveness. In any case, multiple drug therapy is usually required.

Modern stepped care takes account of many individual characteristics and is an essential aid to management. In the view of practising physicians in Britain, it remains the most practical approach to the treatment of hypertension (Waller et al 1990).

BEYOND BLOOD PRESSURE REDUCTION

Antihypertensive therapy reduces the risk of the main complications of hypertension, stroke and myocardial infarction. In preventive medicine, it is often assumed that a successful preventive measure will eliminate entirely the risk of an event. In fact, it can only hope to prevent that proportion of events attributable directly to the risk factor. For stroke, antihypertensive treatment reduces risk by 35–40%, exactly the proportional change predicted from epidemiological data. For coronary heart disease, blood pressure lowering reduces events by about 16% compared with the expected reduction of 20–25%.

These estimates are based on the results of trials with diuretics or β-blockers and there is speculation that with newer drugs the full reduction in coronary heart disease risk attributable to blood pressure might be achieved (i.e. 22.5% instead of 16%). This small improvement in protection will be very difficult to establish unless a very large outcome trial is completed. Even if the results were positive, over 75% of the risk of coronary events would be unaffected.

To make inroads into this requires a strategy beyond blood pressure reduction alone. Attention to the risk factors such as smoking and cholesterol would be beneficial. However, more aggressive blood pressure control using existing drugs would also contribute. Epidemiological data suggest a 'doubling effect', i.e. twice the reduction in blood pressure, twice the reduction in risk (Collins & MacMahon 1994).

Alternatively, newer drugs which interfere with the pathogenesis of the complications of hypertension, independently of blood pressure reduction, might allow greater benefit. As yet, there is little convincing evidence that any drugs provide benefits beyond that due to blood pressure reduction

(Blood Pressure Lowering Treatment Trialists' Collaboration 2000, Staessen et al 2001).

DELIVERY OF CARE

Although the evidence base for the treatment of hypertension is among the strongest in medicine, surveys of management in Britain reveal major short-comings (Colhoun et al 1998). Fewer than a third of individuals with hypertension obtain adequate blood pressure control. In the not too distant past, the management of hypertension could be described as following the 'rule of halves' (Smith et al 1991). Within a population, for example a group of patients in a health centre, half of those with hypertension would be known; of this identified group, half would be treated and, of the treated group, only half would have blood pressure at a normal level. In other words, of all hypertensive patients, only about one in eight was satisfactorily managed. Now, management appears to approximate to a 'rule of two thirds': two thirds aware of diagnosis, two thirds of those are treated and two thirds of those treated achieve target levels of blood pressure $- 2/3 \times 2/3 \times 2/3 = 8/27$, i.e. less than one third with adequate blood pressure control (Colhoun et al 1998).

One contributory factor is failure to develop a management strategy in partnership with the patient. Also, doctors often appear to underestimate the difficulties in achieving blood pressure targets and give the patient unrealistic expectations. The management of hypertension is not easy. It requires lifestyle changes, usually multiple drugs and a sometimes lengthy period of trial, error and tribulation before the best regimen for an individual is identified. Most importantly, it requires perseverance from both the doctor and the patient.

Successful management is only likely if time is taken to develop an understanding, caring doctor–patient relationship leading to a management plan with the patient as the key player. There is no substitute for direct communication. A well-educated nurse is invaluable in sharing this load.

Follow-up visits

Routine follow-up visits can be organized in nurse-run clinics but a doctor needs to be available for advice. At each visit weight and blood pressure should be measured and recorded. A history of current general health should be sought along with an assessment of adherence to pharmacological and non-pharmacological treatment as well as side-effects. Any abnormalities detected need to be investigated.

Clear targets for blood pressure (and other risk factors) help to aid adherence to therapy. Current recommended goal blood pressure is <140/85 mmHg (<140/80 mmHg in diabetes). Care should be taken in discussing blood pressure control. While a fall from 180/100 to 150/90 mmHg is encouraging, it is all too easy to give the impression that control is satisfactory. Rigorous targets are attainable in general practice but only if there is patient and professional compliance with the multiple drug regimens usually necessary.

In a nurse-run clinic, the flowchart in Figure 4.2 suggests guidelines for when to refer the patient to a doctor. Patient education on aspects of

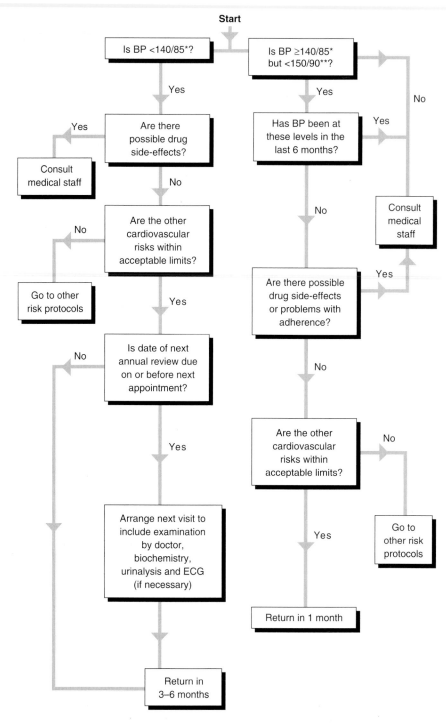

Figure 4.2 Flowchart for the follow-up of treated hypertensive patients. *In patients with diabetes mellitus ≥140/80 mmHg. **In patients with diabetes mellitus <150/85 mmHg.

hypertension and drug treatment can be continued along with discussion of achievable targets for reducing other cardiovascular risks. A return appointment after no more than 6 months is suggested for well-controlled patients, i.e. with a BP less than 140/85 mmHg. However, if systolic blood pressure is 140–160 mmHg or diastolic blood pressure is 86–90 mmHg then a 3-month return visit is suggested so that treatment change can be considered if blood pressure is still high. Similarly, if systolic blood pressure is greater than 160 mmHg or diastolic blood pressure is greater than 90 mmHg, a 1-month return visit is recommended to assess treatment change if blood pressure is still elevated, particularly if end-organ damage is present. Untreated patients can be scheduled in a similar way.

Annual review

The purpose of an annual review is to monitor blood pressure, risk factors and target organ damage. A review of the management of blood pressure and other cardiovascular risk factors may be necessary. It may also be necessary to institute more stringent measures such as an increase in drug treatment or referral to a smoking cessation programme or dietitian.

The procedures recommended at an annual review include:

- brief history including lifestyle, drugs (including over-the-counter preparations) and side-effects
- measurement of blood pressure
- urinalysis for protein
- a random venous blood sample to test for urea and electrolytes, creatinine, urate, glucose, cholesterol and γ-GT.

If the initial ECG is normal, repeat assessment every 3–5 years can identify serious changes. Remember that an earlier ECG may be clinically indicated, e.g. with the occurrence of chest pain. The progression and regression of LVH should be monitored by annual serial ECG. Echocardiography (ultrasound assessment of the heart), although a sensitive index of LVH, is not readily available for hypertensive patients cared for in the community. If physical examination, including funduscopy, is considered appropriate (e.g. persistently uncontrolled blood pressure or evolving target organ damage), review by the general practitioner is necessary.

Overall cardiovascular risk increases with age and reassessment should be carried out annually. As well as antihypertensive therapy, consideration should be given to instituting lipid-lowering treatment or low-dose aspirin.

Audit

The long-term follow-up care by the health team must be of a high standard. By setting standards for management and targets for blood pressure reduction, protocols can be developed to encourage optimum care. This can be achieved most successfully by including adequately educated nursing staff using an agreed protocol with recall facilities for patients who fail to attend (Kenkre et al 1985, Silverberg et al 1982). In a practice of 2500 it is estimated that 162 nurse-hours/year are employed managing 225 mild, 25 moderate and three severe hypertensive patients.

Regular review of the patient registration system for those lost to follow-up helps to identify patients at risk and who need prompting. On diagnosis of hypertension, a standardized READ code, such as G 2, can be recorded in the general practice computer system. Recall can be enhanced by sending a prompt letter to attend for annual blood pressure assessment. Carefully completing documentation for each patient at annual review allows access to data either in the form of a log book, card system or computer program. All or part of the data from completed annual reviews can be evaluated. The proportion of patients with blood pressure reaching audit standards (<150/90 mmHg), weights and the presence of other risk factors can be monitored over the years. Individuals with recorded blood pressure ≥150/90 mmHg can be identified and reviewed. A sample set of forms to facilitate these activities is shown in Figure 4.3. By using such forms, aspects of patient care can be reviewed and discussed with all members of the health-care team.

Referral for specialist advice

Most patients with essential hypertension can be managed in general practice. However, when the clinical evaluation or results of simple investigations suggest a need for further investigation it is usually best to refer for specialist advice, because the additional investigations needed are often difficult to arrange from general practice. Indications for referral for specialist advice or treatment are suggested in Box 4.9.

CONCLUSION

The successful management of hypertension depends on five Rs:

- *Register* – establishment of a register of individuals at high risk from high blood pressure identified by opportunistic but systematic screening of a general practice population.
- *Recall* – development of a robust system for regular assessment of all individuals in the population, with particular attention to those previously identified as having borderline hypertension, and to recall hypertensives lost to follow-up.
- *Review* – regular systematic review of those diagnosed as hypertensive, with monitoring of blood pressure control and compliance with both non-pharmacological and pharmacological treatment.
- *Record* – documentation of follow-up care to allow assessment of interventions for individuals and audit of overall success within the care setting.
- *Rational treatment* – successful treatment depends on appropriated lifestyle changes and rational use of drugs. We now have many effective, convenient and well-tolerated antihypertensive drugs. Choice should be based on these properties but also on the results of long-term experience, prospective trials to evaluate the influence on outcome (events), and on cost. Conventional bendroflumethiazide (bendrofluazide)-based stepped care remains the logical approach to the management of hypertension.

Cardiovascular patient record

Initial assessment   Date _____

Name:			Date of birth:	

Sex:	Ht:	Family history:	Ethnicity:

Initial examination

Weight		BP left arm		Random blood cholesterol		Alcohol units/week	
BMI		BP right arm		High density lipoprotein		Exercise level No of 30-min sessions/week	
Waist circumference		BP erect		Random blood glucose		Smoking status	
% absolute CHD risk over 10 years		Pulse		End organ damage	Yes/No *(Delete as appropriate)*	Diet	

Urinalysis	Fasting lipids	U&Es	Fasting glucose	ECG	FBC	Others

Problem checklist				
Problems	Tick if present	**Date**	**Management**	**Follow-up**
Cerebrovascular accident				
Transient ischaemic attack				
Myocardial infarction				
Heart failure				
Angina pectoris				
Peripheral vascular disease				
Renal disease				
Hypertension				
Hyperlipidaemia				
Diabetes				
Overweight				
Alcohol abuse				
Airways disease				
Thyroid disease				
Others				

Treatment history					
Drug	**Dose**	**Dose change**	**Start date**	**Stop date**	**Side-effects**

Figure 4.3 Hypertension record sheets: (A) patient details.

Cardiovascular patient record

Annual review

Name:		Date of birth:			

(Complete each test as necessary, file results and indicate if abnormal)

Date					
BP & pulse					
Weight					
Urinalysis					
U&Es, LFTs					
Cholesterol					
Glucose					
Diet check					
Smoking check					
Exercise check					
Alcohol check					
ECG results					
Diabetic check					
Funduscopy					
Peripheral pulses					
Neuropathy					
Foot check					
HbAIC					
Microalbuminuria					
Hyperlipidaemia check					
Fasting lipids: trigs					
Chol/HDL ratio					
Calculated LDL					
Other tests/procedures					
Influenza vaccine					
Pneumococcal vaccine					
Exercise tolerance test					
Echocardiography					
Symptoms					
Breathlessness Chest pain (frequency) Ankle swelling Other					

Figure 4.3 Hypertension record sheets: (B) annual review.

Cardiovascular patient record
Follow-up visits

Name:	Date of birth:

Date	Weight	BP & pulse	Check drugs	Blood tests	Risk factor modification	Comments

Additional comments

Figure 4.3 Hypertension record sheets: (C) follow-up record.

■ **BOX 4.9   Suggested indications for specialist referral**

Urgent treatment needed

- Accelerated (malignant) hypertension
- Severe hypertension (e.g. >220/120 mmHg)
- Impending complications (e.g. TIA, left ventricular failure)

Possible underlying cause

- Any clue in history or examination of a secondary cause
- Hypokalemia/increased serum sodium (Conn's syndrome?)
- Elevated serum creatinine
- Proteinuria or haematuria
- Recent onset or worsening of hypertension
- Resistant to a three-drug regimen
- Young age (any hypertension <20 years; needing treatment <30 years)

Therapeutic problems

- Treatment resistance
- Multiple drug intolerance
- Multiple drug contraindications
- Persistent non-compliance
- Treatment declined (the reluctant hypertensive)

Special situations

- Unusual BP variability
- Possible isolated clinic hypertension
- Hypertension in pregnancy

The guidelines outlined in this chapter are suggested as a basis for a blood pressure clinic protocol which should include management and audit. The protocol should include the methods used to:

- standardize blood pressure measurement and assessment of other cardiovascular risk factors
- advise and counsel patients on non-pharmacological methods for reducing blood pressure and overall cardiovascular risk
- provide education on the benefits of long-term follow-up and adherence with therapy
- prescribe antihypertensive drug therapy as necessary after a period of monitoring
- follow up all patients and complete an annual review
- document care by a computer and/or card registration system.

These guidelines are based on national (Ramsay et al 1999) and international (WHO/ISH 1999) recommendations. Each health-care team should devise its own protocol based on these guidelines, taking into consideration local constraints and conditions. Protocols must be revised at regular intervals to incorporate new evidence.

Hypertension is a good example of a condition where exchange of information between health professionals and patients is essential for successful management. The condition is asymptomatic but life threatening. Treatment is not easy and needs to be taken for life. Lifestyle changes and numerous drugs, alone or in combination, may be necessary. It is important that patients are given consistent advice by the health-care team and it is tailored to the level that they can best assimilate. Patients who have bought a home blood pressure device may also need help with interpreting the results obtained and maintaining the machine. Brief information booklets, such as that illustrated in the appendix, can be helpful. However, such aids are no substitute for detailed, careful and repeated face-to-face consultations. Only in this way can a personalized strategy with appropriate targets and support be developed with the patient as the key player.

■ KEY POINTS

- Hypertension is one of a number of cardiovascular risk factors and should be treated not in isolation, but as part of a multiple risk factor strategy.
- Blood pressure lowering decreases cerebrovascular and coronary heart disease morbidity and mortality.
- All those involved in the care of hypertension must be trained to measure blood pressure accurately.
- Secondary causes occur in less than 10% of patients with hypertension. However, protocols should include appropriate screening and guidance on referral for specialist assessment.
- The general practice team is in a key position to improve the identification, follow-up and control of essential hypertension in the community.
- Hypertension should only be diagnosed after careful monitoring of blood pressure over time.
- All identified hypertensive patients should be assessed and followed in the long term using an established protocol developed from national and international guidelines.
- Other cardiovascular risk factors should be identified and interventions instituted where appropriate.
- Non-pharmacological treatment for hypertension should always be considered prior to and along with drug treatment.
- Individualized patient education is an essential component of management.
- Long-term follow-up should include assessment of end-organ damage on a regular basis, generally annually.
- The effectiveness of the protocols and strategies can only be assessed by regular audit.

■ CASE STUDY 4.1

A 49-year-old man comes to the general practitioner for travel immunization. The practice nurse sees him and takes the opportunity to check his blood pressure. It is 154/96 mmHg and his body mass index is 28 kg/m^2. There is no previous history of high blood pressure but his father has angina and his mother recently had a stroke aged 78 years. He has never smoked and used to play a lot of football, but now takes little exercise. He is married and works shifts as a controller in the fire service. At present, he is looking forward to his holiday in Greece in 3 months' time and is keeping well.

Questions

1. This patient needs to have his blood pressure rechecked; how soon would you offer him another appointment?
2. What could he do before his next visit to try to reduce his blood pressure?

Answers

1. Discuss the level of blood pressure and reassure him that this is only one reading, when he was nervous about coming for a painful procedure. It is not an immediate problem but one that should not be ignored, so it is important to check his blood pressure again in 4 weeks' time. If the blood pressure is still at this level at the next two visits, 1 month apart, he should be given an appointment for a baseline physical examination by the general practitioner and initial investigations (routine biochemistry and cholesterol, urinalysis and an ECG).
2. He should consider his diet and exercise patterns. As he is overweight, he should reduce his calorie intake, taking foods high in fibre and vitamin C. Check how much salt, e.g. in convenience food and snacks, and alcohol and coffee he takes. He has a sedentary job so exercise could be a problem and needs to be addressed. He need not worry that this might prevent him from going on holiday.

■ CASE STUDY 4.2

A 59-year-old woman is found to be hypertensive while attending a well woman clinic. There is no relevant history and physical examination is unremarkable other than raised blood pressure and obesity. Blood pressure remains high on repeated measurements. Routine investigations are negative except for a random blood sugar of 12 mmol/l. Calorie restriction results in satisfactory reduction in weight and normalization of non-fasting blood sugar, but blood pressure remains elevated after 3 months' observation.

Questions

1. What antihypertensive drugs would you considered appropriate?
2. If blood pressure does not settle on monotherapy, what would be your preferred treatment option?

Answers

1. Drugs from any of the main classes are now considered appropriate.
2. Monotherapy seldom achieves the rigorous target blood pressure recommended. Inclusion of a diuretic is often necessary.

■ PRACTICAL EXERCISE

It is known from the HOT Study (Hansson et al 1998) that only about one third of patients will require one blood pressure-lowering therapy to control their blood pressure to target. Undertake an audit of patients diagnosed with hypertension in your practice to identify those with blood pressure not controlled to target. A computer search will be able to identify these patients if data entry is well organized. For audit purposes the British Hypertension Society recommends a target blood pressure of 150/90 mmHg (in diabetes 140/85 mmHg). Calculate the percentage of patients with hypertension treated to target. Once patients have been identified determine whether they are on no medication, one, two or three medications to lower blood pressure. This audit will allow you to identify at least three categories of patients for follow-up:

- those with poor adherence to medication
- those requiring more therapy or adjustment to dosage
- those to be referred for a specialized opinion.

To complete the audit cycle set a standard for the percentage of patients treated to target and repeat the audit in 1 year to determine if this has been met. Each year gradually increase this percentage.

REFERENCES

ALLHAT Officers and Co-ordinators for the ALLHAT Collaborative Research Group 2000 Major cardiovascular events in hypertensive patients randomized to doxazosin vs chlorthalidone. The Antihypertensive and Lipid-Lowering Treatment to Prevent Heart Attack Trial (ALLHAT). Journal of the American Medical Association 283: 1967–1975

Bailey DG, Spence JD, Munoz C, Arnold JM 1991 Interaction of citrus juices with felodipine and nifedipine. Lancet 337: 268–269

Barber JH, Beevers DG, Fife R et al 1979 Blood pressure screening in general practice. British Medical Journal 278: 843–846

Berchthold P, Jorgens V, Kemmer FW, Berger M 1982 Obesity and hypertension: cardiovascular response to weight reduction. Hypertension 4 (suppl III): 500–555

Berry C, Brosnan MJ, Fennell J, Hamilton CA, Dominiczak AF 2001 Oxidative stress and vascular damage in hypertension. Current Opinion in Nephrology and Hypertension 10: 247–255

Blood Pressure Lowering Treatment Trialists' Collaboration 2000 Effects of ACE inhibitors, calcium antagonists, and other blood-pressure-lowering drugs: results of prospectively designed overviews of randomised trials. Lancet 355: 1955–1964

Bulpitt CJ (ed) 2000 Handbook of hypertension: volume 20: epidemiology of hypertension. Elsevier Science, London

Colhoun HM, Dong W, Poulter NR 1998 Blood pressure screening, management and control in England: results from the health survey for England 1994. Journal of Hypertension 16: 747–752

Collins R, MacMahon S 1994 Blood pressure antihypertensive drug treatment and the risks of stroke and coronary heart disease. British Medical Bulletin 50: 272–298

Criqui MH, Cowan LD, Heiss G, Haskel WL, Laskarzewski PM, Chambless LE 1986 Frequency and clustering of nonlipid coronary risk factors in dyslipoproteinemia: the Lipid Research Clinics Program Prevalence Study. Circulation 73 (suppl 1): 140–150

Feathers C 2001 Equipment for blood pressure measurement. Professional Nurse 16: 1458–1462

Feher M, Harris-St John K, Lant A 1992 Blood pressure measurement by junior hospital doctors – a gap in medical education? Health Trends 24: 59–61

Fletcher AE, Bulpitt CJ, Chase DM et al 1993 Quality of life with three antihypertensive treatments – cilazapril, atenolol, nifedipine. Hypertension 19: 499–507

Hansson L, Zanchetti A, Carruthers SG et al for the HOT Study Group 1998 Effects of intensive blood pressure lowering and low-dose aspirin in patients with hypertension: principal results of the Hypertension Optimal Treatment (HOT) randomised trial. Lancet 351: 1755–1762

He J, Whelton PK 1999 Elevated systolic blood pressure and risk of cardiovascular and renal disease: overview of evidence from observational epidemiologic studies and randomised controlled trials. American Heart Journal 138: S211–S219

Hjendahl P, Wikland IK 1992 Quality of life on antihypertensive therapy: scientific end point or marketing exercise? Journal of Hypertension 10: 1437–1446

Kannel WB 2000 Risk stratification in hypertension: new insights from the Framingham Study. American Journal of Hypertension 13 (Pt 2): 3S–10S

Kannel WB, Neaton JD, Wentworth D et al 1986 Overall and coronary heart disease mortality rates in relation to major risk factors in 325,348 men screened for the MRFIT. American Heart Journal 112: 825–836

Kenkre J, Drury VWM, Lancashire RJ 1985 Nurse management of hypertension clinics in general practice assisted by computer. Family Practice 2: 17–22

Loscalzo J 1995 Nitric oxide and vascular disease. New England Journal of Medicine 333: 251–253

Luscher TF 1990 Functional abnormalities of the vascular endothelium in hypertension and atherosclerosis. Scandinavian Journal of Clinical Laboratory Investigations 50 (suppl 199): 28–32

MacMahon SW, Norton RN 1986 Alcohol and hypertension: implications for prevention and treatment. Annals of Internal Medicine 105: 124–126

MacMahon SW, Macdonald GJ, Blacket RB 1985 Plasma lipoprotein levels in treated and untreated hypertensive men and women: the National Heart Foundation of Australia Risk Factor Prevalence Study. Arteriosclerosis 5: 391–396

MacMahon S, Peto R, Cutler J et al 1990 Blood pressure, stroke, and coronary heart disease. Part 1, prolonged differences in blood pressure prospective observational studies corrected for the regression dilution bias. Lancet 335: 765–774

McInnes GT 1995 Hypertension and coronary artery disease: cause and effect. Journal of Hypertension 13 (suppl 2): S49–S56

McInnes G 1998 Pocket reference to angiotensin II antagonists. Science Press, London

McInnes GT, Yeo WW, Ramsay LE, Moser M 1992 Cardiotoxicity of diuretics: much speculation – little substance. Journal of Hypertension 10: 317–335

McKay DW, Campbell NRC, Parab LS, Chockalingam A, Fodor JG 1990 Clinical assessment of blood pressure. Journal of Human Hypertension 4: 639–645

Mullen P, Simons-Morton D, Ramirez G et al 1997 A meta analysis of trials evaluating patient education and counselling for three groups of preventive health behaviours. Patient Education and Counselling 32: 157–173

Multiple Risk Factor Intervention Trial (MRFIT) Research Group 1986 Coronary heart disease death, nonfatal acute myocardial infarction and other clinical outcomes in the Multiple Risk Factor Intervention Trial. American Journal of Cardiology 58: 1–13

O'Brien E, O'Malley K (eds) 1991 Handbook of hypertension: volume 14: blood pressure measurement. Elsevier, Amsterdam

O'Brien E, Mee F, Tan KS, Atkins N, O'Malley K 1991 Training and assessment of observers for blood pressure measurement in hypertension research. Journal of Human Hypertension 5: 7–10

O'Brien E, Petrie J, Littler W et al 1993 The British Hypertension Society protocol for the evaluation of blood pressure measuring devices. Journal of Hypertension 11 (suppl 2): S43–S62

O'Brien ET, Petrie JC, Littler WA et al 1997 Blood pressure measurement. Recommendations of the British Hypertension Society, 3rd edn. BMJ Books, London

Petrie J, Jamieson M, O'Brien ET, Littler WA, Padfield P, de Swiet M 1990 Blood pressure measurement (video). BMJ Publications, London

Pickering G 1968 High blood pressure, 2nd edn. J & P Churchill, London

Primatesta P, Falaschetti E, Gupta S, Marmot M, Poulter N 2001 Association between smoking and blood pressure evidence from the Health Survey for England. Hypertension 37: 187–193.

Psaty BM, Heckbert SR, Koepsell TD et al 1995 The risk of myocardial infarction associated with antihypertensive drug therapies. Journal of the American Medical Association 274: 620–625

Ramsay LE, Williams B, Johnston GD et al 1999 Guidelines for management of hypertension: report of the third working party of the British Hypertension Society. Journal of Human Hypertension 13: 569–592

Ray K, Dorman S, Watson R 1999 Severe hyperkalaemia due to the concomitant use of salt substitutes and ACE inhibitors in hypertension: a potentially life threatening interaction. Journal of Human Hypertension 13: 717–720

Sigurjonsdottir H, Franzson L, Manhem K, Ragnarsson J, Sigurdsson G, Wallerstedt S 2001 Liquorice-induced rise in blood pressure: a linear dose response relationship. Journal of Human Hypertension 15: 549–552

Silverberg DS, Baltuch L, Hermoni Y, Eyal P 1982 Control of hypertension in family practice by the doctor–nurse team. Journal of the Royal College of General Practitioners 32: 184–186

Smith WCS, Lee AJ, Crombie IK et al 1991 Control of BP in Scotland: the rule of halves. British Medical Journal 302: 1057–1060

Staessen JA, Wang JG, Thijs L 2001 Cardiovascular protection and blood pressure reduction: a meta-analysis. Lancet 358: 1305–1315

Stein PP, Black HR 1993 The role of diet in the genesis and treatment of hypertension. Medical Clinics of North America 77: 831–847

Swales JD 1994 Overview of essential hypertension. In: Swales JD (ed) Textbook of hypertension. Blackwell Scientific Publications, Oxford

Treatment of Mild Hypertension Research Group 1991 The Treatment of Mild Hypertension Study: a randomized, placebo-controlled trial of a nutritional hygienic regimen along with various drug monotherapies. Archives of Internal Medicine 151: 1413–1423

UK Prospective Diabetes Study Group 1998a Efficacy of atenolol and captopril in reducing risk of macrovascular and microvascular complications in type 2 diabetes: UKPDS 39. British Medical Journal 317: 713–720

UK Prospective Diabetes Study Group 1998b Tight blood pressure control and risk of macrovascular and microvascular complications in type 2 diabetes: UKPDS 38. British Medical Journal 317: 703–713

Waller PC, McInnes GT, Reid JL 1990 Policies for managing hypertensive patients: a survey of the opinions of British specialists. Journal of Human Hypertension 4: 509–515

Wassertheil-Smoller S, Blaufox MD, Oberman AS, Langford HG, Davis BR, Wylie-Rosett J 1992 The Trial of Antihypertensive Interventions and Management (TAIM) Study; adequate weight loss, alone and combined with drug therapy in the treatment of mild hypertension. Archives of Internal Medicine 152: 131–136

Wingfield D, Pierce M, Faher M 1996 Blood pressure measurement in the community: do guidelines help? Journal of Human Hypertension 10: 805–809

Wolf-Meier K, Cooper RS, Banagas JR et al 2003 Hypertension prevalence and blood pressure levels in 6 European countries, Canada and the United States. Journal of the American Medical Association 2003 (28a): 2363–2369

Wood C (ed) 1986 Dietary salt and hypertension: implications for public health policies. Round Table Series Number 5. Royal Society of Medicine Services, London

World Health Organization/International Society of Hypertension 1999 Guidelines for the management of hypertension. Journal of Hypertension 17: 151–183

FURTHER READING

Beevers DG, MacGregor GA 1988 Hypertension in practice. Martin Dunitz, London

O'Brien ET, Beevers DG, Lip GYH 2001 ABC of hypertension. BMJ Publishing Group, London

Tudor Hart J 1993 Hypertension – community control of high blood pressure, 3rd edn. Radcliffe Medical Press, Oxford

APPENDIX: LIVING WITH HIGH BLOOD PRESSURE

What is high blood pressure?

- High blood pressure (also known as hypertension) is one of the most common medical conditions in the UK. As many as 20% of the entire population has high blood pressure.
- High blood pressure is not an illness but, without treatment, it increases the risk of heart attack, stroke and other vascular diseases.
- High blood pressure itself does not cause symptoms and therefore you are likely to feel completely well. This emphasizes the importance of early identification and long-term treatment.
- With effective treatment, someone with high blood pressure can expect to live a full and productive life.

What causes high blood pressure?

- In the vast majority of people with high blood pressure, no cause is found. This is called essential (primary) hypertension.
- A few people with high blood pressure have an underlying cause, usually due to a kidney or glandular (hormonal) problem. This is called secondary hypertension.
- The usual form of high blood pressure (essential hypertension) often runs in families.
- Some lifestyle factors can make matters worse:
  - overeating
  - lack of exercise
  - excessive alcohol consumption
  - too much salt in the diet.

What other things are important?

- High blood pressure is not the only important and correctable risk factor for vascular diseases.
- Other important factors include:
  - cigarette smoking
  - blood fats (cholesterol)
  - diabetes mellitus
  - weight
  - excess alcohol intake
  - lack of exercise.
- Your doctor or practice nurse will want to assess these and other factors to advise you on what needs to be done.

What can we do to control high blood pressure?

- You are not in this alone.
- Your doctor, practice nurse and others are there to help you.

- Effective treatment involves regular visits to your doctor or practice nurse for measurement of blood pressure and other simple tests, to make sure your lifestyle is healthy and, if necessary, for medication.
- At the start, you may need to be seen several times over weeks or months, while lifestyle changes are introduced, before a decision is made about whether medication is necessary.
- Later on, visits every 3 months may be all that is needed.

What lifestyle changes should you make?

Don't smoke

- Smoking harms the heart (and lungs) and can lead to many problems.
- **Stop smoking now!!**
- If you need help talk to your doctor or practice nurse or contact Smokeline on 0800 84 84 84.

Watch your weight

- Being overweight increases blood pressure and the risk of vascular diseases.
- If you are overweight, this does not necessarily mean that you eat excessively. However, it means that you eat more than your body needs for your level of activity.
- Your doctor or practice nurse will advise you on your ideal weight and give you advice on dieting, if necessary.
- There are several things that you can do to reduce weight. The good news is that changing your diet may not be hard work. Small changes made gradually can be included in your daily routine.
- Losing weight to achieve your ideal weight will make you feel better, help to reduce blood pressure and the risk of vascular disease.

Keep fit

- Remain as active as possible.
- Suitable exercise includes walking, cycling, swimming, keep fit classes, bowling, golfing or dancing – the more exercise the better.
- If you are unsure, your doctor or practice nurse will advise you about suitable exercise for you.
- Regular exercise will make you feel better as well as helping to reduce blood pressure and the risk of vascular disease.

Drink alcohol only in moderation

- Excess alcohol increases blood pressure.
- Safe limits for alcohol are:
  - 21 units of alcohol per week in men
  - 14 units of alcohol per week in women.
- One unit of alcohol is equal to:
  - ½ pint of regular beer
  - 1 small glass of wine
  - 1 small measure of spirit.

- Keeping alcohol intake within safe limits will help reduce blood pressure and the risk of vascular (and other) diseases.

Avoid salty food

- We all need some salt but too much salt in the diet increases blood pressure.
- Taste your food before adding salt or, better still, don't add salt at the table.
- Remember that processed foods (e.g. frozen or canned) often contain a lot of salt.
- Reducing your salt intake will help reduce blood pressure.

Eat a healthy diet

- Reduce the total amount of fat, especially animal fat.
- Eat more fish, lean meat and poultry.
- Cut down on pies, sausages and burgers.
- Increase your intake of fibre-rich foods like wholemeal bread, pasta, jacket potatoes, fruit, vegetables, high-fibre breakfast cereals and porridge.
- Cut down on sugar, cakes, sweets and biscuits.

Benefits of successful lifestyle changes

- You will feel better.
- Your need for medicines to reduce blood pressure will be lessened and sometimes these will be unnecessary.
- Your risk of vascular disease will be greatly reduced.

Medicines for high blood pressure

- Most people will require medication to reduce blood pressure. More than half will require two or more medicines. One third will require three or more medicines. So don't be alarmed if you need more than one medicine.
- Many medicines are available to reduce blood pressure. The main groups are:
  - diuretics
  - β-blockers
  - ACE (angiotensin-converting enzyme) inhibitors
  - calcium antagonists
  - α-blockers
  - angiotensin receptor blockers.
- Different medicines act in different ways. Therefore, using medicines together leads to greater reductions in blood pressure.
- Modern drugs for high blood pressure cause few side-effects and these are usually mild. Although many side-effects are listed on the package insert which comes with a medicine, it is important to realize that this list includes every side-effect which *might* have been due to that particular medicine when given to thousands or even millions of people. **Your chance of experiencing a side-effect is very low. Remember that**

symptoms while taking a medicine may not be due to the medicine. If you think you may have a side-effect, contact your doctor or practice nurse immediately.
- Clinical trials in nearly 50 000 people with high blood pressure have shown beyond doubt that treatment with medicines to reduce blood pressure saves lives and prevents heart attacks, strokes and other vascular diseases.

Other medicines
- It is important to control other risk factors for vascular disease and this may mean the prescription of additional medicines.
- Some but not all people with high blood pressure and high blood fat (cholesterol) levels may need medicines to reduce fats (lipid-lowering drugs).
- Some people with high blood pressure, particularly those with previous heart attacks or strokes, may benefit from the use of aspirin.
- Other medicines may also be needed in particular cases, e.g. people with diabetes or after a heart attack.
- Your doctor will assess your personal risk and likely benefits before deciding with you on the most appropriate medication.

Things to remember
- Always keep your appointment to see the doctor or practice nurse.
- Follow lifestyle advice.
- **Take your prescribed tablets every day**.
- Make sure you *never* run out of tablets, especially on holidays or trips away from home.
- Keep taking your tablets until told to stop by your doctor or practice nurse.
- You will probably need to take your medicine for life.
- Do not take over-the-counter medicines without informing your doctor or practice nurse. Some of these may increase blood pressure.

Lifestyle management: smoking

Doreen McIntyre

5

■ CONTENTS

INTRODUCTION

Smoking is the chief avoidable cause of premature death and ill health in the world. It is estimated that worldwide, 4 million people die from smoking every year and if current smoking patterns persist, tobacco will kill 10 million smokers every year by 2030 (World Bank 1999). In the UK, 120 000 people die prematurely from smoking-related diseases each year (HEA 1998). One in four of these smoking-related deaths is from coronary heart disease (CHD) and cigarette smoking is responsible for approximately 17% of all deaths from CHD (HEA 1998).

FACTS AND FIGURES

In 1948, when the first surveys of smoking rates were undertaken by the tobacco companies, 82% of British men smoked, a peak in male smoking prevalence. Since the late 1950s there has been a steady decline in this rate.

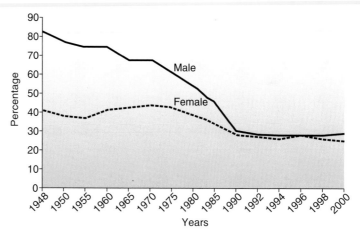

Figure 5.1 Percentages of men and women who smoke (1948–2000).

Smoking prevalence amongst women peaked much later at 45% in the late 1960s and has declined more slowly since then (Wald & Nicolaides-Bauman 1991).

In 1972 when the OPCS started to collect smoking prevalence data, 52% of men and 41% of women aged 16 and over smoked. By 2000, this figure had dropped to 29% of men and 25% of women (ONS 2001), but over the last 20 years the rate of decline has slowed (see Fig. 5.1).

The main concern at the beginning of the 21st century is that smoking is strongly associated with health inequality, with smoking rates highest among the most deprived groups. While smoking rates have declined in affluent groups, they have not in poorer groups although interest in stopping is equally high in all.

WHAT IS SMOKING?

Cigarette smoking is largely a 20th-century phenomenon, when the introduction and promotion of manufactured cigarettes changed the nature of tobacco use to that of a regular consumer activity. The introduction of cigarettes is important from the point of view of health for two main reasons: firstly, the cigarette smoke is directly, deliberately inhaled and secondly, as cigarettes are portable and convenient, tobacco smoking became a social and everyday phenomenon rather than a ceremonial and formal activity. The regular use of cigarettes quickly leads to addiction.

Tobacco smoke contains some 4000 chemicals in the form of particles and gases; 60 of these substances are known or suspected carcinogens (IARC 1986). In the USA, the Environmental Protection Agency (1992) has classified tobacco smoke as a class A carcinogen along with asbestos, arsenic and radon gas.

The main components of tobacco smoke are:

- *tar* – a solid irritant, tar coats the lungs, blocks the airways and causes emphysema and lung cancer. Tar is a complex mixture of toxic substances that include formaldehyde, ammonia and benzene

- *carbon monoxide (CO)* – carbon monoxide is absorbed via the lungs into the bloodstream where it binds to haemoglobin, replacing oxygen. The level of CO in a smoker's body depends on the number of cigarettes smoked and how they are smoked. Carbon monoxide causes heart and arterial disease

- *nicotine* – this is the addictive component of tobacco smoke, which diffuses into the bloodstream very quickly. The nicotine in each puff of inhaled smoke reaches the brain in less than 7 seconds. Nicotine is not a benign substance – in pure form it can be highly toxic – but the amounts delivered by cigarette smoking, or particularly in medicinal treatments like nicotine replacement therapy (NRT), are not sufficient to cause major physical harm in themselves.

SMOKING AND HEALTH

As early as the 1920s, doctors noticed an increase in the frequency of lung cancer in patients who smoked heavily. But it was not until the 1950s that widespread awareness of the problem developed following studies by Doll & Hill (1950) on smoking and lung cancer.

Doll et al's 1994 report updated 40 years' observation of 35 000 British doctors. It concluded that about half of all smokers will be killed by their smoking. Of those killed in middle age, the average loss of life expectancy is 20–25 years.

The main diseases caused by smoking are CHD and lung cancer; 26% of smokers die from lung cancer and 25% from CHD. Other forms of cardiovascular disease and emphysema are the other main causes of smoking-related deaths, at 15% each (OPCS 1991), and about 11% of stroke deaths are smoking related (Shinton & Beevers 1989).

Smoking has also been linked to cancers of the mouth, oesophagus, larynx, bladder and pancreas. Stroke, chronic bronchitis and circulatory problems are also caused by smoking. Research continues to find links between smoking and many other disease risks including premature menopause, complications in pregnancy, impotence, premature ageing and reduced fertility.

Passive smoking

Passive smoking is breathing other people's tobacco smoke. Tobacco smoke consists of sidestream smoke from the burning tip of the cigarette and mainstream smoke that has been inhaled and then exhaled by the smoker; 85% of the smoke from a cigarette is emitted as sidestream smoke (US DHHS 1986).

As well as the short-term effects of passive smoking such as eye irritation, headaches, sore throats and coughing, research has found longer term, more serious health risks. The British government's Independent Scientific Committee on Smoking and Health (ISCSH 1988) found an increased risk of lung cancer in non-smokers exposed to passive smoking of between 10% and 30% and a 23% increase in the risk of heart disease.

Smoking and coronary heart disease

Smoking has been called 'the most important of the known modifiable risk factors for CHD' (US DHHS 1990). The death rate for all cardiovascular disease for smokers is 2–3 times that of non-smokers and between 35% and 40% of these deaths occur before retirement age (RCP 1983).

Smoking rapidly increases the heart rate and constricts blood vessels, while simultaneously reducing the blood's capacity to carry oxygen.

Smoking is associated with both aspects of atherosclerosis; it promotes the development of lesions, thus creating sites susceptible to blockage, and promotes the occurrence of triggering events that lead to blockages (US DHHS 1989).

Evidence has more recently linked passive smoking with CHD. In the short term, passive smoking decreases the ability of the heart to receive and process oxygen. In the longer term, it promotes the build-up of plaque and the development of atherosclerotic lesions (Wells 1994). In a review of recent literature, Glantz & Parmley (1995) concluded that passive smoking reduces the ability of the blood to deliver oxygen to the myocardium and reduces the ability of the myocardium to use the oxygen it does receive effectively. The study reports that the effects of passive smoking on the cardiovascular system are a result not of a single component in tobacco smoke but of many elements, including carbon monoxide and nicotine.

Benefits of stopping

Approximately 13 million adults in the UK are ex-smokers (ONS 2001). Therefore, people do stop smoking and the US Surgeon General's review of evidence (US DHHS 1990) found both significant short- and longer term benefits of doing so.

Short-term benefits of stopping

As soon as a smoker stops smoking the body starts to eliminate tobacco constituents. Within 8 hours nicotine levels will be reduced by half and within 24–48 hours of stopping, the smoker's carbon monoxide level will be comparable with that of a non-smoker. The oxygen level gradually returns to normal and the heart beat slows.

The lungs start to clear the tar, the cilia recover and the ex-smoker feels less wheezy and breathless. Within a few weeks the senses of smell and taste improve, teeth are whiter and breath fresher.

Longer term benefits of stopping

The longer term benefits to cardiovascular risk are very considerable and these benefits occur at all age groups and at all stages of cardiovascular disease.

The excess risk of CHD from smoking reduces by half within 1 year of stopping smoking. After 15 years, the risk reverts to about the same level as that of someone who has never smoked. As would be expected, the level to which the risk drops varies between individuals and depends on how long the person smoked, how heavily he or she smoked and the other risk factors present.

For an individual who already has heart disease or who has had a heart attack, giving up smoking reduces the risk of premature death or another heart attack by up to 50% or more.

For lung cancer, smokers who stop after less than 20 years can reasonably expect their risk of developing lung cancer to fall to that of a lifelong non-smoker after approximately 10 years' cessation.

WHY DO PEOPLE START SMOKING?

In order to advise patients who smoke and help them in any attempt to stop, it is important to have an understanding of smoking, separating out why people start, why they continue and why they decide to stop. Your understanding can then help to facilitate smokers' own understanding of their smoking behaviour and ultimately help them to stop.

Until about the age of 10, children accept the fact that smoking is bad for health. But as they approach adolescence, many of these children start smoking. Many factors combine to influence children's uptake of smoking:

• *Peer pressure*. Adolescence is a time of change, characterized by aspiration to join the adult world. Smoking can be used to gain acceptance by peers and an increased feeling of maturity. When smoking is perceived to be common and unrestricted in a child's immediate environment, it will be seen as an appropriate behaviour to adopt. Parental and sibling smoking is strongly associated with uptake by children.

• *Transitional times*. Significant increases in uptake are seen in the age groups in which children move from primary to secondary education and again when they move from secondary education to further training or into employment. This is probably associated again with aspiration to join a more adult group.

• *A desire to rebel*. Smoking is presented as an adult behaviour not allowed in children, making it seem like an act of defiance to those in authority.

• *Out of curiosity or suggestibility*. This is of course a natural childhood characteristic, leading to early experimentation.

• *Promotion of tobacco*. Direct advertising of tobacco products was banned in the UK from 14 February 2003. However, until that time tobacco advertising tended to use humour and puzzles to portray cigarettes as interesting and stylish. Children particularly enjoy this type of advertising and smoked the most heavily advertised brands. Cigarette brands were also advertised through sponsorship, for example of sport, art and entertainment events, and indirect promotions. Tobacco sponsorship of international sport events like Formula 1 racing will continue to be allowed until 2006.

Uptake of smoking is largely a teenage phenomenon, with most smokers having established regular smoking by age 18.

WHY DO SMOKERS CONTINUE TO SMOKE?

Very quickly after starting to smoke, dependent behaviour often sets in. Symptoms of nicotine addiction have been identified in children after just four or five cigarettes, but the most evident sign is the establishment of a regular daily smoking pattern. Smokers become accustomed to a regular nicotine level in their bloodstream and smoke the requisite daily number of cigarettes to maintain those levels without discomfort.

Most smokers are well aware that smoking is harmful to health and most will readily name cancer, especially lung cancer, as the main smoking-related disease. They are less likely to name CHD as an outcome of smoking, despite its relatively higher likelihood, particularly in combination with other common lifestyle issues like overweight and lack of exercise. There is some understanding of other risks of smoking, e.g. bronchitis and emphysema, and of the more recently documented health risks of smoking, e.g. complications to pregnancy, circulatory diseases, premature menopause and ageing. Awareness of health effects is, however, insufficient and smokers often rationalize their continued smoking in a number of ways. Denial is one response.

- 'It won't happen to me'
- 'I can give up any time'
- 'I will stop in 5 years'

Part of the problem is that many serious ill effects of smoking usually do not become apparent until later. Smokers who feel healthy now do not believe any damage has or will be done and cannot actually see the damage being done to their lungs or arteries. Relative risk can also be a difficult concept to understand – people will on the one hand cling to the hope of a lottery win despite extremely high odds against it but at the same time believe that 50–50 chances of dying of a smoking-related illness are good odds: they will be the lucky one. Knowing the facts, then, is not enough; some very powerful drivers keep people smoking.

Drug dependence

The main reason for not giving up even when a smoker wants to is the addictive nature of nicotine.

Nicotine reaches the brain approximately 7 seconds after the first puff on a cigarette and an average of 10 inhalations is taken on each cigarette; a very high frequency of 'shots' makes smoking a very overlearned behaviour.

Most people smoke to obtain nicotine; a smoker will often subconsciously take more frequent, deeper puffs on a so-called low-tar cigarette to keep the level maintained. (The term 'low tar' is misleading as these cigarettes deliver just as much tar and carbon monoxide to human smokers as regular cigarettes. The filter holes that are intended to dilute the smoke become clogged or covered when a smoker draws on the cigarette, rendering them ineffective. They should never be recommended as a safer option.)

Withdrawal symptoms from nicotine can be serious, e.g. cravings, irritation, sleep disturbance and anxiety. These symptoms are a main reason for relapse, but they can be greatly relieved with the use of an appropriate pharmacological therapy.

Enjoyment

Many smokers enjoy the taste and ritual handling of their cigarettes. They may reward themselves with a smoke after a difficult task or at the end of a work shift.

Cigarettes also have a social function and can act as ice breakers, be used as time fillers and to deal with boredom.

However, most people smoke not for enjoyment but because they feel miserable if they do not smoke. The urge to smoke is often the urge to relieve nicotine withdrawal, but has subconsciously become associated with other pleasures. Similarly, the urge to smoke can be prompted by ritual in the same way that one might always have a coffee at a particular time of day; being deprived of that can feel disturbing.

Relaxation

Smokers learn to use cigarettes as a means of relieving stress and believe that cigarettes 'calm the nerves'.

In fact, nicotine is a powerful stimulant and what actually happens is that withdrawal symptoms emerge when a smoker has not smoked for a while. The next cigarette alleviates these symptoms and the smoker feels better and 'relaxed'.

Concentration

Some smokers smoke to aid their concentration but again this is more a result of habit and association. The smoker deliberately chooses to use a cigarette to help him or her concentrate (and to ward off withdrawal restlessness) and therefore feels more concentrated – a self-fulfilling prophecy. Again, any real physical effect is likely to be coming from regulating nicotine levels, removing the distraction of withdrawal-related discomfort.

Health beliefs

Smokers are very good at denial or adopting a fatalistic approach to the consequences of smoking.

- 'I could get knocked down by a car tomorrow' or 'I'm going to die anyway.' Out of 1000 young male smokers, one will be murdered, six will be killed on the roads and 250 will be killed by tobacco (Peto 1980).
- 'My uncle is 92 and smoked 40 a day.' Forty percent of smokers do not collect their pension as they die before retirement, compared with only 15% of non-smokers. One in two smokers dies from smoking and loses on average 23 years of life (Doll et al 1994).
- 'I'll have stopped by the end of next year.' Most smokers regret starting and start wanting to stop from an early stage, but in fact most ex-smokers report having smoked for 20 years or more. It is important to encourage cessation attempts as soon as smokers express regret about starting.

Weight control

Fear of gaining weight is a very powerful obstacle to stopping, particularly amongst young women who are under constant social pressure to be thin.

Nicotine has a small metabolic effect that can account for 2–3 lb of weight gain on stopping smoking. However, when ex-smokers experience weight gain, most of that is attributable to extra eating – snacks and sweets instead of cigarettes are the usual culprits.

Mood control

Smokers feel that cigarettes control their temper and moods. Smoking calms them down and prevents them from being irritable and bad tempered. Conversely, they can feel cheered up and revived when they have a cigarette. Women in particular tend to say they depend on cigarettes for mood control.

Fear of failure

The fear of failure is probably the single biggest obstacle to stopping smoking. It is true that most smokers will need several attempts before they are able to stop for good, but with appropriate support and pharmacological treatment their chances of success can be at least doubled. The most important factor is to plan the attempt.

Components of smoking behaviour

Smoking is a complex behaviour which may be summarized as a blend of three components:

1. pharmacological addiction
2. learned behaviour becoming an automatic habit
3. psychological/emotional dependence.

Pharmacological addiction

When the nicotine falls below an accustomed level the smoker feels the desire to smoke. The need to smoke to maintain the level of nicotine in the blood is an addiction.

Plasma nicotine levels fall rapidly so a cigarette is usually needed every waking hour to maintain the smoker's preferred level – most smokers smoke 15–20/day. One easy way to gauge a smoker's level of addiction is to ask how soon after waking he or she has the first cigarette of the day. The majority will light up within an hour of waking, but highly addicted smokers will do so within a few minutes of waking or even report waking during the night in order to smoke.

Learned behaviour becomes an automatic habit

Smoking is a behaviour acquired with social reinforcement, usually during the teenage years.

Inhaling tobacco smoke is initially repugnant, but each puff gradually increases the physical tolerance and smoking becomes easier. The nicotine addiction is gradually built up until the act of smoking itself produces enough reinforcement without social pressure. Smoking then becomes associated with routine daily activities, e.g. smoking and drinking coffee, smoking and driving, and smoking after a meal.

These links are established over many years in some cases and can be difficult to break; they usually become so automatic as to be subconscious. Most smokers would not be able to identify every cigarette smoked during the day, only the significant ones, e.g. first thing in the morning, one after lunch, etc.

Psychological/emotional dependence

Smokers use cigarettes to cope with stress and to combat negative feelings of anxiety, frustration and anger.

Smokers may experience exaggerated emotions when trying to stop because they have previously used cigarettes to subdue these feelings. Some smokers feel on stopping that they have lost something – a friend or a prop.

WHY DO SMOKERS STOP SMOKING?

Just as people start to smoke and continue to smoke for different reasons, the decision to stop is a very personal one and may be the result of a number of different factors. The vast majority of smokers express regret about starting and the reasons they give fall into five main categories. Most of the quitters you will have contact with in your work will fall into the first two categories below.

Awareness of health risks

Although the majority of smokers are aware of the health risks of smoking, such as lung cancer and heart disease, a smoker may acquire new information or become aware of a risk to his or her own health, e.g. a pregnant woman reads about the complications caused in pregnancy by smoking or a smoker with a persistent cough realizes that smoking makes it worse. Advice from a GP or practice nurse can be a powerful motivator for a smoker to stop smoking. For instance, a patient with CHD may be told about the link between smoking and his or her heart disease and advised to stop smoking to improve prognosis and recovery. It is important to help smokers explore their knowledge of the impact of smoking on their personal health and correct any misinformation they may have.

Financial considerations

Increases in the price of cigarettes or greater demands on finances can make the cost of smoking more apparent to a smoker. The savings made by stopping smoking can be a significant reward for a quitter to maintain motivation to stay stopped. Cost can, however, be a sensitive issue, particularly for poorer smokers, who may be spending significant proportions of their household income on cigarettes. Many smokers will express feelings of guilt about this.

Addiction

Smokers, especially young smokers, can become aware of the hold cigarettes have on their lives and dislike this feeling. They want to regain a sense of control.

Disgust

Some smokers express feelings of shame and disgust about the smell and mess created by smoking.

Restrictions and social pressure

Smoking is becoming more and more restricted in public places, workplaces and social settings and a smoker may feel antisocial and decide to stop. Encouragement from the family, particularly young children, can be a powerful reason to stop smoking. Becoming a parent or a grandparent for the first time can also be a trigger.

HOW DO SMOKERS STOP AND HOW CAN YOU HELP THEM?

There are two models that can be used to understand why smokers stop and how they can be helped. These are known as the Health Belief Model and the Prochaska & Diclemente Cycle of Change model and are discussed in greater depth in Chapter 8.

Health Belief Model

This model (Becker 1974) helps to explain what determines whether or not people follow treatment regimens or take any necessary preventive action. This theory can be used to understand whether a smoker will try to stop and how he or she might go about doing so.

Behaviour is seen as determined by:

- the value placed on achieving a goal, in this case stopping smoking
- a belief in the likelihood that a particular action will achieve that goal, e.g. smokers may be convinced that attending a hypnotherapist or following the advice in a quitter's pack will help them stop.

Whether an individual takes action depends on the following factors:

- Perceived susceptibility or vulnerability to disease/illness – 'Will I suffer ill health from smoking?'
- Perceived severity of the results of contracting the disease – 'How ill will I be?'
- Perceived benefit of taking the preventive action – 'Will stopping now make any difference to my health?'

- Perceived cost of taking the action, the time and money invested – 'Do the benefits outweigh the costs?'
- Health motivation level – the extent to which the individual is generally interested or concerned with health; this can depend on a number of factors including age, sex, social class, circumstances, etc.
- Cue to action – the stimulant or trigger required for the individual to take action, e.g. pregnancy, increased price, work policy.

Smokers may fail to take action to stop smoking because of their beliefs at any of a number of points. For example, a smoker may smoke fewer than 20 cigarettes a day and mistakenly believe this to be a safe level or a smoker may recognize the personal seriousness of the risk of smoking but believe that the effort of giving up outweighs the benefits of stopping.

It is therefore important to explore smokers' beliefs about smoking and health, and discuss their motivations, before giving any information about stopping.

Cycle of Change Model

According to this model (Prochaska & Diclemente 1983), stopping is not a single simple act but a process involving a series of changes leading towards the final stage of maintained abstinence (see Fig. 5.2). The move through the cycle can take weeks, months or even years and may be repeated more than once before the smoker stops for good.

Before you can give any help to the smoker, you need to know where the smoker is in the cycle to determine the appropriate approach to take.

- A smoker may believe smoking is not harming him and even feel better when he has a cigarette. This is the 'contented smoker' stage and a change in attitude is needed. The smoker's positive beliefs about smoking need to be explored and challenged with discussion and relevant corrective information.
- A smoker may know the risks of smoking and can feel the ill effects on his health. This smoker has passed the 'contented' stage but now needs to

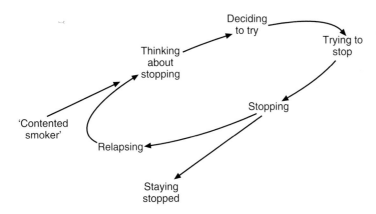

Figure 5.2 The Cycle of Change Model (adapted from Prochaska & DiClemente 1983).

be convinced about the personal benefits of stopping. This will encourage a move into the 'intention to stop' stage.

• A smoker has made the decision to stop. A stop day should be fixed and the smoker will then need some advice on what preparations to make, what to do on the day and what to expect afterwards.

The health professional's role: practical aspects of intervention

Since 1999, a network of specialist NHS services for smokers has been developed in the UK. Smokers can self-refer to these centres or be referred by their own health-care professionals. It is important, however, that non-specialist health professionals understand and play their role in encouraging their patients to stop either by using these services, on their own, or with other sources of help.

A major review of the strength of evidence for smoking cessation interventions resulted in comprehensive guidelines for health professionals in primary health care, hospitals and community trusts and specialist smoking cessation clinics (West et al 2000).

Patients expect health professionals to ask about their smoking and can interpret professional silence as tacit condoning of smoking. Nurses and other health-care staff are therefore in a unique position to help their patients stop, by virtue of their skills, their standing, patient expectations and the context in which their patient contacts take place.

Target patient groups

Most patient contact occasions provide opportunities to intervene on smoking. Consider the various patient groups you might meet and how smoking might be an issue for some of the less obvious ones:

• Young children – may be living in a smoky atmosphere, aggravating respiratory problems.

• Teenagers – may be experimenting with smoking or already presenting with smoking-related symptoms; by age 16, around 25% are likely to be regular smokers.

• Young women seeking the contraceptive pill, whose side-effects are greatly complicated by smoking.

• Pregnant women.

• Parents – may be smoking around the house, aggravating children's health problems as well as their own and increasing the likelihood that their children will grow up to be smokers; there is an added household safety risk when young children have access to smokers' materials.

• Adults with smoking-related conditions (heart, respiratory or circulatory disease, ulcers, gum diseases, cancers).

• Adults in general – around 30% are likely to be smokers, more in areas of deprivation where smoking prevalence can be well over 50%.

The care of CHD patients provides an even more potentially fruitful context for stop-smoking interventions. These patients have had dramatic personal proof of the health consequences of smoking and the challenge to their carers is to enable them to accept and learn from the experience. Compared with other serious smoking-related illnesses, health gain from stopping smoking is seen most rapidly in this group.

The professional's role in a stop-smoking intervention

The aim of a stop-smoking intervention with patients from any group is to encourage and enable the patients to make health-enhancing behaviour changes for themselves. This may involve work on motivation, skill building and confidence building and it will certainly demand the best of communication skills. The role of enabler is a subtle one; it does not involve treating or teaching patients in a traditional sense but working with them to help them identify solutions and strategies for themselves. It can be hard for professionals to take on this role, which can feel like handing over responsibility or expertise, but this is exactly what must be done for a successful intervention. It is the smokers who give up smoking, not their counsellors.

What is minimal intervention?

A minimal intervention involves effective and efficient use of health professionals' time to equip patients with the knowledge and motivation they need to make health-enhancing behaviour change later. Drawing on Prochaska & Diclemente's cyclic model of behaviour change (see Fig. 5.2), minimal intervention aims to move a patient towards behaviour change one stage at a time. In the context of smoking cessation, a minimal intervention will not necessarily result in instant successful stopping but it will help the patient move towards it through understanding his or her own smoking behaviour and devising a relevant action plan. The evaluation implication for health professionals should be reassuring – the professional is not expected to produce a successful quitter in one go every time.

In a minimal intervention, responsibility for successful behaviour change remains with the patient, as does control of the process. This approach is highly acceptable to smoking patients, who need to make their own decision to stop, in their own time, to have the best chance of success. Moreover, the approach is highly cost effective. Good-quality minimal intervention with a large number of patients results in far more ex-smokers than the equivalent amount of time spent in more intense interventions with smaller groups of patients, e.g. in stop-smoking clinics.

Macleod Clark's research with coronary patients suggests that there is a best time to intervene to maximize the chance of successful stopping, ideally after their first coronary event (Macleod Clark et al 1990). This may be because of the type of smoker involved: it is possible that smokers who go on smoking even after the onset of related disease are a particularly 'hard-core' group. This is even more likely to be true of patients who are still smoking after more than one coronary event.

The same research suggests that interventions should be considered with recent ex-smokers too. Coronary patients seem to be slightly more likely to relapse later than other ex-smokers who, if they stay abstinent for a year, usually stay smoke free for good. It is therefore worth asking all coronary patients if they have ever been smokers and reinforcing cessation among ex-smokers.

Having established that minimal interventions are recommended in most situations, there are some patients who will need more sustained interventions. The main group of such patients will be the 'contented smokers': those who, for whatever reason, do not associate their smoking with health damage or long-term relapsed quitters who have resigned themselves permanently to smoking. Using Becker's theory, explained earlier in this chapter, exploration of a patient's health beliefs will reveal whether either of these situations applies. However, with scarce time resources, it are more efficient simply to raise the subject opportunistically with these patients and concentrate interventions on those who express interest in stopping.

Another group of patients who might need a longer intervention are people with low self-efficacy – patients who do not feel that they have the skills to give up smoking and who seek the support of other people to help them do it. Again, exploration of the patient's health beliefs about the perceived costs of giving up smoking should reveal this.

A final group who might need more sustained support are people who have little personal or social support. People who come from households or social groups with a high smoking prevalence and low interest in stopping might come into this category. In these circumstances it is not uncommon for other smokers to undermine an attempt to stop, making it extremely difficult for a smoker to succeed. While some population sectors may be particularly prone to this problem, e.g. some deprived communities with high unemployment, the issue of family and social support should always be explored.

Motivational interview techniques for smoking cessation

The core skill of motivational interviewing is active listening – the use of open questioning, reflecting patient responses and picking up on cues. The important thing is to help the patient resolve ambivalence and avoid provoking resistance in the patient. It can be helpful to plan an intervention like this in the same way as one would plan for other health promotion or educational interventions – by identifying aims, objectives, methods and desired outcomes, which will in turn help suggest appropriate evaluation methods. The aims and objectives in such an intervention plan might therefore read as follows:

- *Aim* – to increase the patient's motivation to make a behaviour change.
- *Specific objectives*:
  - to identify the patient's position in the cycle of change
  - to establish the patient's health beliefs about stopping smoking
  - to enable the patient to progress to the 'deciding to stop' stage.
- *Desired outcome* – patient will name a stop date.

The method to use in pursuit of these objectives is one which will involve the patient in doing most of the talking and all the decision making. Remembering that most smokers wish that they could stop, even if they do not readily express this desire, 10–15 minutes should be enough, if the subject is raised appropriately, to allow the conversation to progress quickly to the process of stopping. A conversation outline might be as follows:

1. Raise the subject – ask the patient whether he or she smokes or has recently stopped. Depending on the patient's smoking status:

   • congratulate a non-smoker on their status – reinforcement of this positive behaviour encourages them and can act as an example to others, as patients tend to tell everyone when they meet approval! Record non-smoking status in notes: writing things down emphasizes their importance. You may wish to consider asking if the patient spends much time in smoky atmospheres as this can be particularly health damaging for patients with other cardiovascular risk factors

   • congratulate an ex-smoker on their achievement and explore any anticipated problems with staying stopped. As with non-smokers, explore the patient's exposure to passive smoking. Again, record ex-smoker status in notes

   • ask smokers how they feel about their smoking – this opening strategy will give you a very rapid insight into the patient's position in the cycle of change and allow you to start an exploration of health beliefs about smoking and stopping. It is not really very useful to ask detailed questions about how long patients have been smoking or how much they smoke; all this does is give you a few more facts, when the important one is that they smoke at all. It can also be risky to get into conversations about the number of cigarettes smoked – patients can interpret this as implying there is a safe or acceptable level of smoking.

2. After raising the subject, ask one or two open questions, for example:
   • 'How do you feel about your smoking?'
   • 'How do you see it relating to your heart condition?'
   • 'What might be putting you off having a go at stopping?'

You will be able to position the patient within the cycle of change and you should have gained a few insights into useful avenues to explore with the patient.

How the conversation proceeds depends on the patient's starting point, as follows.

'Contented smoker' patients

There should be very few of these and it need not be assumed that contented smokers are necessarily hard-core, determined-to-continue smokers. It may just be that they don't know enough about smoking and how to stop. However, there is a possibility that remaining smokers amongst cardiac patients may well be hard-core smokers, denying the risks of smoking and refusing to accept the need to stop. You will know this from responses to your initial open questions.

For these smokers, your minimal intervention will be aimed at simply moving them into thinking about stopping; a more intensive intervention will be required to move them further if indeed they agree to proceed.

Hard-core smokers in denial will need to be encouraged to accept the scientific evidence about smoking and the benefits of stopping. Common reactions from this group will be reliance on the example of the immortal smoker or quoting facts about every other risk factor, i.e. ignorance of relative risk. The health professional's role in these cases is:

- to correct misinformation – it can be useful to have simple, relevant fact sheets or booklets to hand for back-up and make it absolutely clear that the evidence on smoking is conclusive
- to give clear advice that the patient should stop smoking as soon as possible, personalizing the danger of continuing and the benefit of stopping
- to warn the patient of follow-up enquiry, but leave the patient with information on where and how to get help.

The contented smoker who simply has not thought about stopping smoking before is of course easier to deal with and many can quickly be moved on to the 'deciding to stop' stage. A few more open questions to explore health beliefs and establish that denial is not a problem should indicate that it is more likely to be a case of ignorance of the benefits of stopping or concern about the perceived 'costs' of stopping, e.g. fear of failure, anxiety or weight gain or lack of social support.

Again in this case, it can be helpful to have simple relevant patient education literature to hand for reference. If patients express an interest in thinking about stopping smoking, it may be appropriate to arrange a special follow-up appointment but if not, make a point of raising the subject again at the next routine visit. Make it clear that your unequivocal advice is to stop smoking as soon as possible and leave the patient with information on where and how to get help.

'Thinking about stopping' patients

Most patients who smoke will already have progressed at least to this stage, which you will be able to tell from their responses to your subject-raising questions.

- 'I know I should stop …'
- 'It's a stupid habit …'
- 'I've only myself to blame …'
- 'The damage is done now …'

These patients have started to think negatively about their smoking, so it is the professional's role to reinforce that thought process, correct any misinformation and encourage them to believe that stopping would be both beneficial and possible. Use open questions to explore beliefs about stopping, for example:

- 'Can you think of any ways in which stopping smoking might do you good?'
- 'What's putting you off having a go at stopping?'
- 'How confident would you feel about having a go at stopping?'
- 'What could I do to help you have a go at stopping?'

These will help the patient to talk through concerns and identify positive beliefs or actions to build on.

Having helped the patient to establish that stopping would be personally beneficial, the professional's role is to encourage the patient to name a stop day, thereby moving on to the next stage in the cycle.

'Deciding to stop' patients

These patients will need reinforcement of their positive decision and beliefs, together with clear guidance on how to go about stopping. The procedure can be described as seven steps, which are summarized in the patient handout in Box 5.1.

Step 1: Name a day A named day is essential, as is the intention to stop completely on that day rather than start cutting down. Cutting down is rarely useful as it can reinforce dependence on the remaining cigarettes and can provide a false sense of reassurance that health gain has ensued. In fact, most smokers who cut down tend to smoke their remaining cigarettes harder (longer, deeper, more frequent puffs), thereby maintaining their overall exposure to smoke. Some smokers may, however, feel they have to cut down first as part of the preparations for a named stop day; if this is the case, then encourage them to keep the cutting-down period to a minimum and to learn consciously about each cigarette they eliminate from the daily routine. The patient should allow at least 1 week to prepare properly and choose a day which will be relatively free from other major stresses. Many people like to choose a significant day like New Year, a birthday or No Smoking Day, but this does not really matter as long as the day becomes a target day to stop completely.

Step 2: Consider the benefits of stopping versus the costs The smoker should think through all his or her personal reasons for stopping – the expected gains – and identify any reasons why smoking should continue. Honesty about both is important as many smokers still cling to underlying positive beliefs about smoking and unless these are dealt with openly, they can sabotage a stop attempt. Encourage the smoker to explore any remaining perceived benefits of smoking and identify how else those benefits might be attained.

Step 3: Encourage the smoker to keep a cigarette diary for a day or two The aim of this is to enable the smoker to understand his or her own smoking patterns. By recording each cigarette and the circumstances in which it is smoked, the smoker will be able to identify those cigarettes which are

■ **BOX 5.1 How to become a non-smoker in seven simple steps**

1. Name a quit day, a few days or weeks away, and use the in-between days to prepare for quitting.
2. Make a list of your reasons for quitting, and any reasons you might have for continuing to smoke. Make sure that you really want to quit this time.
3. Keep a cigarette survey sheet for a day or two to analyse your smoking pattern.
4. Work out what you will do in different smoking situations:
   - what distractions or substitutes will you have around for when the cravings come?
   - do you need to practice a relaxation exercise?
   - what will you say if someone offers you a cigarette?
   - will you need to arrange to be able to talk to a friend in any desperate moments?
   Write down your plans somewhere handy, and keep looking back at your reasons to quit for motivation.
5. The night before your quit day, have your last cigarette, but make sure you don't enjoy it – smoke an old stale one, or smoke out in the rain – just make sure it isn't a happy memory. Then get rid of all your smoking equipment – ashtrays, lighters and any spare cigarettes.
6. On quit day – think positive! You've made your plans for coping, so put them into action. Make a note of any particularly difficult moments during the day, and rethink your plans if you need to.
   Drink lots of water or fruit juice (try to avoid caffeine) and have some low-calorie nibbles on hand. At the end of your first day, reward yourself, even if no-one else does! Spend your cigarette money on a treat and enjoy it – you deserve it.
7. Later days – repeat Step 6 as long as you need to. Go back to your list if your will-power flags, and keep rewarding yourself for every smoke-free day. Don't panic about the odd lapse – simply review your plans for the difficult moments and change them if necessary.
   Start calling yourself a non-smoker – YOU ARE!

smoked out of addiction and those which are prompted more by habit. Each type can then be tackled separately.

Step 4: Develop coping strategies The patient needs to think about ways to deal with the different smoking situations identified in the diary – coping strategies like relaxation exercises for stressful moments, refusal techniques for dealing with unexpected offers, distractions or substitutes like low-calorie snacks or glasses of water to deal with nicotine cravings. The health professional should have a stock of these tips, which are listed in most self-help literature, but the important thing is for smokers to decide on the ones they feel will work for them.

Step 5: The night before the stop day The smoker should have a final cigarette and then dispose of all smoking materials. It can be helpful to make sure that the last cigarette is not a positive experience which the smoker may later remember with fondness. A hurried, stale cigarette in uncomfortable surroundings can act like aversion therapy. Most smokers then find it helpful to get rid of all ashtrays, lighters and cigarettes but some say they prefer the reassurance of keeping a packet of cigarettes to hand in case of desperation.

Step 6: The stop day Coping plans are put into action. Ideally the day will be a relatively stress-free one, when the smoker will have access to exercise opportunities, fresh fruit and cool drinks, and any social support needed. However, some smokers prefer to make the day as normal as possible, to get used to facing real-life situations and stresses without cigarettes. Some kind of personal treat will be important to celebrate a first day off smoking; often, smokers don't get this kind of positive feedback from other people or themselves but it can really boost motivation.

Step 7: The maintenance step Repeating the coping strategies identified at Step 6 until a new set of health-enhancing behaviours is learned, reviewing progress and rethinking any relapse situations. Relapses should be seen as isolated incidents rather than failures; they usually occur in unforeseen or extra-stressful situations or in off-guard moments (particularly in social settings and when alcohol is involved).

'Staying stopped' patients

This group of patients will include recent quitters, who may need continued reassurance and reinforcement in the early weeks (most relapses occur within the first 3 months), and longer term ex-smokers. Most quitters who abstain for a full year end up as permanent ex-smokers, but relapse sometimes happens after very long intervals. For example, women who stop smoking during pregnancy sometimes go back to smoking when their children start school.

Very late relapse is also encountered among some CHD patients, who may feel that the danger of a further attack has passed. It is therefore always worth reinforcing the continuing benefits of permanent cessation for all ex-smoker patients.

'Relapser' patients

This patient group can be treated in a similar way to patients who are 'contented smokers' or 'thinking about stopping', as appropriate, with the modification that the previous experience of stopping should be drawn on. It may be that the previous experience of stopping was a bad one, leaving the smoker with negative health beliefs that can be explored and modified. Or the stopping process itself was satisfactory but sabotaged by a relapse incident, in which case there is considerable scope to build on positive experience.

In summary, the motivational interview approach to smoking cessation interventions involves the health professional in helping smokers to understand and control their own stop-smoking process.

The communication skills involved are open questioning, active listening to explore ambivalence and avoid resistance, and the sparing provision of relevant information.

The expression of continuing interest by a health professional can enhance motivation and boost patient cessation rates.

Common questions and answers

Smokers will express concerns, doubts and objections to your advice throughout the process of change. They may just be expressing doubt to seek reassurance or be testing you to find an excuse to reject your advice. However, there are ways to respond to this without needing to be an expert on every aspect of smoking. Here are some of the most common questions raised by smokers, with suggested approaches to answering them.

'There's no point in giving up smoking – I'm already ill, too old ...'

There are very few patients for whom stop-smoking advice is really inappropriate and it is unlikely that you will come across them in normal care circumstances. Even if a patient's existing health problem is irreversible, there will be health benefits of some kind to everyone: easier breathing, less strain on the heart, fresher tasting mouth, improved circulation, better wound healing, etc.

Care should be taken with CHD patients, though, to acknowledge and avoid aggravating other potential risk factors like excessive weight gain, additional anxiety and increased use of other drugs like caffeine and alcohol. The benefit of stopping smoking does, however, greatly outweigh the extra risk that might be posed by these factors, to the extent that for many, stopping smoking would remove them from the risk band that would require statin treatment.

All smokers will benefit financially and even if there is nothing at all the patient would like to do with the substantial cash savings, including charitable donation, there is the comfort of not swelling the tobacco industry's profits. You might also appeal to patients' sense of responsibility – reducing other people's exposure to passive smoking, reducing the number of bad examples children see, etc.

'What's the point – everyone else in the house smokes'

The example of other smokers is a big problem for people giving up smoking. It is a fair point that exposure to passive smoking is health damaging, although it is not as bad as active smoking. However, a successful ex-smoker can become an example of good practice, possibly inspiring other smokers to have a go too. Ideally, other smokers in the household should be approached to consider stopping at the same time or at least to avoid undermining the smoker's attempt.

Convalescence is a good time to address the problem of passive smoking in the home, say by restricting smoking to certain rooms or times in the house.

'But it's the only thing that calms me down'

While many people use tobacco to relieve stress, nicotine is in fact a stimulant. A discussion of alternative ways to relax or, better still, to tackle the source of stress can help. Non-smokers get stressed too and have similar but less harmful responses. The point of dealing with stress in this way is not so much that the response is a real relief but simply that in most cases the 'ritual' provides a distraction from the stressful situation. Making a cup of coffee, eating a bar of chocolate or having a cigarette is no more than an excuse for a 5-minute break, which is what relieves the stress. Much better stress relievers are those which involve bodily relaxation – a short walk, a breathing or muscle control exercise, a warm bath or lie down, etc.

'I gave up smoking before and put on 2 stones'

This is a particularly common fear among women and is also an important concern for CHD patients, who must avoid excessive weight gain. We can eliminate the myth that cigarettes are a weight-control method. The only way to gain weight when stopping is to consume more calories than the body uses. The only way to control weight is to adjust that balance. When people gain weight on stopping smoking, it is almost always because they are replacing cigarettes with food. The patient should avoid calorie-laden snack items or compensate by increasing levels of activity.

The average long-term weight gain is only 2–3 lb, which in most cases will have no health consequences. Small weight gains can easily be dealt with at a later date, after the smoker is safely off cigarettes. For most patients it would take a weight gain of 3 stones to cancel out the health benefit to the heart of stopping smoking.

'I've tried everything – hypnosis, groups – nothing works'

There is no magic treatment to make smokers stop. All the therapies, pharmaceutical or otherwise, are no more than aids to cessation; the real work has to be done by the smokers themselves. A smoker who attributes success or failure to a therapy does not understand the stopping process, so an explanation of the different components of smoking can help. However, there is reliable evidence that nicotine replacement therapy (NRT) and bupropion (trade name Zyban) can double a smoker's chance of success and these products should be considered for any smoker who does not have clear contraindications.

'What about the patches?'

Properly used, patches and other forms of NRT can double the likelihood of successful stopping among nicotine-addicted patients who are motivated and supported to stop. Current guidelines suggest that although NRT has traditionally not been recommended for CHD patients, it is considerably safer than continuing to smoke and should therefore be offered to this group too.

'I've heard Zyban is really dangerous'

Zyban (bupropion) is safe and effective when used under medical supervision. It acts differently from NRT, affecting the brain's reaction to nicotine.

It belongs to the family of antidepressant drugs and carries a small seizure risk for some identifiable patient groups; for this reason it is a prescription-only drug. Many smokers have been put off using the drug by media reports of deaths among its users. These reports have been based on misunderstanding of the circumstances of the cases and are not reliable as an indicator of the drug's safety. As with NRT, the drug is considerably safer than continued smoking which carries a 1 in 2 risk of death. The National Institute for Clinical Excellence (NICE 2002) provides clear guidance on the use of both bupropion and NRT for smoking cessation.

Creating the climate for cessation

The whole-practice approach

Even the best smoking cessation and prevention programmes need to be set in a supportive context if they are to succeed. Education programmes commonly fail when their recipients do not have their lessons reinforced by experience. In the smoking cessation context, quitters often relapse in the face of unrestricted smoking by their peers and workmates.

It is therefore essential to pay attention to the context in which any smoking cessation intervention is delivered. In the health-care setting, this can pose less of a problem, as most facilities are already completely smoke free. If this is not the case, a policy should be introduced as soon as possible.

Interventions have the best chance of success when they are understood, accepted and reinforced by everyone associated with the environment in which the intervention is taking place. In a hospital or primary care setting, it is important to ensure that all staff sectors are involved. This applies particularly to reception and auxiliary staff who by virtue of their less formal contact with patients often have a crucial communication role. Any smoking action plan should therefore acknowledge and clarify all staff groups' roles. Areas to consider in planning a comprehensive approach to smoking include the following:

- Rules about staff, patient and visitor smoking on the premises
  - What are they?
  - How will staff, patients and visitors know what they are?
  - Who will enforce the rules and how will breaches be dealt with?
- Intervention procedures
  - How will smokers be identified on registration with the practice and subsequently?
  - What arrangements will be made for proactive opportunistic or systematic interventions?
  - Will any particular patient groups be targeted (e.g. symptomatic patients, pregnant women, parents of infants)?
  - What arrangements will be made to cater for smokers who make spontaneous requests for help (and to encourage them to do so)?
  - What records will be kept to document, evaluate and review interventions?

- Promotion of non-smoking as the norm
  - What patient education materials, e.g. leaflets and posters, will be displayed?
  - How will tobacco promotional material be avoided, e.g. consider whether waiting-room magazines, etc. have tobacco advertisements in them?
  - How will staff and patient interest be maintained, e.g. participation in national and local no-smoking campaigns?
- Liaison with specialist services
  - What information is available on local specialist services?
  - Who is responsible for communication with those services?
  - How will patients be referred to them?

The development of a comprehensive approach to smoking in a health-care setting need not be arduous, but it is a process which will demand careful communication and wide representation. It can be helpful to include an intervention procedure so that smokers are not missed – sample protocols for hospital and primary care settings are given in Boxes 5.2 and 5.3.

When developing intervention procedures, it is important to be aware of different client groups and their specific needs, e.g. CHD patients will need to be approached very differently from teenage patients or pregnant women. Consider too whether you have any literacy or cultural issues to consider among different patient groups.

The secret of success in the design and implementation of comprehensive programmes is responsibility: named individuals should have responsibility for overall co-ordination and specific aspects of the programme, but everyone involved should understand and accept their personal role. Care should be taken over colleagues who smoke: they have a useful contribution to make both in being seen to abide by the rules on smoking and by using their experience as smokers to work sympathetically with patients.

A further secret of success is 'lightness of touch'. While the smoking issue is an extremely serious one, the approach taken needs to be light-hearted, practical and supportive rather than doom-laden scare tactics. While fear-arousing messages can act as motivators to some smokers, they must be balanced with the message that stopping smoking is both beneficial and possible. Patients must be confident that you are there to support, not criticize, when they come forward for help.

Finally, measure, record and celebrate success. If realistic programme goals are set, it should be possible to document considerable achievement in tackling patient smoking. Bearing in mind that minimal interventions are not immediately concerned with long-term cessation as an outcome, success should be measured in terms of moving patients round the cycle of change: moving a contented smoker to thinking about stopping is a successful outcome! An attempt to stop which ends in relapse is still a successful outcome, as most smokers need a few attempts before they stop for good.

The health-care professional needs to analyse the large-scale task of helping patients stop into all its component parts, from setting up a

■ **BOX 5.2   Suggested smoking cessation protocol for hospital settings**

General environment

- Smoking should be banned completely or restricted to separately ventilated, designated areas which are not used for any other purpose.
- Supplies of suitable stop-smoking literature and posters should be maintained on each ward.

Proactive intervention

- A named coordinator should be identified on each ward – normally the ward sister/charge nurse.
- Sufficient staff members on each ward should be adequately trained to deliver a simple stop-smoking intervention.

Suggested admission, care and discharge procedure

- Admission:
  - record each patient's smoking status on admission document
  - remind patient about hospital rules on smoking
  - liaise with coordinator to arrange separate counselling session for all suitable patients.
- Delivery of advice:
  - introduce subject by reminding patient why the hospital has a policy on smoking
  - invite patient to consider stopping smoking, or to discuss concerns about difficulty coping with restrictions on smoking while in hospital
  - talk patient through short-term coping strategies
  - remind patient about personal benefits of stopping for good
  - discuss strategies for ensuring visitors' support
  - invite patient to discuss the subject again if required
  - leave patient with self-help pack
  - record intervention in patient notes.
- Discharge – where notes show that stop-smoking advice has been given:
  - congratulate patient on time off smoking
  - remind patient where to get more help with staying stopped
  - refer to intervention on GP discharge letter
  - tell patient that the primary health-care team will be asked to continue working on stopping smoking
  - ensure patient has self-help pack on departure.

system to identify patients to removing tobacco advertisements from the waiting room. Evaluate success in terms of the extent to which you have completed your own tasks – each one is a contribution to the big picture.

■ BOX 5.3   Suggested smoking cessation protocol for primary care settings

General environment

- Smoking should be banned completely or restricted to separately ventilated, designated areas which are not used for any other purpose.
- Supplies of suitable stop-smoking literature and posters should be maintained and displayed routinely.
- Waiting room materials should be free of tobacco advertising.

Proactive intervention

- A named coordinator should be identified – normally a practice nurse.
- All practice staff should be briefed on the practice's policy on smoking, and trained to deliver interventions appropriate to their normal role.
- Patient record systems should incorporate reference to smoking status and interventions undertaken.
- Practice information leaflets should make reference to the main points of the smoking policy, including availability of cessation advice.

Suggested opportunistic intervention procedure

- Ensure that all case notes have prominent mark of patient's smoking status.
- Routinely ask all patients if smoking status has changed.
- Point out any relationships between smoking and patient's presenting condition.
- Offer self-help information on quitting, or a planned appointment to discuss smoking at a later date.

■ KEY POINTS

- Smoking is the chief cause of avoidable premature death and ill health in the world; 120 000 people die each year from smoking-related disease in the UK alone.
- One in four of these deaths is from CHD and cigarette smoking is responsible for 17% of all deaths from CHD.
- In 2000, 29% of men and 25% of women over 16 smoked in the UK.
- Tobacco smoke contains a cocktail of over 4000 chemicals, 60 of which are known or suspected carcinogens. Cigarette smoke is an important cause of CHD in smokers. Evidence shows that passive smoking also causes CHD.
- There are significant benefits of stopping. Immediately after stopping the body clears itself of poisons. Nicotine levels reduce by half within 8 hours and 24–48 hours after stopping, carbon monoxide is down to the level of a non-smoker.

- Within 1 year of stopping the excess risk of CHD from smoking reduces by half. After 15 years the risk is down to about the same as in someone who has never smoked. For an individual who has heart disease or who has had a heart attack, the risk of premature death or another attack reduces by up to 50% or more.
- People usually start to smoke in adolescence as a result of peer pressure, rebellion or out of curiosity.
- Smokers continue to smoke for a number of reasons including enjoyment, relaxation, concentration, health beliefs and mood control. The main driver of continued smoking is dependence on nicotine, a very powerful drug.
- The three main components of smoking are pharmacological addiction, habit and psychological dependence. All three need to be addressed in an attempt to stop.
- Health professionals have high credibility with smokers and can be effective in helping them to stop for good.
- Most patient contacts provide an opportunity to intervene on smoking. The most effective intervention strategy for health professionals is minimal intervention, backed up with referral to specialist services.
- Minimal intervention aims to equip patients with the knowledge and motivation they need to change behaviour, one stage at a time.
- Motivational interviewing techniques should be used in discussing smoking with patients, involving open questioning and active listening, with the patient doing the decision making. Advice and information offered should be relevant to what the patient says.
- The whole practice can be involved in creating the climate for cessation. Rules about staff, patient and visitor smoking should be in place. Smokers should be identified on registration and procedures outlined for interventions. Non-smoking should be promoted as the norm throughout the practice.

■ PRACTICAL EXERCISE

Set up a reference file for local support services.

It is important to offer smokers a choice of support options both to ensure that they get the type of help that will suit them best and to ensure that your practice time is used efficiently. Appoint yourself resource investigator for the practice, and find out:

- the address, opening times and services offered by specialist stop-smoking services for your area. In the UK, you can get the contact number from the national telephone helpline
- the name of your health authority's smoking cessation lead officer – there may be resources and training available to help your work

- the names of any local pharmacists who are willing to support smokers using any medication during their attempt to stop smoking
- contact details for any local providers of support for specialist groups – speakers of other languages or deaf/blind services
- website addresses for online help – there are many excellent sites that could suit smokers who prefer to go it alone. There is an annotated list of reputable sites on www.ash.org.uk.

Try out the helpline and clinic services for yourself – identify yourself as a health professional and see what they can offer. If you have visited a clinic or spoken to helpline operators yourself, you will be better able to explain them to potential clients.

Get some sample packets of NRT products and bupropion to show patients when you are talking to them. Familiarize yourself with them so that you can explain properly how to use them.

REFERENCES

Becker MH 1974 The health belief model and personal health behaviour. Health Education Monographs 2: 324–508

Doll R, Hill A 1950 Smoking and carcinoma of the lung. British Medical Journal 2: 739–748

Doll R, Peto R, Wheatley K, Gray R, Sutherland I 1994 Mortality in relation to smoking: 40 years' observations on male British doctors. British Medical Journal 309: 901–911

Environmental Protection Agency 1992 Respiratory health effects of passive smoking: lung cancer and other disorders. Office of Health and Environmental Assessment, Washington DC

Glantz SA, Parmley WW 1995 Passive smoking and heart disease. Journal of the American Medical Association 273(13): 1047–1058

Health Education Authority (HEA) 1998 The UK smoking epidemic: deaths in 1995. Health Education Authority, London

Independent Scientific Committee on Smoking and Health (ISCSH) 1988 Fourth report of the Independent Scientific Committee on Smoking and Health (Chairman Sir Peter Froggatt). HMSO, London

International Agency for Research on Cancer (IARC) 1986 IARC monographs on the evaluation of the carcinogenic risk of chemicals to humans. Volume 38. IARC, Lyon

Macleod Clark JM, Haverty S, Kendall S 1990 Helping people to stop smoking: a study of the nurse's role. Journal of Advanced Nursing 16: 357–363

National Institute for Clinical Excellence (NICE) 2002 Technology Appraisal Guidance No 39 – guidance on the use of nicotine replacement therapy (NRT) and bupropion for smoking cessation. NICE, London. www.nice.org.uk

Office for National Statistics 2001 Living in Britain – Results from the 2000 General Household Survey. HMSO, London. www.statistics.gov.uk

Office of Population Censuses and Surveys (OPCS) 1991 Deaths by cause. HMSO, London

Peto R 1980 Editorial. Health Education Journal 39: 45–46

Prochaska JO, Diclemente CC 1983 Stages and processes of self-change of smoking: towards the integrative model of change. Journal of Consulting and Clinical Psychology 51(3): 390–395

Royal College of Physicians (RCP) 1983 Health or smoking. Pitman, London

Shinton R, Beevers G 1989 Meta-analysis of relation between cigarette smoking and stroke. British Medical Journal 298: 789–794

US Department of Health and Human Services (DHHS) 1986 The health consequences of involuntary smoking: a report of the Surgeon General. DHHS Publication No. (PHS) 87-8398. US Department of Health and Human Services, Washington DC

US Department of Health and Human Services (DHHS) 1989 Reducing the health consequences of smoking: 25 years of progress. A report of the Surgeon General. DHHS

Publication No. (CDC) 89-8411. US Department of Health and Human Services, Washington DC

US Department of Health and Human Services (DHHS) 1990 The health benefits of smoking cessation. A report of the Surgeon General. DHHS Publication No. (CDC) 90-8416. Office on Smoking and Health, Atlanta, GA

Wald N, Nicolaides-Bauman A 1991 UK smoking statistics, 2nd edn. Oxford University Press, London

Wells AJ 1994 Passive smoking as a cause of heart disease. Journal of the American College of Cardiology 24: 546–554

West R, McNeill AD, Raw M 2000 Smoking cessation guidelines for health professionals: an update. Thorax 55: 987–999

World Bank 1999 Curbing the epidemic. Governments and the economics of tobacco control. World Bank, Washington DC

FURTHER READING

Royal College of Physicians 2000 Nicotine addiction in Britain. Royal College of Physicians, London

Tobacco Control. A quarterly journal from the BMJ Publishing Group, containing the latest peer-reviewed papers, news and editorial on all aspects of tobacco control. On-line and hard-copy subscription is available.

www.ash.org.uk. An invaluable web resource containing up-to-date information, analysis and links to resources on all aspects of tobacco control, including cessation.

Lifestyle management: diet

Bruce A. Griffin   *Kirsten A. Whitehead*

6

CONTENTS

INTRODUCTION

Hyperlipidaemia, obesity, diabetes and hypertension are recognized as major risk factors for coronary heart disease (CHD). Dietary modification has an important role to play in the management of these risk factors. It is not uncommon for individuals to present with one or more of these conditions. Dietary management must therefore be planned on an individual basis and will vary from person to person. This chapter will focus on the rationale and guidelines associated with the management of hyperlipidaemia and obesity. The dietary management of hypertension and diabetes is discussed in Chapters 4 and 12.

HYPERLIPIDAEMIA

Definition and classification of hyperlipidaemia

Hyperlipidaemia refers to a raised level of blood lipids (neutral fats and cholesterol). This can be caused by both genetic and environmental factors and, most importantly, through interactions between our genetic make-up and lifestyle factors such as diet. A phenotypic classification of hyper-lipidaemia based on the relative increases in cholesterol and/or blood fat (triglycerides) is required in a clinical setting in order to identify the principal targets for dietary intervention. The most simple classification identifies three categories as defined by the European Atherosclerosis Society Task Force (1992):

- hypercholesterolaemia (raised cholesterol)
- hypertriglyceridaemia (raised fat)
- combined (mixed) hyperlipidaemia (raised cholesterol and fat).

The above presents only a broad surface picture of a more complex collection of underlying metabolic and genetic abnormalities. Each hyper-lipidaemia may have a variable aetiology. Thus, whilst the classification is useful as a first approach, it is often necessary to characterize further the metabolic and/or genetic defect before selecting the most appropriate dietary treatment.

What are dietary fats?

The bulk of edible fats in our food are triglycerides (TG) or triacylglycerols (TAG) (80–100 g/day), which consist of a backbone of glycerol to which are attached three fatty acids. The melting point of different dietary TG and thus their 'hardness' increase with the chain length (number of carbon atoms) of their constituent fatty acids and number of double bonds (degree of saturation). Therefore, TG containing predominantly saturated fatty acids (SFA) with no double bonds will be hard at room temperature whilst those with predominantly polyunsaturated fatty acids (PUFA) will be oils.

Cholesterol is a steroid that is essential for the structure and function of cells and for the production of steroid hormones (oestrogen, testosterone, cortisol), vitamin D and bile acids. For further information on the metabolism and composition of dietary fats and cholesterol in foods, refer to Gurr (1993).

Principles of a lipid (cholesterol)-lowering diet:
fat quantity versus quality

The most important underlying principle of a lipid-lowering diet over the past 10–20 years has been to reduce the absolute quantity of total dietary fat to below the recommended value of 35% of total energy intake (DoH 1994). The rationale behind this recommendation is an attempt to correct the adverse effects of the chronic, overconsumption of high energy-dense foods which increase body weight and cause obesity. Fat intake, however, has fallen in the last 10 years in countries such as the UK without any decrease in the prevalence of obesity, which suggests physical inactivity rather than dietary excess as a primary cause. Studies have also shown that in many cases a reduction in total fat is insufficient to influence blood lipids and must be accompanied by a modification in the quality of fats to achieve favourable effects on these and other risk factors for coronary disease.

Table 6.1 Dietary unsaturated fatty acids

Fatty acid	Class*	Example/ dietary source	Principal lipid effect
Polyunsaturated (PUFA)	n-6	Linoleic acid/corn and sunflower oils	LDL-cholesterol ↓
	n-3 (long chain)	EPA, DHA[†]/fish oils	Serum TG ↓
		Linolenic acid/rape & flax seed oils	Unknown
Monounsaturated (MUFA)	n-9	Oleic acid/olive & rape seed oils	LDL oxidation ↓

*n = number of carbon atoms before first double bond.
[†]EPA & DHA = eicosapentaenoic and docosahexaenoic acids.

The cholesterol-raising properties of saturated fats, chiefly palmitic and myristic acids, lie behind the recommendation to reduce dietary SFA intake to less than 10% energy and add further weight to the question of the most appropriate macronutrient to replace this fat.

As a substitute for fat, complex carbohydrates (starch and non-starch polysaccharides) will lower total serum and LDL-cholesterol. However, dietary carbohydrate, especially in its refined form (containing sucrose), can increase serum TG and lower HDL-cholesterol, most notably in patients with initially high serum TG. To avoid these unfavourable effects whilst maintaining the reduction in cholesterol, SFAs may be replaced with unsaturated fatty acids (MUFA and PUFA) and the common practice has been to use n-6 PUFA of vegetable origin. A consequence of this has been an overemphasis on dietary linoleic acid from corn and sunflower oils at the expense of other more metabolically active n-3 PUFA (Table 6.1).

Saturated fat is responsible for raising serum cholesterol and not dietary cholesterol. Whilst the amount of SFAs in our diet has fallen with the consumption of leaner meat and low-fat dairy products, their quantity still greatly exceeds that of dietary cholesterol and as such, it is the former rather than the latter that exerts a major impact on serum cholesterol. Since eggs represent the major source of dietary cholesterol, they have carried a label of being inappropriate for coronary health. Nevertheless, numerous intervention studies have shown that the consumption of 1–2 eggs per day has no clinically significant impact on blood cholesterol levels (serum cholesterol increased by only about 0.1 mmol/l for every 100 mg of dietary cholesterol).

Recommendations for the consumption of dietary n-3 and n-6 PUFA

The substitution of SFAs with n-6 PUFA (linoleic acid) from corn, sunflower, safflower oils and soya is unequivocally associated with decreases in the concentration of total serum and LDL-cholesterol. However, current guidelines suggest intake of PUFAs should be restricted to below 10–13% of energy as levels above this may lower HDL, increase the oxidation of LDL, a prerequisite step in the deposition of cholesterol in arteries, and increase the risk of gall stones by increasing the lithogenicity of bile. For this reason it was concluded that the safety of n-6 PUFA levels above 6% of total energy (estimated as the current intake) 'remains untested' (DoH 1994).

In contrast to the guidelines for n-6 PUFA, in 1994 the government recommended doubling the intake of long-chain n-3 PUFA, which at present is estimated to be 1% of our energy intake. This figure translates into an increase of 0.1–0.2 g/day or the equivalent of eating two meals of oily fish per week. The basis for this advice lies in the potent metabolic effects of these fatty acids in preventing the more acute endpoints of CHD, namely myocardial infarction and cardiac arrhythmia, rather than their effects on atherosclerosis. The latter, which would include reducing serum TG, is of greater relevance to members of the free-living population who are 'at risk' of developing CHD; that is, in a primary rather than a secondary prevention setting (see below).

Diets enriched with moderate levels of long-chain n-3 PUFA (1 g/day equal to 100 g tinned pink salmon or 30 g sardines) increase the capacity to clear dietary TG from the blood after a fat-containing meal (postprandial lipaemia) and can reduce fasting serum TG by up to 60%. The metabolic origin of these effects may lie in the ability of n-3 PUFA to increase the insulin sensitivity of certain tissues. Whether through effects on blood lipids, thrombosis or cardiac arrhythmia, a moderate intake has proven clinical benefits in terms of reducing CHD mortality (GISSI 1999). Dietary long-chain n-3 PUFA are thus effective agents for the treatment of hypertriglyceridaemia (2–3 g/day) and can be equally effective in lower doses (1 g/day) when in combination with an HMG CoA reductase inhibitor for the treatment of mixed hyperlipidaemia (Contacos et al 1993).

Dietary PUFA and the oxidation hypothesis of atherosclerosis

Fats in foods oxidize in air and 'go off' or become rancid. Fats in membranes and circulating lipoproteins, and in particular PUFA, also undergo oxidation. The oxidation of PUFA in LDL, the principal transport vehicle of cholesterol in blood (see Chapter 3), facilitates the retention of cholesterol in the artery wall. Conversely, antioxidant processes, which prevent this, are thus likely to protect against cholesterol deposition and atherosclerosis. Diets enriched with PUFA increase the levels of the same fatty acids within LDL and thus increase its oxidative potential. This naturally raised concern that dietary PUFA, and in particular the most abundant n-6 PUFA, may actually accelerate atherosclerosis. An upper limit of 6% energy has been recommended for dietary n-6 PUFA until this issue has been fully resolved.

Monounsaturated fatty acids (MUFA)

Countries in the Southern Mediterranean, notably Greece and southern Italy, demonstrate a significantly lower incidence of CHD than the rest of Europe. A dietary factor implicated in this relative protection against disease is their high intake of MUFA in the form of olive oil (24% total energy), which is nearly twice that consumed by Northern Europeans. Dietary MUFA produces only moderate effects on blood lipids, lowering serum cholesterol and raising HDL. A more likely source of this cardioprotection is through the effects of MUFA on LDL against oxidation, which is minimal as a result of the single (mono) double bond. Moreover, the first-press or 'virgin' olive oil contains a number of polyphenolic compounds derived from the skin of the olive that are also known to act as potent antioxidants.

Dietary *trans* fatty acids and CHD risk

The prefixes *trans* and *cis* are chemical terms that describe the configuration or 'shape' of a molecule or, in this case, of unsaturated fatty acids. SFAs have straight chains and as a result pack tightly into membranes and lipoproteins. Conversely, PUFA and MUFA in the *cis* configuration have bends or 'kinks' in their chains that give them greater flexibility in membranes and lipoproteins. Unsaturated fatty acids in the *trans* configuration lack these kinks and tend to behave like SFAs. The hardening of vegetable oils in the manufacture of margarines and related products (biscuits and pastries) by the widely adopted practice of partial hydrogenation results in the removal of double bonds and reconfiguration of many of the fatty acids into *trans* acids. Evidence from a number of cross-sectional and prospective studies (Stender et al 1995) suggested that *trans* fatty acids may be more responsible for the link between dietary fat and CHD than SFAs. This view stems from the finding that high intakes of *trans* (~7%) were associated with raised LDL and low HDL. The intake of *trans* fatty acids in most balanced diets, i.e. excluding high intakes of biscuits, cakes and other shortenings, is considerably less (~2% energy) than that associated with these adverse effects on blood lipids and as such, *trans* fats are not a major cause for concern.

The effects of dietary fibre (non-starch polysaccharides) and alcohol

Non-starch polysaccharides (NSP) are major components of the plant cell wall and include cellulose and non-celluloses (pectins in fruit and vegetables, glucans in oats and barley and gums in food additives). Cellulose, which is insoluble, has an indirect effect in lowering serum cholesterol by displacing saturated fat from the diet. The non-celluloses, which are mainly soluble compounds, produce a more pronounced lowering of serum cholesterol through the binding and prevention of the reabsorption of bile acids in the small intestine (interruption of the enterohepatic circulation). However, despite the reported effects of soluble NSP, the health benefits associated with a high-fibre diet may not be due to the NSP itself but to some other dietary constituent in a diet 'characterized' by a high level of NSP (DoH 1994).

Alcohol

A strong inverse relationship exists between the moderate consumption of alcohol (30 g alcohol/day: 1–2 drinks for women, 2–3 drinks for men) and incidence of CHD. This apparent protective effect of alcoholic beverages against CHD has been ascribed to properties of the alcohol itself and not other components of specific drinks. As much as 50% of this benefit is thought to be due to the capacity of alcohol to increase HDL and reduce thrombotic tendency, effects which may be mediated through an increase in the ratio of oestrogen to testosterone. In addition, red wine contains natural antioxidant compounds (polyphenols) that may also contribute to cardioprotection. In sharp contrast to these favourable effects of alcohol, it is well known that intakes above a moderate level are associated with increased CHD, a variety of cancers and other socially deleterious effects.

Role of antioxidant micronutrients

The oxidation hypothesis of atherosclerosis is based on the principle that LDL must be oxidatively modified before it can deposit cholesterol in the artery wall. The oxygen free radicals responsible for generating the oxidative stress that damages lipids in membranes and lipoproteins may be regarded as reactive fragments of molecules produced as byproducts of metabolic reactions. The body has evolved antioxidant defence mechanisms to prevent this oxidative damage, which take the form of enzyme systems located within cells and aqueous and lipid-soluble antioxidant micronutrients present in cell membranes and circulating in blood and in lipoproteins. Examples of antioxidant micronutrients (vitamins) include ascorbic acid (vitamin C), α-tocopherol (an active form of vitamin E) and β-carotenoids (derived from vitamin A).

Epidemiological studies support the oxidation hypothesis by showing that low plasma levels of essential antioxidants are associated with increased coronary risk. They also suggest that antioxidants from dietary sources should, at least in theory, be able to provide protection against this increased risk if plasma levels of antioxidants can be made to exceed 'threshold' values (Gey 1993). The word 'threshold' in this context means optimum levels for the prevention of free radical-mediated damage to lipids and other biological molecules. Dietary intake values required to exceed these optimum levels must clearly be above recommended daily amounts (RDA), figures for which are established on the basis of much lower plasma levels that are sufficient to prevent symptoms of vitamin deficiency (Table 6.2).

Table 6.2 Recommended dietary intake of antioxidant vitamins necessary to achieve optimum antioxidant status in plasma

Vitamin	Recommended daily intake	Threshold plasma level (μmol/l)
C	60–250 mg (1–4 × RDA)	40–50
E	60–100 IU (4–6 × RDA)	28–30
A	1 mg (=RDA)	2.2–2.8
β-carotene	6–15 mg	0.4–0.5

Unfortunately, human intervention trials have failed to confirm the efficacy of optimal antioxidant levels in CHD prevention, largely because the high doses of purified vitamin supplements used in clinical trials could not reproduce the biological effects of real foods. However, the existing evidence is still considered to be sufficient to warrant modification of current dietary recommendations. The target levels indicated in Table 6.2 are regarded as being 'safe' and should be achieved through the consumption of a diet rich in vegetables, fruits, nuts and seeds, with saturated oils being replaced by less saturated oils.

Current research into the antioxidant potency of a number of other compounds, such as carotenoids other than β-carotene (e.g. lycopene) and a group of substances known as the phenolic flavonoids (e.g. catechins) present in red wine, tea and fruits and vegetables, may reveal an important supplementary role for these compounds in conferring further protection against CHD.

Phytoprotectants: plant sterols, isoflavones and lignans

Plant sterols (and stanols) have received a great deal of attention as additives to margarines that can lower serum cholesterol. These compounds closely resemble cholesterol in chemical structure, but are not actively absorbed and compete effectively with the reabsorption of dietary and biliary cholesterol in the small intestine. This reduced reabsorption of cholesterol increases the activity of LDL receptors in the liver, which lowers serum LDL cholesterol (see Chapter 3). As little as 2 g of either of these compounds (an average daily intake of spread ~21 g) can reduce LDL-cholesterol by up to 14% over a period of months. Plant sterols are naturally present in small amounts in our diet. Despite having the potential to reduce the availability of fat-soluble carotenoids and vitamin E by some 25% and 8% respectively, they are safe and have been described as an 'important innovation' in the prevention of coronary disease through diet (Law 2000).

A number of naturally occurring compounds in plants exert weak oestrogen effects in the body and as such are referred to as phyto-oestrogens. Soya contains phyto-oestrogens known as isoflavones. Daily intake of textured vegetable (soyabean) protein containing just 45 mg of isoflavones has been shown to influence the level of female sex hormones and alter the menstrual cycle. Soya thus offers a potential alternative therapy for the treatment of menopausal symptoms and other hormone-dependent conditions such as cancer, coronary disease and osteoporosis (Cassidy & Griffin 1999). Oestrogens confer protection against coronary disease through stimulation of LDL receptors and a lowering of LDL-cholesterol, protection that is lost after the menopause. In the same way, the well-known cholesterol-lowering effect of soya can be explained by the oestroegenic effect of its isoflavones. Lignans are another important group of phyto-oestrogens found in fibre-rich foods, which can exert similar effects to the isoflavones in soya. Together, these phyto-oestrogens are likely to make a significant contribution to the lower incidence of coronary disease associated with vegetarian diets.

■ **KEY POINTS**

For lowering serum cholesterol

- Reduce total fat intake to <35% total energy intake and saturates to <10% energy, substitute with n-6 PUFA (<6% energy) and MUFA (rape and olive oils) and complex carbohydrates (soluble and insoluble starches).
- Consider increasing consumption of 'phyto-protectants': plant sterols or stanols (functional margarines), isoflavones (soya), lignans (high-fibre cereals, flaxseed).

For lowering serum TG

- Increase intake of n-3 PUFA (oily fish) at the expense of n-6 PUFA (corn and sunflower oils).
- Reduce total fat intake to ≤30% total energy intake and saturates to <10% energy.
- Avoid high intakes of carbohydrates (particularly refined sucrose) that raise serum TG.

Serum triglycerides (TG): a major but modifiable CHD risk factor

Serum cholesterol alone provides an inadequate scientific basis on which to explain the relationship between diet, blood lipids and CHD in free-living populations. It is a fact that, within populations such as the UK, the majority of people who succumb to premature CHD do not have distinctly raised serum cholesterol. Hence, whilst a measure of serum cholesterol is of diagnostic and prognostic importance in the management of patients with clinically defined hyperlipidaemias, its value in a population approach to the prevention of CHD through dietary modification is extremely limited. The greatest source of risk that can be attributed to an abnormality in blood lipids within free-living populations is raised serum TG. The most common lifestyle factors to predispose to increased coronary risk, an increase in body weight and physical inactivity, are closely associated with serum TG, through an inappropriately high intake of energy and poor efficiency of energy utilization. As a result, serum TG is highly responsive to changes in lifestyle and thus provides a more rational therapeutic target for reducing CHD risk through dietary modification. A moderately raised fasting level of serum TG (>1.5 mmol/l) produces abnormalities in plasma lipoproteins that increase coronary risk and are known collectively as an atherogenic lipoprotein phenotype (ALP) (Box 6.1). An ALP forms part of the insulin resistance syndrome, otherwise known as the polymetabolic syndrome or syndrome X.

An ALP is a common phenomenon with a predicted population frequency of about 25% in adult men and postmenopausal women in Northern Europe and the United States. It is associated with a 3–4-fold increase in the relative risk of CHD but is highly responsive to appropriate changes in diet

■ **BOX 6.1   Features of an ALP**

- Low HDL-cholesterol (<1.0 mmol/l): impairs the capacity to remove cholesterol from the body.
- Predominance of small, dense LDL particles: an atherogenic form of LDL.
- Intolerance to dietary fat after a fat-containing meal (impaired clearance of postprandial lipaemia): accompanied by an increase in the number and residence time of atherogenic TG-rich lipoprotein remnants in the blood.
- Total serum cholesterol is unremarkable, often lying between 5.2 and 6.5 mmol/l, and is of no diagnostic value in this case.

(see Key points for lowering serum TG, above). Lifestyle measures which reduce fasting serum TG to below a critical threshold of ~1.5 mmol/l, including weight loss, exercise and dietary modification, may be effective in correcting the lipoprotein defects associated with this high-risk lipid profile.

OBESITY

Coronary heart disease is the main cause of the excess mortality in obese people and overweight individuals have a twofold increase in the risk of developing CHD (BNF 1999). Obesity is usually based on the calculation of the body mass index (BMI), which relates weight to height.

$$\text{BMI} = \frac{\text{Weight (kg)}}{\text{Height (m}^2)}$$

The classification in Table 6.3 is generally accepted, although the World Health Organization (1997) and the Scottish Intercollegiate Guidelines Networks (SIGN 1996) suggest a BMI range of 18.5–24.9 and 18.5–25 respectively as a healthy weight and a reasonable target, and <18.5 as underweight.

BMI is applicable to adults but is not satisfactory for children, adolescents or the elderly in whom the proportion of lean body mass (LBM) is changing.

As BMI increases above 25, risk of all-cause mortality increases. Hypertension, type 2 diabetes and congestive failure are all significantly more common among obese people than among people of normal weight (BNF 1999). Obese people also have abnormalities of blood-clotting factors that increase the risk of thrombosis and MI (Meade et al 1993). Weight loss in obese people leads to improvements in lipid profile, glucose tolerance, blood pressure and clotting factors.

Android obesity, i.e. a central distribution of excess adipose tissue, is associated with metabolic changes that confer greater risk of CHD than peripherally distributed fat, gynoid obesity (Donahue et al 1987, Larsson et al 1984). Males and females with a waist:hip ratio (WHR) of >1.0 and >0.8 respectively are considered most at risk. However, it is now becoming clear that waist measurements alone can become a good measure of intra-abdominal fat and that reduction of waist circumference is associated with improvements in cardiovascular risk factors (Han et al 1997). Weight reduction is

Table 6.3 Grades of obesity		
Grade	**BMI**	
0	<20	Underweight
1	20–24.9	Normal weight
2	25–29.9	Overweight
3	30–39.9	Moderately obese
4	>40	Severely obese

required when waist circumference is >102 cm in men and >88 cm in women (Lean et al 1995, 1998).

BMI takes no account of body fat distribution. It is therefore more useful to measure BMI and either WHR or waist circumference in order to identify overweight individuals most at risk of CHD, than to use BMI alone. These are simple, cheap and reliable techniques suitable for use in clinical settings.

Prevalence of obesity

In the UK the incidence of obesity and consequently the risk of CHD is increasing. Surveys showed that between 1984 and 1990, obesity within the population had increased from 32% to 36% in females and 40% to 45% in males (Gregory et al 1990, Knight 1984). In a survey conducted in 1993, 16% of females and 13% of males were identified as obese (BMI >30) (OPCS 1995). These figures highlight clearly a need for cost-effective treatment of obesity and preventive strategies to avoid individuals becoming overweight.

Management of obesity

Genetic, hormonal, metabolic, psychological and social factors play an aetiological role in the development of obesity, but fundamentally an imbalance between energy intake and energy expenditure is the pathophysiological disturbance, which results in increased body fat deposition (Garrow 1981).

The aim of any weight loss programme is to achieve, and maintain, a target weight. Active treatment should be geared to those people with grades 3 and 4 classified obesity who are most at risk of serious medical and psychological problems and who should be able to achieve a healthy weight. It is also recommended that those in grade 2 are treated, particularly those with a high central fat deposition, if they are young or have additional medical complications and risk factors, to prevent their progression to grade 3 or 4.

Any treatment of obesity will only be successful if an energy deficit is created by reducing energy intake and/or increasing energy expenditure, which leads to loss of body fat whilst meeting all other nutrient requirements. Factors necessary for a safe weight loss programme are shown in Box 6.2.

In practice, treatment of obesity is often difficult and there is a vast array of diet aids, slimming programmes and publications readily available to the general public. Many rely on gimmicks and fail to address the complex

---

■ **BOX 6.2**   **Factors associated with safe weight loss programmes**

- Maintains muscle and organ protein stores, i.e. lean body mass (LBM).
- Promotes loss of body fat.
- Delivers essential nutrients necessary for the conversion of stored fat to energy.
- Maintains fluid, electrolyte and pH balance.
- Maintains micronutrient status.
- Incorporates nutritional recommendations to decrease risk of chronic diseases.
- Incorporates behavioural modification to encourage long-term healthy behaviour.

---

issues which lead to weight gain, and as such may be associated with adverse effects (Lissner et al 1991).

Conventional diet therapy

Most weight loss programmes based upon dietary manipulation alone advise a daily energy deficit of between 500 and 1000 kcal (3500 and 7000 kcal in a week), as a safe and acceptable target. This should lead to the optimal rate of weight loss, which is between 0.5 and 1 kg per week; 1 kg of adipose tissue stores approximately 7000 kcal. A more rapid rate of loss is undesirable due to accompanying breakdown of LBM. Everybody has a different requirement for energy, which will vary from day to day, largely depending upon activity levels. As a guide, the average man and woman attempting to lose weight will require a diet plan providing a daily intake of about 1500 kcal and 1200 kcal respectively to achieve the recommended rate of weight loss.

Other therapies for the management of obesity

Very low calorie diets   Very low calorie diets (VLCDs), popular in the 1970s and 1980s, involve the use of meal replacement formulas and bars to provide <1000 kcal, and sometimes as little as 400 kcal, daily. The general public can easily obtain them, as they are not controlled by medical prescription. They often achieve an initially fast weight loss but at the expense of LBM and accompanying fluid losses. Side-effects include fatigue, nausea, dizziness, constipation, muscle cramps and depression. The first VLCDs were not nutritionally adequate and combined with loose medical supervision resulted in a number of deaths.

'Yo-yo dieting' or weight cycling frequently occurs when normal eating practices resume after a period of dieting. This in part may be due to a fall in the resting metabolic rate (RMR) through loss of LBM and also the failure to educate the individual on healthy eating and physical activity practices for life. VLCDs should only ever be used under medical supervision for extreme obesity where life is threatened. The COMA Report on *The use of very low calorie diets in obesity* (DoH 1987) recommends that VLCDs be used for periods of no more than 4 weeks, under medical supervision and in obese individuals with a BMI greater than 30 who have not succeeded in losing weight with moderate dietary interventions. VLCDs are not suitable for use by those with other medical complications or anyone who merely has a desire to be thinner. They carry the risk of both physical and psychological side-effects and therefore cannot be regarded as promoting healthy lifestyle changes.

Surgical interventions There are advantages and disadvantages to surgical interventions for obesity. To some extent when patients consent to surgery they are giving control over to the medical staff. The outcome has less to do with the patient's ability to change their diet and lifestyle and more to do with the skill of the surgeon. Depending on the type of surgery performed, the patient may have to adopt a restricted diet to avoid symptoms such as vomiting or diarrhoea. There are two main types of surgical intervention: malabsorption techniques such as jejuno-ileal or gastric bypass and techniques to restrict intake, e.g. jaw wiring, stapled gastroplasty and extragastric banding.

Surgical procedures should be reserved for those who are severely obese (BMI >40) and who have failed non-surgical treatment. Experienced surgeons in specialist centres should perform the operations and lifelong monitoring is required postoperatively (BNF 1999). In the UK there are currently few specialist centres for the management of obesity but as the prevalence of obesity increases and the awareness of its importance as a medical condition improves, this situation is likely to change.

Pharmacotherapy The primary treatment for weight reduction and weight maintenance is a combination of diet, physical activity and behaviour modification (BNF 1999). Drug treatment may be considered for those with a BMI of 30 or greater who have failed to lose 10% of their body weight by dietary management over a period of at least 3 months. The decision to use drug therapy should consider the individual medical history and the risks of continuing obesity (BNF 1999). Drugs used to treat obesity are predominantly those that act on either the gastrointestinal system or central nervous system.

There are now two drugs licensed in the UK for the treatment of obesity. Guidelines for their use have been produced by the National Institute for Clinical Excellence (NICE). *Orlistat* is a pancreatic lipase inhibitor which leads to a decrease in ingested triacylglycerol hydrolysis. Adherence to a low-fat diet is essential to avoid adverse effects such as loose stools, faecal urgency and oily discharge owing to fat malabsorption. The ability to adhere to a low-fat diet must be shown prior to the prescription of the drugs. Fat-soluble vitamins can be lost and vitamin status should be monitored. *Sibutramine* inhibits the reuptake of the neurotransmitters that control food intake (serotonin and noradrenaline). This helps patients to feel satisfied with smaller portions so that they eat less. Adverse effects may include dry mouth, constipation, insomnia and loss of appetite.

Whichever type of treatment is used for obesity, long-term monitoring and follow-up are needed. Whether drugs or surgical interventions are used, it is still essential to empower the patient to make changes to diet and lifestyle.

Physical activity and lifestyle modification Much of the increased prevalence of obesity is thought to be due to a huge drop in physical activity and increasing sedentary behaviour. Combining dietary restriction with increased physical activity is becoming increasingly popular as a dual approach to treating obesity. Exercise alone appears to add only small amounts of weight loss but has been shown to lead to greater loss of fat mass and conservation of fat-free mass. Randomized controlled trials (RCTs) of physical activity promotion in free-living healthy adult populations have shown that sustained high levels of participation shared some common features (Hillsden et al 1995):

- home-based programmes
- unsupervised, informal exercise
- frequent professional contact
- walking as the promoted exercise
- moderate-intensity exercise.

While it is easy, at least in theory, to reduce energy intake by 500 kcal by controlling food intake, it is more difficult to increase energy output by increasing physical activity. For example, 30 minutes of steady breast-stroke swimming will expend little more than 250 kcal. However, even if exercise contributes to only a little negative energy balance, it benefits by promoting physical fitness (Box 6.3).

Therefore, for the overweight individual a combined approach to weight loss and maintenance shows encouraging results that are likely to confer significant benefits in reducing the risk of CHD. Evaluations of weight management services suggest that sustained clinically significant weight reduction in obese patients is rare (Hughes & Martin 1999). However, there are some factors associated with success (Box 6.4).

There is growing evidence for the effectiveness of lifestyle interventions, including diet and exercise, for decreasing cardiac risk factors (Campbell et al 1998a, b, Steptoe et al 1999) but few projects appear to meet all of their aims. Long-term intervention and follow-up increases success, but significant and sustained weight loss remains an elusive goal for many. The National Obesity Forum (www.nationalobesityforum.org.uk) has produced simple, easy-to-use guidelines for the management of obesity in primary care.

■ **BOX 6.3 Beneficial effects observed from closely monitored combined diet and exercise programmes**

- Loss of body fat (particularly centrally deposited fat) whilst maintaining LBM
- Maintenance of desirable body weight
- Prevention of 'yo-yo dieting'
- Reduced hypertension
- Increased insulin sensitivity
- Improved self-esteem

■ **BOX 6.4   Factors associated with successful weight loss**

- High CHD risk factor status (health-related anxiety motivates change).
- Emphasis on lifestyle changes to decrease energy intake and increase energy expenditure.
- Programmes adapted to the needs of the individual.
- Regular appointments, either one-to-one or in groups, continuity of programme and practitioners. Unsuccessful patients cite infrequent contact and lack of continuity as causative.
- Patients attending group sessions were more likely to achieve weight loss.
- Dietary interventions combined with exercise sessions resulted in weight losses greater than those achieved by diet alone.
- Dietary advice aimed at all the family so that the patient's dietary changes are readily incorporated into the family's eating pattern, which appears to improve compliance.

SAVING LIVES

In *Saving lives: our healthier nation* (DoH 1999), poor diet, containing too much fat and salt and not enough fruit and vegetables, is identified as an important cause of CHD and particularly a problem for many low-income families who may have difficulty accessing shops with a variety of affordable foods.

Saving lives does not make detailed dietary recommendations but outlines the principles of dietary changes needed:

- increased consumption of fruit and vegetables and oily fish (particularly amongst the worst off)
- control of body weight to keep at the right weight for height
- avoiding drinking alcohol to excess.

There are also guidelines for how local partnerships and national government can enable individuals to choose the healthier options, e.g. by promoting healthy catering in schools and hospitals, developing national standards for school meals and enabling access to food outlets.

There are three chapters of the National Service Framework for Coronary Heart Disease (DoH 2000) in which the need for dietary changes is clearly stated.

- Chapter 1 – Reducing heart disease in the population (Standards one and two)
- Chapter 2 – Preventing CHD in high-risk patients (Standards three and four)
- Chapter 7 – Cardiac rehabilitation (Standard twelve).

The importance of a healthy diet has a much higher profile than before and there are many opportunities for community projects to improve food provision and dietary habits. Health Action Zones, Healthy Schools Initiatives,

Healthy Workplaces and Healthy Neighbourhoods are all part of the drive to create partnerships and to deliver shared health goals. State registered dietitians together with nurses and other health-care professionals have an important role in initiating, co-ordinating and supporting projects to promote healthy eating in the local community and in partnership with other agencies. They need to be able to translate the nutritional guidelines into consistent dietary messages which the general public understand, thereby enabling them subsequently to make healthy choices more easily. *Saving lives* places a much greater emphasis on the key role of primary care and public health in improving health.

RECOMMENDED DIETARY GUIDELINES

The NACNE (1983) and COMA (DHSS 1984, DoH 1994) reports clearly outlined nutritional requirements for health. In 1990, the British government published a document, *Eight guidelines for a healthy diet* (MAFF 1990), reinforcing these recommendations in a booklet suitable for use by the general public, which offers simple suggestions to implement the guidelines stated below.

1. Enjoy your food.
2. Eat a variety of different foods.
3. Eat the right amount to be a healthy weight.
4. Eat plenty of foods rich in starch and fibre.
5. Don't eat too much fat.
6. Don't eat sugary foods too often.
7. Look after the vitamins and minerals in your food.
8. If you drink, keep within sensible limits.

Further guidance on making healthy diet choices has been outlined in *The balance of good health,* a national food guide produced by the Health Education Authority (1994) in partnership with the Department of Health and Ministry of Agriculture, Fisheries and Food (MAFF, now DEFRA) after extensive consumer research. It aims to give consistent and practical advice and visual displays of food types and portion sizes for a healthy well-balanced diet. It is based on the five commonly accepted food groups, which are:

- bread, other cereals and potatoes
- fruit and vegetables
- milk and dairy foods
- meat, fish and alternatives
- fatty and sugary foods.

Its key message is to consume a variety of foods in the proportion shown by the different areas occupied by each of the food groups in the visual display. It is not necessary to achieve the balance shown at every meal, or even every day, although this may be the most sensible and practical approach. Balance can be achieved over a period of a week or two. The guide encourages people to eat more portions of fruit and vegetables than most currently do (five or more portions a day is recommended) and it also suggests that they eat increased amounts of bread, other cereals and potatoes. Specific guidance about portion sizes is included. A range of number of portions is given for bread, other cereals and potatoes as this will depend on individual requirements.

It is anticipated that everyone will be able to use the national food guide to make balanced food choices whether at home, planning meals or writing a shopping list, or in a supermarket or restaurant. However, *The balance of good health* is also an excellent teaching tool for use by all health professionals involved in promoting healthy eating practices to groups and individuals.

FOOD LABELLING

With an expanding market for new product ranges and greater varieties of food items, especially pre-packed and convenience foods, it is becoming increasingly difficult for the consumer to identify healthy food choices. Many manufacturers guide consumers by highlighting healthier options with nutritional claims such as 'low fat' or 'lower in fat' but these can be misleading, e.g. a bag of 'low-fat' crisps contains less fat than the usual variety but is still a high-fat snack, and many of these products may prove to be more expensive than nutritionally similar options.

Teaching clients to read food labels may be a useful way of guiding sensible food choices but it may raise more questions than it answers and is not a suitable tool for all. Box 6.5 shows how to use information on food labels.

■ **BOX 6.5   Using the information on food labels**

- Read the list on the label, which gives the ingredients in descending order of weight.
- If fat is in the top three or listed several times by various names then the food is probably high in fat. This will also apply to sugar and salt.
- Fat may be hidden under the following aliases: vegetable fat, vegetable oil, animal fat, hydrogenated fat, shortening, lard, cream, butter, margarine.
- Sugar may present in many forms, e.g. honey, glucose syrup, sugar cane and molasses.
- Salt (sodium) may also be disguised as it is incorporated into many ingredients, e.g. sea salt, monosodium glutamate, soya sauce, tomato puree, garlic salt.

IMPLEMENTING DIETARY CHANGE

Preparing your client for change

Before giving any dietary advice you will need to establish whether your client is prepared to make any lifestyle changes. An initial consultation to assess motivation is an effective use of time. If your client is ready and eager to make changes then a routine dietary assessment, the setting of realistic goals and constructive dietary advice can follow. However, it is widely recognized that even highly motivated individuals such as those with risk factors will continue to require support and guidance to succeed.

Motivation often wanes, as clients feel cheated because immediate benefits are not observed. At this stage it will be necessary to remotivate to prevent your client giving up. For those clients identified as having risk factors and not yet prepared to make changes, giving detailed dietary advice at this stage is likely to alienate them even further. It is better to have an informal session explaining simple ways to achieve a healthier lifestyle and potential short-term benefits relevant to that individual, e.g. being able to fit into favourite clothes or go for a long walk without being out of breath. It is important to stress that a healthy lifestyle is a balanced one achieved by realistic and gradual change. Many people are discouraged from attempting change if they feel it means having to give up everything they enjoy in life.

Assessing dietary habits

Before attempting to offer any constructive dietary advice it is essential to know what your clients eat and why they choose to eat particular foods. Only then can you offer useful tips and suggestions that will help them to adapt their diet.

You will also need to consider the many factors which influence food choices. Recognition of the factors affecting an individual's eating habits will enable the provision of personal and motivating dietary advice. For example, if cost is a major concern, then advice on cheap healthy meals is required but it would not be appropriate for the businessman needing ideas for healthy options for eating out.

The main methods of dietary assessment include:

- 24-hour recall
- food (record) diary or questionnaire
- 7-day weighed food inventory
- diet history.

24-Hour recall

Advantages
- A quick method of obtaining information on dietary intake.
- No commitment other than memory is required from the client.

Disadvantages
- Tends to be inaccurate as people generally have great difficulty in recalling the previous day's intake.
- The previous day may not be typical.
- There is known to be variation between weekdays and weekend days.

Main uses The main use of the 24-hour recall is in clinic or home situations where an assessment of nutritional intake is needed on which to base advice.

Daily food record or questionnaire

Advantages
- Gives a reasonable overall idea of types of food eaten and frequency of intake.
- Establishes meal pattern and possible lifestyle factors, e.g. number of meals out.
- Gives a reasonable estimate of nutritional intake and adequacy of diet.

Disadvantages
- No idea of portion sizes.
- Difficulties in assessing accurate energy intake.
- Time consuming for client, which may be reflected in inaccurate records.
- Method may not appeal to all social groups.

Main uses
- To give a general idea of diet in an area or within a population group.
- Assessment of frequency of certain food items consumed upon which simple advice can be based.

Seven-day weighed food inventory

Advantages Accurate nutritional assessment of foods documented.

Disadvantages
- Time consuming, requiring a high degree of motivation from the client.
- Underreporting of food intake.
- Alteration of usual food intake.

Main uses In research and population surveys of nutritional intakes.

Diet history

Dietitians routinely use diet histories to gain a subjective assessment of a person's eating habits. A diet history gives a limited knowledge about a person's eating style and habits but is simple and quick to perform, especially if one simply wishes to gain an insight into the regularity of meals, snacking habits, cooking methods and favourite food choices. Knowledge of these factors will give a rough appreciation of energy and fat intake and consumption of fruit and vegetables.

Steps in taking a diet history The length of the session will vary according to time available, the information you wish to obtain and your client's attention span.

Stage 1 Establish what is consumed on a 'typical' day. Determine meal and snack pattern, foods usually chosen, approximate quantities consumed, work and exercise routine.

Stage 2 Establish the weekly pattern. Consider weekend differences, meals out, extra snacks and alcohol.

Stage 3 Fill in any other relevant details, e.g. shopping and cooking arrangements, cooking techniques, frequency of any specific foods consumed.

Stage 4 Clarify and crosscheck. Food models and photographs are particularly useful in clarifying types of foods and quantities consumed.

Assessing diet histories After taking a diet history you should be able to:
• give an overall assessment of the client's eating pattern and habits
• assess what changes need to be made
• prioritize the changes and agree short- and long-term goals with your client.

Giving dietary advice

For most people, changing lifelong habits is a gradual process requiring frequent sessions for further advice, new ideas and continuing support. Providing too much advice initially will often lead to confusion and distract from the individual's immediate priorities.

Use of a simple action plan (Box 6.6) clearly identifies immediate targets. Targets set should be agreed as realistic and achievable within a specified timespan and regularly reviewed. The decision on how much information is offered and the number of sessions in which it is given will vary with each client and the priorities of the health professional. Usually it is preferable to hold frequent appointments, i.e. monthly, until the client has achieved the agreed short-term targets and is confident enough to be monitored less often.

Dietary advice should be practical and appropriate to the individual's medical condition, lifestyle, financial status and food preferences.

Once a target has become a regular habit, it can be ticked off and a new target set. This will help to develop a healthy lifestyle without too many drastic changes at once.

Advice should be relevant and practical

In dealing with individuals or groups, whether overweight or hyperlipidaemic or at a slimming club, you need to be able to offer constructive advice that is practical and can easily be followed.

■ BOX 6.6   **Examples of agreed dietary targets**

Date	Change	Achieved
2 Feb.	Eat breakfast each morning before work	
1 Mar.	Use semi-skimmed instead of full-fat milk	
7 Mar.	Eat three pieces of fruit daily	
14 Mar.	Try cooking a new 'healthy' recipe each week	
28 Mar.	Go for a brisk walk before dinner every day	

Although medical and social conditions, and therefore requirements, will vary from person to person the dietary issues relevant in reducing risk of CHD can be summarized as follows:

1. Eat a variety of foods.
2. Reduce fats and oils. In particular, decrease saturated fats and choose monounsaturated or polyunsaturated fats whenever possible (see Box 6.7).
3. Increase complex carbohydrates.
4. Eat more fruit and vegetables.
5. Increase fibre intake.
6. Reduce sugar intake.
7. Reduce salt intake.
8. Drink sensible amounts of alcohol.

There are a number of 'healthy eating' brochures and leaflets available from the Food Standards Agency, large supermarket chains and your local community dietitians, which are a useful source of additional practical information.

It is important to note that not all individuals will need or be able to make these changes but most will require practical hints and tips to guide gradual change.

■ **BOX 6.7 Modifying the type of fat in the diet**

- Eat fish more often, replacing meat with tuna, mackerel or sardines.
- Use less meat in dishes by adding beans and pulses to stews, chilli con carne, shepherd's pie, spaghetti bolognese and casseroles.
- Use unsaturated spreading fats and oils in cooking and dressings, e.g. sunflower, safflower, rapeseed, olive and peanut oils.
- Cut back on biscuits and cakes.

Hints for healthier eating

Reducing fats and oils Fat is an essential component of the diet, a concentrated energy source that makes meals tasty, palatable, satisfying and rich in texture, and the sole source of essential fatty acids and fat-soluble vitamins in the diet.

Recent UK surveys show that most of the fat in the diet comes from meat and meat products, spreading fats and oils, dairy products and cakes and biscuits. Therefore, most people should be able to reduce their fat intakes by eating less of these products and making use of low-fat alternatives (see Box 6.8).

Products containing plant sterols There are now a variety of products available containing added plant sterols, such as spreads, cream cheese-style spreads and yogurts. These can be used as an adjunct to diet and exercise but not as an alternative. In order for them to have a clinically significant effect they need to be consumed 2–3 times a day. This may be

■ BOX 6.8 Hints for reducing fat in the diet

Protein and dairy foods

- Choose lean cuts of meat and chicken and fresh fish or seafood.
- Choose tinned fish not canned in oil or drain off the oil.
- Trim all fat and skin from meat and chicken, preferably before cooking.
- Choose low-fat varieties of processed meats, avoiding high-fat sausage and luncheon meat products.
- Whether meat, chicken or fish, serve a small portion as an accompaniment to a high-carbohydrate food.
- Make use of low-fat dairy products, e.g. skimmed milk, cottage cheese, yogurt, fromage frais.
- Cheese is the highest fat dairy food; even the low-fat hard cheeses are still high in fat and therefore you still need to limit the serving. Grating cheese or using a cheese slicer to cut cheese thinly helps. Avoid adding additional cheese to dishes such as spaghetti bolognese.

Added fats and oils

- Learn to use cooking methods that require little fat. Grill, bake, microwave, steam, stir fry or 'dry fry' in a non-stick pan.
- Enjoy fresh bread, crackers, scones with only a small scrape of spread or better still 'continental style' without any at all.
- Use salad dressings and sauces which are fat free or low in fat, e.g. herb, vinegar and yogurt dressings. Avoid butter- or cream-based sauces and sour cream; make use of low-fat yogurt and fromage frais.

Snack foods and takeaways

- Keep away from crisps and chips. Enjoy lower fat snacks such as pop corn, raw vegetables, crackers and toasted pitta bread which are all low-fat alternatives and easy to prepare.
- Most takeaways are high in fat. Choose only occasionally and select lower fat options such as chicken or grilled burgers and follow with fresh fruit. Try to avoid deep-fried, battered or pastry items.

Processed foods

- Learn to read the labels and select those which are lower in fat. There are lower fat alternatives for many foods, e.g. scones and bagels instead of croissants (see Box 6.9).
- You can make your own 'healthy' recipes by reducing the amount of fats and oils and other high-fat ingredients.
- Enjoy a small amount of sweets, chocolate, pastries and cakes as a treat occasionally.

■ **BOX 6.9** Low-fat carbohydrate replacements for high-fat carbohydrate foods

High-fat carbohydrate food	*Lower fat alternative*
Lasagne	Pasta with a small amount of meat/beans and tomato sauce
Pasta with rich creamy sauce	As above
Croissant	Bagel or bread roll
Pizza with everything	Thick-crust pizza with seafood or vegetables and less cheese
French fries	Jacket potato
Doughnut	Scone, crumpet or teacake
Toasted ham/cheese sandwich	Toasted banana or baked bean sandwich using thick-sliced bread and scrape of spread
Chocolate bar	Plain muesli bar, low-fat brands

useful if it fits into an individual's lifestyle, but for those who do not eat all their meals within the home or do not eat much of this type of product, profound changes in daily routine may be necessary. Labelling on the packets states the portion sizes recommended. It is important to remember that these products still contain calories and this must be considered if weight management is an issue. Low-fat varieties are available for some products. Another consideration for many people is cost as these products are much more expensive than other yogurts and spreads.

Increasing unrefined carbohydrates Traditionally, sources of carbohydrate have been classified in terms of simple (sugars) or complex (starches). Sugars contain few other nutrients except energy (calories) and have little satiety value. In contrast, complex sources are usually filling foods and good sources of a variety of vitamins and minerals as well as fibre and lignans. *The balance of good health* clearly reflects current dietary guidelines to consume complex carbohydrates as the major energy source.

A common mistake is to assume that carbohydrate-rich foods are high in calories (energy) and are therefore fattening. They only become fattening if they are eaten with additional oil or spreads, e.g. chips, garlic bread, doughnuts, etc. An excessive intake of complex carbohydrate foods is unlikely as they are bulky and promote early satiety.

Clients should be encouraged to turn typical eating habits inside out. Carbohydrate foods should become the base of all meals and snacks (Box 6.10). Advice must be constructive to encourage people to change attitudes and become creative with rice, pasta, bread and potatoes that have traditionally been considered as an accompaniment or afterthought in our meal planning. An added incentive to make these changes is that meals are generally cheaper.

■ **BOX 6.10   Increasing the complex carbohydrate in the diet**

- Plan each meal around a carbohydrate food, making it the centre of attention and adding the rest of the meal around it, e.g. add filling to a sandwich, sauce to pasta, topping to jacket potato or rice. Alternatively, take half your usual protein portion and fill up with a generous serving of starchy foods and vegetables.
- Choose breakfast cereals that are low in sugar and high in fibre. These are also ideal as snacks at any time during the day. Be careful with toasted mueslis and similar cereals, which are high in fat and sugar. Hypertensive patients may be advised to look at labels for the salt content as some cereals are high in salt and lower salt cereals are available.
- Eat plenty of all types of fruit, be it fresh, canned, stewed or baked.
- Enjoy different types of bread and rolls.
- Replace rich cakes and puddings with scones, muffins or crumpets, particularly wholemeal varieties.
- Experiment with root vegetables; add extra parsnips, carrots, swede, turnip and try out pumpkin and squash, which are all filling and cheap foods.
- Be adventurous with cooking, try out new recipes and make cereals, grains, pulses and vegetables the focus of the meal.

Increasing consumption of fruit and vegetables Controversy exists over the protective role of antioxidant supplements, but evidence supports health benefits from a high daily intake of fruit and vegetables. In addition, all fruit and vegetables are low-fat, high-fibre foods, promoting satiety, and therefore ideal food choices for people attempting to lose weight. Many of the suggestions discussed earlier will promote an increased intake of fruit and vegetables. Box 6.11 shows ideas for how to increase fruit and vegetable intake.

Increasing dietary fibre (non-starch polysaccharides) Many of the suggestions listed above will promote an increase in both water-soluble and insoluble NSP. Box 6.12 shows additional suggestions for increasing NSP intake.

Reducing sugar intake Sugar is the popular name for sucrose, the most commonly occurring simple sugar in the Western diet and the most refined of all carbohydrate foods, with all other nutrients removed during processing. Sugar and related substances appear in many forms in the diet, e.g. honey, molasses, maltodextrins, glucose, corn syrup, fructose, and all provide energy (calories) and little else.

It is now recognized that sugar is not the direct cause of disease, apart from its contribution to tooth decay. It is more by association that sugar is related to health problems. Sugar is a compact and delicious form of calories, especially in the form of sugar-coated fats such as chocolate, cake and ice cream. This combination of high calories and fat, lacking fibre, vitamins and minerals, has the potential for overuse and subsequent health

■ BOX 6.11   How to increase fruit and vegetable intake

- Aim to eat five portions or more of any fruit and vegetable each day.
- Eat all types of fruit: fresh, tinned, dried, stewed, baked and juice.
- Eat fruit as a healthy, filling snack.
- Eat fruit as part of a main course, e.g. in stir fries or curries, or add to salads for variety and colour.
- Be adventurous with desserts; enjoy fresh whole fruits or fruit salads or baked fruits with low-fat yogurts and fromage frais.
- Use seasonal fruits or tinned fruits for summer pudding.
- Select fruit-based desserts for dinner parties or when eating out, instead of rich creamy cakes and desserts. Serve at least two vegetables in addition to potatoes at meal times.
- Serve a side salad with all meals and eat smaller portions of the main course, especially with pizza, lasagne and other dishes, which are frequently eaten without vegetables.
- Experiment with vegetarian dishes such as stuffed vegetables, e.g. marrow, courgettes, peppers, tomatoes, as the main part of a meal.
- Try out stir fries based on oriental vegetables as a quick and easy meal.
- Don't be put off by the price of fresh vegetables. Choose those in season, which tend to be cheaper, and make use of tinned and frozen vegetables, which are just as good nutritionally.
- Add vegetables to casseroles and composite dishes, e.g. shepherd's pie, chilli con carne.
- Choose fruit and vegetable-based starters as fillers to meals at home or when eating out, e.g. grapefruit, melon, corn on the cob, crudités.

■ BOX 6.12   Additional hints for a healthy fibre intake

- Select wholegrain breads and breakfast cereals, wholemeal pastas and brown rice.
- Cook with wholemeal flour or a mixture of white and wholemeal.
- By choosing foods naturally high in fibre you will not need to add additional bran, which can impair absorption of other nutrients.
- Increase intake of soluble fibres by enjoying more fruit and vegetables and eating the skins and seeds where appropriate.
- Experiment with beans and pulses in cooking.
- Include oat-based cereals and foods.

disadvantages. Box 6.13 identifies some ways in which to decrease sugar intake.

Reducing salt intake Salt in the diet is provided as sodium chloride but only the sodium component is a health concern due to its regulatory effect on blood pressure and volume, and fluid balance.

■ **BOX 6.13   Ways to consume less sugar**

- Gradually reduce the amount of sugar added to drinks and breakfast cereals.
- Select 'unsweetened' and 'no added sugar' brands.
- Use less sugar in traditional recipes or replace it with an artificial sweetener.
- Make use of low-calorie artificial sweeteners but where possible get used to a less sweet taste. Be careful as not all sweeteners are low in calories.
- Choose processed foods with less sugar by learning to read labels and recognizing sugar by its other names.

■ **BOX 6.14   How to use salt wisely**

- Use salty sauces and flavourings sparingly, e.g. soya sauce, stock cubes, yeast extracts.
- Experiment with herbs, spices, lemon juice, garlic and other salt-free flavourings.
- Reduce your intake of salty snack foods, processed foods and takeaways, which are often high in fat and calories too.
- Learn to read labels to check the salt content of processed foods; look for new varieties with reduced salt or low-sodium content.

Sodium is found naturally in many foods but recent dietary habits have distorted sodium intake through the large amounts of salt added to meals and snack foods. For most people cutting out the salt added to their meals at the table and that used in cooking will still leave their intake above the recommended level of 5–6 g per day as manufactured foods are the main source of sodium. However, gradual changes are needed as your taste adapts to a lower salt intake. Box 6.14 shows how to use salt wisely.

Drinking alcohol sensibly Drinking alcohol in moderation and within the recommended limits is not considered detrimental to health. Most people should be encouraged to keep to sensible limits and drink no more than 1–2 units daily with 2–3 alcohol-free days every week.

All alcoholic beverages are high in calories and drinking often promotes a carefree attitude towards eating a sensible diet. People who are trying to lose weight or attempting to alter dietary habits should minimize their alcohol intake. For many this may be difficult, as alcohol is a major source of relaxation and social focus, and much encouragement is needed to succeed. Box 6.15 shows some tips for sensible drinking.

The cost of eating healthily: poverty and diet

There is much evidence to show that a healthy diet costs more than a less healthy diet. Some healthier options are cheaper, e.g. skimmed milk and

■ **BOX 6.15   Tips for sensible drinking**

- If you choose to drink alcohol, enjoy one or two on an occasion and avoid binges.
- Organize social events which do not involve drinking, e.g. tenpin bowling, cinema, ice skating, sporting activities.
- Use tricks to make the alcohol go further. Drink low-alcohol beers, mix your wine with water to make a spritzer, make shandies with a low-calorie lemonade and use a large low-calorie mixer to dilute a measure of spirit. Try out many of the new non-alcoholic beverages and alternate with an alcoholic one.
- Only drink in company.
- Offer to drive to the pub as an excuse not to drink at all.
- If you need to restrict your energy intake, treat alcohol as a luxury. There are far more nutritious and tasty ways to consume calories.

low-fat spreads tend to be less expensive than their full-fat counterparts, but wholemeal bread is more expensive than white bread.

The effects of poverty on diet are more far reaching than simply adapting the amount and choice of foods bought. Cooking and storage facilities are both limited, whilst access to supermarkets to buy cheaper foods may mean expensive bus or taxi fares.

High earners spend considerably less of their available income on food and are able to travel to supermarkets, buy in bulk and enjoy a greater choice of foodstuffs obtainable at a lower cost. Lower income shoppers on the other hand may avoid supermarkets because the temptations on offer are difficult to resist, resulting in overspending on essential items and not just luxuries.

For many, health considerations may not be a priority, the provision of cheap, filling food being of far greater importance. Emotional and social issues manifesting as low self-esteem, depression and feelings of despair may in turn lead to smoking or drinking or eating 'junk' foods. It is rather simplistic to expect these clients to substitute their sweets, chocolates or biscuits for 'healthier' options. A 'client-centred' approach is needed where clients are able to discuss their needs and wants and practical individual advice is offered. *Saving lives* has suggestions to promote healthier neighbourhoods, including access to healthier foods. This is also a priority for many Health Action Zones. There are ways to make healthier choices on a lower income and some are shown in Box 6.16.

With care, planning and a willingness to try new recipes, healthy eating need not be more expensive. By following *The balance of good health,* expensive items such as meat, cheese and dairy products will be eaten in smaller quantities and replaced with cheaper staple items such as cereals, bread and potatoes and legumes.

■ **BOX 6.16   Practical shopping tips**

- Make a shopping list of essential items and avoid buying extras.
- Look for the supermarket's own-label lines, which are usually cheaper than leading brand names.
- Stock up on special offers.
- Cheaper fruit and vegetables are available at local markets rather than supermarkets.
- Fruits and vegetables in season will be cheaper than less available varieties. Buy in bulk and store foods if possible.
- Do not attempt to replace usual food choices with more expensive 'low-fat', 'low-sugar' and 'reduced-salt' alternatives but focus purchases on cheaper filling items such as pasta, potatoes, rice, bread, beans and pulses.
- Reduce costs in other ways by cutting down on transport costs and fuel bills, for example:
  - cook meals that require using only one or two hobs, such as spaghetti bolognese or stew and rice
  - boil only the amount of water you need in a kettle
  - boil vegetables in only a small amount of water
  - a toaster uses less electricity than a grill so is a better choice for toasting bread, crumpets, etc.
  - use the oven to the full, e.g. serve jacket potatoes with any oven-cooked dish and braise vegetables in water in the oven.

Convenience foods

Convenience foods can contribute to a healthy diet and, whilst there are many high-fat and salty varieties sold, they do not have to be unhealthy. There are many nutritious, economical convenience foods available.

Tins and packet foods
- Tinned beans and pulses
- Tinned vegetables, particularly tomatoes and sweetcorn
- Tinned fruit, preferably in juice rather than syrup
- Instant mashed potato – rich in vitamin C
- Tinned fish, e.g. mackerel, pilchards, sardines, salmon, preferably canned in brine or sauce
- Dried milk powder or UHT low-fat liquid milk
- Wholemeal or rye crackers

Frozen foods
- All types of frozen fruits or vegetables
- Fish fingers and frozen fish portions
- Packs of chicken and other lean meat portions and minced meat

Ready-made meals may be useful but many are very high in salt and are best served with additional salad or vegetables.

■ KEY POINTS

- Diet plays an important role in a variety of disease processes.
- Plasma lipid levels may be influenced by dietary changes and current recommendations by national bodies suggest specific dietary strategies to lower plasma lipid levels and in turn reduce CHD risk.
- The composition of dietary fats as well as their quantity must be taken into account in assessing any diet.
- Modern dietary guidelines emphasize the importance of increased fruit and vegetable intake. This provides increased dietary fibre as well as potentially important antioxidant vitamins.
- Obesity is the result of an imbalance between energy intake and expenditure.
- The BMI is a useful tool in assessing levels of obesity in adults but also measuring the waist will give a better idea of coronary risk.
- A variety of weight loss programmes exist and all approved programmes should be gradual and, where appropriate, performed under supervision. Whenever possible, dietary changes and increased physical activity should be combined.
- Dietary advice should be tailored to the individual and should be based on detailed dietary assessment and understanding of the client's lifestyle.

REFERENCES

British Nutrition Foundation Task Force 1999 Obesity. Report of the British Nutrition Foundation Task Force. Blackwell Science, Oxford

Campbell NC, Ritchie LD, Deans HG, Rawles JM, Squair JL 1998a Secondary prevention in coronary heart disease: a randomised trial of nurse led clinics in primary care. Heart 80: 447–452

Campbell NC, Thain J, Deans HG, Ritchie LD, Rawles JM, Squair JL 1998b Secondary prevention clinics for coronary heart disease: randomised trial of effect on health. British Medical Journal 316: 1434–1437

Cassidy A, Griffin BA 1999 Phyto-oestrogens: a potential role in the prevention of CHD? Proceedings of the Nutrition Society 58: 193–199

Contacos C, Barter PJ, Sullivan DR 1993 Effect of pravastatin and w-3 fatty acids on plasma lipids and lipoproteins in patients with combined hyperlipidaemia. Arteriosclerosis and Thrombosis 13: 1755–1762

Department of Health 1994 Diet and risk. Report of the Committee on Medical Aspects of Food Policy (COMA). HMSO, London

Department of Health 1999 Saving lives: our healthier nation. Stationery Office, London

Department of Health 2000 National Service Framework for Coronary Heart Disease. HMSO, London

Department of Health and Social Security 1984 Diet and cardiovascular disease. Report on Health and Social Subjects 28 (COMA Report). HMSO, London

Department of Health and Social Security 1987 The use of very low calorie diets in obesity. HMSO, London

Donahue RP, Abbott RD, Bloom E, Reed DM, Yano K 1987 Central obesity and coronary heart disease in men. Lancet 1: 821–824

European Atherosclerosis Society Task Force 1992 Prevention of coronary heart disease: scientific background and new clinical guidelines. Recommendations of the European Atherosclerosis Society prepared by the International Task Force for the Prevention of Coronary Heart Disease. Nutrition, Metabolism and Cardiovascular Diseases 2: 113–156

Garrow JS 1981 Treat obesity seriously: a clinical manual. Churchill Livingstone, Edinburgh

Gey KF 1993 Prospects for the prevention of free radical disease, regarding cancer and cardiovascular disease. British Medical Bulletin 49: 679–699

GISSI-Prevenzione Trial Investigators 1999 Dietary supplementation with n-3 polyunsaturated fatty acids and vitamin E after myocardial infarction; results of the GISSI-Prevenzione trial. Lancet 354: 447–455

Gregory J, Foster K, Tyler H, Wiseman M 1990 The dietary and nutritional survey of British adults. HMSO, London

Gurr M 1993 Fats. In: Garrow JS, James WPT (eds) Davidson's Human nutrition and dietetics, 9th edn. Churchill Livingstone, Edinburgh, pp 77–103

Han TS, Richmond P, Avenell A, Lean MEJ 1997 Waist circumference reduction and cardiovascular benefits during weight loss in women. International Journal of Obesity 21: 127–134

Health Education Authority (HEA) 1994 The balance of good health. HEA, London

Hillsden M, Thorogood M, Antiss T, Morris J 1995 Randomised controlled trials of physical activity promotion in free living populations: a review. Journal of Epidemiology and Community Health 49: 448–453

Hughes J, Martin S 1999 The Department of Health's project to evaluate weight management services. Journal of Human Nutrition and Dietetics 12 (suppl 1): 1–8

Knight I 1984 The heights and weights of adults in Great Britain. HMSO, London

Larsson B, Svardsudd K, Weln L, Bjornturp P, Tubblin C 1984 Abdominal adipose tissue distribution, obesity and risk of cardiovascular disease and death: a 13 year follow up of participants in the study of men born in 1913. British Medical Journal 288: 1401–1404

Law M 2000 Plant sterol and stanol margarines and health. British Medical Journal 320: 861–864

Lean MEJ, Han TS, Morrison CE 1995 Waist circumference as a measure for indicating the need for weight management. British Medical Journal 311: 158–161

Lean MEJ, Han TS, Seidall JC 1998 Impairment of health and quality of life in people with large waist circumference. Lancet 351: 853–856

Lissner L, Odell PM, D'Aigostino R et al 1991 Variability of body weight and health outcomes in the Framingham population. New England Journal of Medicine 324: 1839–1844

MAFF, DoH, HEA 1990 Eight guidelines for a healthy diet. Food Sense, London

Meade TW, Ruddock V, Stirling Y, Chakrabati R, Milloer GJ 1993 Fibrinolytic activity, clotting factors and long term incidence of ischaemic heart disease in the Northwick Park Study. Lancet 342: 1076–1079

NACNE 1983 Discussion paper on proposals for nutritional guidelines for health education in Britain. Health Education Council, London

OPCS 1995 Health survey for England 1993. HMSO, London

Scottish Intercollegiate Guidelines Network (SIGN) 1996 Obesity in Scotland: integrating prevention with weight management. Royal College of Physicians, Edinburgh

Stender S, Dyeberg J, Holme RG, Ovesen L, Sandstrom B 1995 The influence of trans fatty acids on health: a report from the Danish Nutrition Council. Clinical Science 88: 375–392

Steptoe A, Doherty S, Rink E, Kerry S, Kendrick T, Hilton S 1999 Behavioural counselling in general practice for the promotion of healthy behaviour among adults at increased risk of coronary heart disease: randomised trial. British Medical Journal 319: 943–948

World Health Organization 1997 Obesity: preventing and managing the global epidemic. WHO, Geneva

FURTHER READING

Hunt P, Hillsden M 1996 Changing eating and exercise behaviour. Blackwell Science, Oxford

Wilkinson RG, Marmot M 1998 The solid facts: social determinants of health. WHO Europe, Copenhagen

Lifestyle management: exercise

Gillian E. Armstrong

7

INTRODUCTION

Physical activity has a key part to play in improving health and well-being. It helps to prevent coronary heart disease, stroke and some forms of cancer – some of the leading causes of morbidity and mortality in the United Kingdom.

EXERCISE AND CORONARY HEART DISEASE

It has been calculated that 37% of CHD deaths in those under 75 are attributable to physical inactivity (British Heart Foundation 2002).

Secondary prevention of coronary heart disease

Data from two published and widely cited meta-analyses (O'Connor et al 1989, Oldridge et al 1988) of over 4000 patients have demonstrated that patients randomized to exercise-based cardiac rehabilitation after MI have a statistically significant reduction in all-cause and cardiac mortality of about 20–25% compared to patients receiving conventional care. No significant effect on non-fatal reinfarctions was found. Most of the patients were middle-aged low-risk males.

A Cochrane review (Joliffe et al 2000) has recently identified a further 27 trials, most of which were published after the original meta-analyses of the late 1980s. These trials included angina patients as well as post myocardial infarction, percutaneous transluminal coronary angioplasty and coronary artery bypass surgery. A greater percentage of females and older patients was included.

The main findings were that patients randomized to exercise-only cardiac rehabilitation had, over an average of 2.4 years, a reduced all-cause mortality of 27% (random effects model OR 0.73 (0.54, 0.98)) and cardiac death of 31% (random effects model OR 0.69 (0.51, 0.94)). Once again there was no effect on rates of non-fatal reinfarction.

The Cochrane review found that compared to exercise-only trials, there appeared to be no additional benefit from comprehensive cardiac rehabilitation (which included an educational and psychological component as well as exercise training).

The reasons for the differences between exercise-only rehabilitation and comprehensive cardiac rehabilitation are unclear but may in part be dependent on when the trials were carried out. Most of the exercise-only trials were conducted in the prethrombolytic era and when secondary prevention medications such as statins, ACE inhibitors and β-blockers were not standard treatment, whereas most of the comprehensive rehabilitation trials were published in the 1990s. It is also conceivable that the exercise-only participants received ad hoc education while exercising.

Peripheral versus central adaptations

The increase in physical work capacity seen in cardiac patients following exercise training is primarily the result of peripheral adaptations (improved efficiency of the active skeletal muscles), rather than a consequence of improved myocardial efficiency. Skeletal muscles that are able to extract and utilize oxygen more effectively place fewer demands on the cardiovascular system.

Exercise training not only results in desirable changes in muscle strength, it delays the onset of anaerobic metabolism in skeletal muscle, reverses the impairment of peripheral vasodilatation and improves blood flow to exercising muscles (Uren & Lipkin 1992).

Cardiovascular and respiratory responses to acute exercise

Cardiovascular responses

Aerobic metabolism can only take place for as long as there is sufficient oxygen available to the muscles to fully meet their oxygen demands during exercise. The cardiovascular responses to exercise are:

- an increase in cardiac output
- a redistribution of blood flow to the active muscles.

Increase in cardiac output from rest The amount of blood ejected from the left ventricle each minute is called the *cardiac output*. This is the product of heart rate and stroke volume.

During exercise, cardiac output rises as a result of increases in heart rate and stroke volume. Only heart rate increases in direct proportion to oxygen consumption. This is because as the exercise becomes harder and the heart rate is higher, the length of diastole shortens. This reduces ventricular filling time and therefore stroke volume reaches a plateau.

Fitter people have a lower resting pulse and are thus able to perform their day-to-day activities at a lower percentage of their maximum heart rate. The fitter myocardium results in a larger stroke volume with every beat. This means that the same cardiac output is achieved with a lower heart rate.

The heart muscle receives its blood supply during diastole. As the heart rate increases, the period of diastole shortens and the time for coronary perfusion is therefore reduced. For cardiac patients, exercise training could make the difference between disabling angina and no angina during activities of daily life.

Selective distribution of blood flow to the active muscles The regulation of blood flow is achieved by both local metabolic and centrally mediated autonomic changes.

At rest, only 15–20% of the total cardiac output is distributed to the muscles, with the majority going to the brain and abdominal viscera. During exercise, blood is shunted away from the gut, liver and kidneys, so that as much as 85% of the total cardiac output is directed to the exercising muscles. Oxygen is then only delivered to those areas where it is principally needed.

Respiratory responses

As well as the cardiovascular changes, in order to match increased oxygen consumption, both the rate and depth of breathing increase. During light to moderate exercise, there is a linear relationship between ventilation and workload. During vigorous exercise there will come a point when the cardiovascular system is working to capacity. Metabolism then switches to anaerobic pathways. With the onset of anaerobic metabolism, blood levels of lactic acid rise, stimulating a disproportionate rise in ventilation (Fig. 7.1).

The effect of different types of muscular activity on the cardiovascular system

Muscles work in one of two ways, depending upon the specific task being performed.

Isotonic exercise

Isotonic exercise involves the rhythmical movement of the arms, trunk and legs against a low resistance. This type of muscular activity greatly increases the demand for oxygen in the blood and is often referred to as 'aerobic exercise'. Examples include brisk walking, jogging, cycling, swimming and keep fit classes.

During isotonic exercise, the blood vessels within the exercising muscles vasodilate as a result of the action of local metabolites on the vascular smooth muscle, whereas vasoconstriction occurs in the inactive muscles. The combined effect is to cause a greater amount of blood to flow through the active muscles where it is needed most.

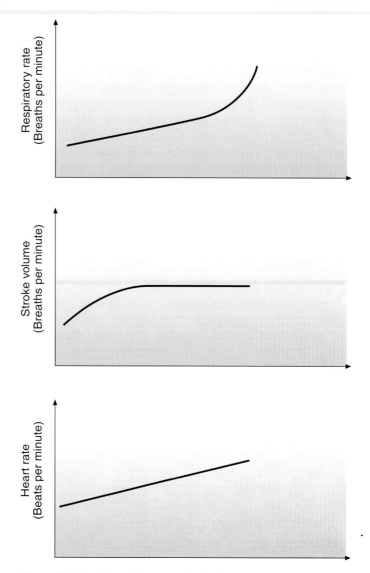

Figure 7.1 The effects of increasing levels of exercise on respiratory rate, stroke volume and heart rate.

When the exercise involves a sufficiently large muscle mass, the net effect is a lowering of peripheral vascular resistance and reduction in afterload. Since:

$$\text{arterial blood pressure} = \text{cardiac output} \times \text{peripheral vascular resistance}$$

systolic blood pressure then rises only moderately, despite large increase in the cardiac output.

If, on the other hand, the exercise involves smaller muscle groups (e.g. during arm exercises), then there is relatively more vasoconstriction (within the inactive leg muscles) and therefore peripheral vascular resistance and systolic blood pressure are relatively greater. Blood pressure is therefore higher during isotonic upper body exercise than during isotonic leg exercise.

One final difference between isotonic arm and leg exercise is in the contribution made by the heart's stroke volume during the activity. Isotonic exercise of the upper body involves a smaller muscle mass, resulting in a lower rate of venous return and therefore a smaller stroke volume. This means that at the same percentage of VO_2max, the heart rate is higher during isotonic arm exercise than during isotonic leg exercise.

Since myocardial O_2 consumption is greater when the heart is working against a pressure load rather than a volume load, the combination of a higher blood pressure (BP) and heart rate (HR) during arm exercise led to fears about myocardial ischaemia and ventricular arrhythmias if the arms were raised above the head for long periods of time. According to Balady (1993) these fears are unfounded because the increased diastolic blood pressure during arm exercise augments diastolic coronary perfusion.

Isometric exercise

Isometric muscle work means that the muscles are contracting without any movement of the joints. For example, lifting and carrying a heavy object requires a lot of isometric muscular work around the neck, shoulders and trunk.

When the muscles are in a constant state of tension, the arterial vessels are compressed, thereby greatly reducing blood flow through the muscle. As a result, isometric exercise is primarily anaerobic and therefore cannot be sustained for long periods of time without muscle fatigue.

Cardiovascularly, if an exercise or activity requires a lot of isometric or static muscle work, then arterial BP (systolic and diastolic) increases markedly in a *pressor response*. The magnitude of this response is dependent upon the muscle mass involved in the activity and how hard these muscles have to work.

Wall motion abnormalities in the myocardium may be aggravated by isometric exercise. Patients with a dilated left ventricle should be discouraged from heavy isometric activities because of the excessive level of myocardial pressure work associated with it.

To make matters worse, during isometric activities, there is a tendency for people to hold their breath and strain. This is referred to as a *Valsalva manoeuvre*, the immediate effect of which is a substantial rise in BP and a reduction in venous return. This could result in serious arrhythmias and ischaemia, particularly in patients with poor left ventricular (LV) function.

EXERCISE PRESCRIPTION

Not all cardiac patients have access to specialist advice from a physiotherapist. It is therefore essential that all health-care professionals can offer patients accurate advice and support to promote physical activity. Many factors need to be taken into consideration. Simply telling someone to take more exercise is not sufficient. The exercise prescription should take account of the FITT principle.

F   Frequency (refers to the number of occasions per week that activity should be undertaken)

I   Intensity (refers to the amount of exertion required)

T   Type (refers to the mode of physical activity being recommended)

T   Time (refers to the actual time spent performing an activity)

A two-stage model for adoption of a progressively more active lifestyle has been proposed to facilitate public and patient education on physical activity. The two stages reflect the weekly goal standards for physical activity and cardiovascular fitness.

Step 1: for improved health

Daily accumulation of at least 30 minutes of moderate-intensity routine activities

Position stands in both the US (Pate et al 1995) and the UK (HEBS 1997) affirm that many health gains may be acquired through exercise or physical activity outside formal exercise programmes. Over 43 epidemiological studies (cited by Leon 1997) have found an inverse relationship between total energy expended in leisure-time physical activity and health outcomes, which include:

- decreasing the risk of cardiovascular disease mortality in general and of CHD mortality in particular. Physically inactive people have about double the risk of CHD
- preventing or delaying the development of high blood pressure and reducing blood pressure in people with hypertension (by about 10 mmHg in men and women with mild hypertension)
- decreasing the risk of stroke. The risk of having a stroke is three times higher in those who do little or no exercise
- improving blood lipid profile, in particular HDL-cholesterol
- helping people to reduce and maintain their body weight. Walking a mile burns up at least 100 kcal.
- reducing the chance of developing non-insulin dependent diabetes
- improving bone health and maintaining strength, co-ordination, cognitive functioning and balance, thereby reducing the risk of osteoporosis, falls and associated fractures
- enhancing the immune system and reducing the risk of colon cancer
- reducing the risk of depression, with positive benefits for mental health including reducing anxiety and enhancing mood and self-esteem.

The term 'sedentary' is usually defined as a person doing less than one 30-minute session of continuous moderate-intensity physical activity per week. Due to the large numbers of people who are currently classed as sedentary, the potential for health gain through physical activity is great.

Population surveys show that the majority of adults exercise only sporadically or not at all. The *Health Survey for England 1998* (DoH 1999) found that around six out of 10 men and seven out of 10 women were not reaching recommended levels of physical activity. Although the greatest absolute health benefit is amongst those who exercise vigorously, Figure 7.2 shows a dose–response curve of the relationship between physical activity (dose) and health benefit (response). The lower the baseline physical activity status, the greater will be the health benefit associated with a given increase in physical activity.

Frequency

Many of the beneficial effects of exercise are short-lived (e.g. increase in insulin sensitivity and glucose uptake and reductions in blood pressure and plasma triglyceride levels) hence the need for physical activity on a daily basis rather than on an irregular basis (Leon 1997).

Intensity

For convenience, exercise intensities can be classified as follows:

- *Light intensity* – easily within an individual's current exercise capacity, placing very little demand on the oxygen transport system.
- *Moderate intensity* – within an individual's current exercise capacity, but causing an increase in respiratory and pulse rates.
- *Vigorous intensity* – intense enough to represent a substantial challenge to a person's cardiorespiratory system (ACSM 1998).

Results from the Harvard Alumni Study indicate that low-intensity activities were not associated with a reduction in all-cause mortality, whereas moderate-intensity activities were beneficial and high-intensity activities were highly correlated with reduced mortality (Lee & Paffenburger 2000). Moderate intensity includes any type of physical activity with an energy expenditure of between 5 and 7.5 kcal/min (HEBS 1997). For healthy sedentary people this is the equivalent of brisk walking (3–4 mph) across level ground. Other studies have not found any additional advantage from vigorous rather than moderate-intensity physical activity. From a health

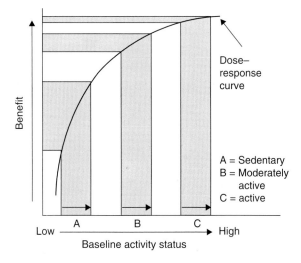

Figure 7.2 Relationship between physical activity (dose) and health benefit (response) (Journal of the American Medical Association 1995, 273: 402–407).

point of view, the major advantage of promoting moderate rather than vigorous exercise is that it is a more achievable goal, with less likelihood of injury or cardiovascular complications (see section on exercise safety below) and with a greater likelihood of long-term adherence.

Time

A day's exercise can, if need be, be broken up into multiple shorter bouts in order to fit in with the individual's lifestyle. DeBusk (1990) found that men who exercised for three 10-minute sessions a day, in lieu of the more usual single session of 30 minutes, showed a significant reduction in body mass and a 7.6% improvement in their aerobic fitness. This improvement would have been sufficient to move them out of the 'low fit' category associated in observational studies with an increased risk of all-cause and cardiovascular mortality (Blair et al 1996). Murphy et al (2000) and Murphy & Hardman (1998) compared long-bout and short-bout brisk walking on health-related outcomes. They noted superior adherence in the group assigned to the frequent short-bout programme.

The 30 minutes referred to in the position statement is the suggested minimum 'dose' of activity which sedentary people *should add to their normal activity.*

Type

Physical activity has been defined as 'bodily movement produced by skeletal muscles that requires energy expenditure and produces progressive health benefits', while exercise has been described as planned physical activity with bodily movements that were structured and repetitive performed for the purpose of improving or maintaining physical fitness. Analysis of epidemiological data has shown that the type of physical activity itself did not appear to influence the health benefits attained (Leon 1997). Therefore occupational, leisure-time physical activity and everyday activities, many of which are performed on an intermittent basis, are considered equally effective when the goal is health related as opposed to fitness related. Some considerations relating to the type of physical activity are detailed later.

Walking (outdoor and treadmill) Walking is a natural form of exercise for all ages and because it is within the physical capabilities of the majority of people, it is an excellent introduction to exercise for sedentary and unfit individuals. It is a low-impact physical activity, making the risk of injury low, even in those with orthopaedic problems.

Walking paces vary from a leisurely stroll to power walking. Maximum benefit is obtained from brisk walking, i.e. at a pace sufficient to leave a person feeling warm and slightly out of breath.

The Allied Dunbar Fitness Survey (1992) found that over 30% of men and 60% of women cannot maintain a speed of 3 mph up a moderate slope. This included most men over 55 years of age and women over 35 years of age.

Most patients tend to overestimate their walking speed and distance. Outdoor walking is self-paced and is therefore subject to individual perceptions and motivation. A pedometer could be used to provide feedback and encouragement.

The main drawback to outdoor walking is, of course, the weather. Cardiac patients with low cardiorespiratory fitness should avoid prolonged periods of exercising outdoors when it is extremely cold or windy, since this is more likely to precipitate angina.

Treadmill walking is a suitable alternative, although it necessitates equipment only usually found in sports centres and hospitals. Visual displays of distance covered, time and even calories burned provide powerful motivation.

Unlike outdoor walking, the main advantage of treadmill walking is that, once programmed, the walking speed is set by the machine so the exercise intensity can be much more accurately controlled.

For those unaccustomed to the treadmill, an inefficient gait increases energy expenditure. Likewise, gripping too tightly on the handrail causes undesirable isometric work. During walking, the likelihood of injury is very low in comparison to other modes of exercise.

Jogging Jogging provides a much higher intensity form of aerobic exercise and is therefore only suitable for those with very good exercise capacity. Jogging is a high-impact activity, making musculoskeletal injuries much more likely. Proper footwear is essential. Joggers should be advised to avoid cement and asphalt surfaces and keep to shock-absorbing surfaces like running tracks. Grass is a reasonable alternative provided the surface is not too rough or uneven. When recommending jogging as an exercise, it is usual to advise that after a warm-up, short periods of jogging should be interspersed with equal periods of walking (conversational jogging). This form of interval training allows less fit individuals to exercise for a longer duration than would otherwise be possible.

Mini-trampoline rebounding Mini-trampolines can be a good alternative to jogging for those with minor lower limb orthopaedic problems since they reduce the shock transmitted through the joints. This type of exercise may not be suitable for people with poor balance, unless the trampoline incorporates a handrail.

Stair climbing/step-ups Exercise should be an integral part of everyday life, yet if given the choice between using the stairs or using an escalator, few opt to use the stairs.

Blamey et al (1995) found that 'Stay Healthy, Save Time – Use the Stairs' posters strategically placed in an underground station resulted in significantly greater stair usage. Provided that it is done slowly at a level well within the person's capabilities, stair climbing is an aerobic activity. However, for patients with weak thigh muscles or congestive heart failure, the activity may become anaerobic. For less fit individuals it is usually better to make use of the step at the foot of the stairs, to step up and down from. This will allow a relatively constant effort to be maintained for the duration of the exercise, as opposed to strenuous effort when ascending several steps followed by much easier effort when descending.

Repetitive stepping, especially from a high step/platform, may exacerbate lower limb orthopaedic problems.

Cycling Cycling works the large muscle groups of the legs in a steady aerobic manner. Cycling, like walking, is an easy activity to maintain at a steady level for the duration of the activity, an important consideration where precise control of exercise intensity is indicated. Cycling is an excellent form of non-weight bearing exercise and is suitable for a wide range of fitness levels since the intensity can be altered by adjusting the pedalling speed or the terrain. The saddle height should be set so that the knee is only slightly bent at the downstroke; this ensures that the muscles work through a large range of movement, thus increasing the efficacy of the exercise.

In 1995, the British government signalled a welcome shift in its transport policy, pledging more money to improve the facilities for inner-city cyclists. At present only about 2.5% of all journeys are done by bicycle. Bhopal & Unwin (1995) found that 62% of all car trips are under 5 km in distance and could quite easily be done by bicycle. Exercise bicycles are popular pieces of equipment bought for using at home. Unfortunately, most of these people give up once the novelty has worn off and the boredom has set in. Watching a favourite television programme while exercising can be good distraction therapy.

Exercise bicycles were once the cornerstone of many of the early cardiac rehabilitation programmes. However, cycling is a skill which uses muscles in a way not frequently used in day-to-day life. Training specificity refers to the adaptations that occur in response to exercise, which take place only in the muscles being exercised. Since most of the improvements that occur after moderate-intensity training come about as a result of peripheral adaptations in the muscles rather than enhanced cardiac function, exercise training which uses a single modality such as cycling is unlikely to improve upper body endurance, something which is necessary for many activities of daily living.

Rowing machines The advantage of a rowing machine over other modes of exercise is that it combines the use of upper and lower limb muscle work. This makes the oxygen costs greater when compared with cycling. Most rowing machines also allow the participant to use legs only or arms only, making them useful for those with disabilities. They are generally not suitable for those with knee problems. Work rate can be adjusted by altering the resistance or increasing the velocity of each stroke. The equipment is of course expensive, which makes it inaccessible to some.

Swimming Swimming incorporates upper and lower limb aerobic muscle work and as such can be a good form of exercise for those having already completed an exercise-based cardiac rehabilitation programme. For those who are unable or find it difficult to participate in weight-bearing exercise because of orthopaedic limitations or obesity, the buoyancy of the water greatly reduces joint loading. The hydrostatic pressure of the water coupled with the horizontal position of the body also enhances venous return. Many elderly people do not go swimming because they are frightened of slipping on wet floors and falling.

The wide variation in skill levels with swimming makes it a difficult mode of exercise for which to quantify individual training intensity accurately. For example, poor swimmers may not be able to attain an effective training stimulus because they are continually stopping. Similarly, highly skilled swimmers may find swimming is too easy, making it difficult to get enough cardiovascular exercise.

The temperature of the pool is a particularly important consideration. In a cold pool, to prevent excessive heat loss, a widespread peripheral vasoconstriction occurs with a resultant rise in arterial blood pressure. There is also an increase in the heart and respiratory rates. For cardiac patients this could precipitate ischaemic symptoms.

Rope skipping Skipping is a high-impact, high-intensity exercise which also requires significant co-ordination and as such, is not recommended for cardiac patients. Skipping can be used as one of the exercises in a supervised cardiac rehabilitation circuit programme, providing it is reserved for those with good exercise tolerance at least 12 weeks post event.

Callisthenics Callisthenics is the name given to light mobilizing exercises of the upper and lower limbs designed to promote general fitness. Callisthenics are most often used in the inpatient setting for stable, uncomplicated cardiac patients, since the exercises represent a low demand on the cardiovascular system (somewhere in the region of 2–3 metabolic equivalents (METs). When planning the exercises, the therapist should alternate between leg and arm work to prevent local muscle fatigue.

Callisthenics should not be confused with 'Callanetics'. Callanetics are small, repetitive end-of-range movements, localized to individual muscle groups and designed to improve muscle tone. These exercises contain a large isometric element and as such are less suitable for cardiac patients, particularly ones with uncontrolled hypertension.

Dancing The aerobic benefits of dancing will vary considerably depending on the type of dance and the tempo of the music. Dancing is usually very sociable and enjoyable and as such may not be looked upon as 'exercise'. This makes it a good activity for those who think that exercise is the preserve of the fit and sporty.

Aerobic/keep fit exercise classes Provided that the class is well structured and kept to low-impact moves, exercise classes can be very enjoyable. One of the disadvantages of exercise classes is that most participants try to keep up with the pace set by the instructor, rather than pacing themselves. Prolonged bouts of exercise with the arms above the head will increase the work of the cardiovascular system, so it is wise initially to encourage participants to modify the exercise, by keeping their arms below chest height. Participants should be encouraged to work at their own pace. Exercise classes can be very daunting for beginners who think they are not co-ordinated. A good instructor can offset this by building up sequences of movements from two or three basic steps, rather than simultaneously changing arms and legs. The Register of Exercise Professionals (www.reps-uk.org) is a system of self-regulation for all instructors involved in exercise and fitness. Registration is achieved and maintained through the gaining of qualifications and training, which are nationally recognized and linked to National Occupational Standards for the area of exercise and fitness. Phase 4 exercise classes should be staffed by chartered physiotherapists or appropriately qualified fitness instructors (NVQ Level 3). Participants usually require medical confirmation (e.g. from their GP) of their suitability.

Exercise videos for home use Cardiac patients should be guided to a low-impact/low-intensity version of aerobic exercise, which includes a distinct warm-up and cool-down. Patients should not be expected to exercise unsupervised at home until they have been taught the various components (frequency/intensity/duration) of an exercise prescription and how these factors interrelate. Most commercially available exercise videos are unsuitable for unfit people who have co-existing morbidity.

Racquet games By nature, racquet sports are highly variable in their intensity. If the participants are of a low skill level, then they could spend most of their time walking slowly or hanging about waiting for others. On the other hand, if the opponents are not equally matched in terms of skills, then the game may be far more demanding for one of them. Games like squash may require explosive bursts of energy, with resultant high cardiovascular demand. Instead of playing to get fit, the best advice is to get fit first and then take up a sport.

Canadian Airforce 5BX and XBX physical fitness programme Despite the fact that some early researchers have used this programme with cardiac patients, it is not one that the author recommends. The plan consists of five different exercises which should be completed in 11 minutes. Although the principles of graduated progression are emphasized, the authors of the programme claim that an additional warm-up is unnecessary. Exercise duration is kept fixed and progression is made by increasing the intensity. High-intensity, short-duration exercise is not suitable for symptomatic individuals. In addition, the exercises themselves, if performed in the manner described, could result in musculoskeletal/back injury (e.g. sit-up with legs straight and feet hooked under a chair).

Competitive exercise Highly competitive exercise should be discouraged, since participants will be much less able to self-monitor and regulate their levels of exertion. If people feel that their team is relying upon them, they will not slow down even if they develop symptoms such as palpitations, breathlessness or chest pain.

Exercise referral schemes Exercise referral schemes involve health professionals recommending that individuals who would benefit from becoming more active and who fit agreed criteria attend locally provided physical activity opportunities. A national Quality Assurance Framework for Exercise Referral Systems has been published which contains guidelines for best practice and best value (DoH 2001).

Step 2: for optimal cardiovascular fitness

This involves longer periods of physical activity, including a more formal exercise programme with three structured 20-minute sessions of moderate-intensity aerobic training.

Frequency

Improvement in aerobic fitness increases with frequency of training, but the magnitude of change is smaller and tends to plateau when frequency of training is increased above 3 days per week (ACSM 1998).

Exercise intensity

The aim of an exercise programme should be to gradually expose the individual to an amount or level of exercise sufficient to bring about a cardiovascular training effect. This level is known as the *training threshold*.

If the exercise intensity is too low, i.e. it is below the threshold, then no improvements in aerobic capacity will take place. In general, the less fit an individual is, then the lower the exercise intensity should be at the start of the programme. For most deconditioned cardiac patients, the threshold intensity lies around 40–50% of the maximum oxygen uptake reserve (ACSM 2000). This corresponds to 55–65% of maximum heart rate (HRmax).

Controlling the exercise intensity Various methods can be used to prescribe and monitor exercise intensity. Clinically, amongst the most useful are:

- heart rate
- patient-perceived exertion
- breathlessness
- METs.

Target heart rate As previously stated, there is a linear relationship between heart rate and oxygen consumption. The lower and upper limits of the target heart rate can be calculated as follows.

> Lower limit of target HR = (HRmax − HRrest) multiplied by
> 0.4 plus HRrest
> Upper limit of target HR = (HRmax − HRrest) multiplied by
> 0.65 plus HRrest

The HRmax is the heart rate at which maximal oxygen uptake is achieved. If the patient has recently undergone a graded maximal exercise test, then the peak heart rate on exercise should be used to calculate the training heart rate. Where no recent exercise test has been done, an estimated HRmax can be made on the basis of the person's age. A different calculation is required for patients taking β-blocker medication (Brodie et al 1998).

Special considerations for patients with angina Myocardial ischaemia manifesting as horizontal or downsloping ST segment depression and/or angina pectoris requires careful review when generating the exercise prescription. The exercise prescription is developed using the method described above; the HRmax is taken as the heart rate at which the patient developed significant ST changes. This ensures the designated training heart rate is below the identified threshold of ischaemia. In general, the heart rate prescription should be a minimum of 10 beats/min below the heart rate at which the abnormality occurs (Fletcher et al 2001).

Whatever method is used, patients need to be taught how to take their own pulse. Usually the radial artery is easy to palpate. The beats are counted over a 15-second period, then multiplied by four, to give a measure of the heart rate.

When individuals first embark on an exercise programme, they will have little idea of what level of exercise corresponds to their training heart rate. This means that heart rate measurements should be taken frequently if exercise intensity is to be reliably regulated.

■ KEY POINTS WHEN USING HEART RATE AS THE SOLE METHOD FOR CONTROLLING EXERCISE INTENSITY

- An individual's signs and symptoms are overriding factors when prescribing the intensity of an exercise. For example, patients with COAD may be unable to maintain the exercise intensity calculated using only the heart rate guidelines, because they become short of breath.
- Commonly prescribed cardiac drugs considerably lower a patient's maximum heart rate (Pollock & Schmidt 1995), for example β-blocking medications.
- Patients with an irregular pulse need to count for an entire minute.
- Patients have to interrupt their exercise session to find and check their pulse.
- If the heart rate is fast, this makes it difficult to count every beat.
- Patients with poor perfusion to their fingers will have difficulty finding a strong radial pulse.
- Patients can become obsessive about counting their pulse during activities, possibly increasing anxiety amongst certain individuals.

Patient-perceived exertion In the 1970s, Gunner Borg discovered that subjective perception of effort or exertion could be used to predict heart rate during a graded exercise test. He developed a visual analogue scale from 6 to 20 used to describe the intensity of effort being put into an activity (see Box 7.1). This has been tested extensively using both normal individuals and cardiac patients. A rating of perceived exertion (RPE) of 12–13 has been found to be highly correlated to 60% HRmax, while an RPE of 16 corresponds to 85% HRmax (Birk & Birk 1987). Consequently, most individuals will achieve a training effect by exercising at a 'somewhat hard' level (RPE 12–13).

At the onset of an exercise programme, individuals can be instructed to exercise at a specified heart rate and to self-monitor the RPE at that intensity. Once they have learned to recognize the feeling that arises when the exercise intensity is at the right level then there is no need for them to stop exercising

■ Box 7.1   Rating of perceived exertion (RPE) scale

6	
7	Very, very light
8	
9	Very light
10	
11	Fairly light
12	
13	Somewhat hard
14	
15	Hard
16	
17	Very hard
18	
19	Very, very hard
20	

in order to check their pulse. RPE can be successfully used by patients who have difficulty checking their own pulse accurately, in patients taking β-blockers and after heart and heart lung transplant. It should be remembered, however, that a small percentage of individuals cannot use the scale with any accuracy and instead tend to select unrealistic RPE scores (Hall 1993).

Breathlessness 'Sing–talk–gasp' (Hall 1993). This is probably the simplest yet most effective means of teaching exercise participants the skills of self-monitoring. If they are able to sing as they exercise, then the intensity should be increased. If they do not have enough breath to sing yet are still able to talk in sentences as they exercise, then they are achieving the correct intensity. If they are unable to talk in sentences and are gasping for breath, they are working at too high an intensity and need to decrease the pace at which they are exercising.

METs Metabolic equivalents (METs) are the unit of measurement used to describe the oxygen costs of an activity. One MET equals the oxygen costs of resting metabolism.

$$1 \text{ MET} = VO_2 \text{ at rest} = 3.5 \text{ ml/kg/min}$$

MET values for common leisure activities are listed in Table 7.1. Once a person's peak MET is known, then a mode of exercise equivalent to approximately 65% of that can be selected. A person's peak MET is usually reported in the exercise tolerance test results.

For example, a person with a maximum MET of 5 should choose an activity from the tables that corresponds to an MET of around 3. This would include activities such as walking (3 mph), leisurely cycling and ballroom dancing. If on the other hand a person's MET was 10, then he or she should

Table 7.1 Estimated energy requirements of selected activities (Fletcher et al 1990)

Activity	METs	Activity	METs
Light intensity		Mowing the lawn	3.0
Baking	2.0	(power mower)	
Billiards	2.4	Playing drums	3.8
Bookbinding	2.2	Sailing	3.0
Canoeing (leisurely)	2.5	Swimming (slowly)	4.5
Conducting an orchestra	2.2	Walking (3 m.p.h.)	3.3
Ballroom dancing	2.9	Walking (4 m.p.h.)	4.5
Golf (with cart)	2.5		
Horseback riding (walking)	2.3	**Vigorous intensity**	
Playing a musical instrument:		Badminton	5.5
accordion	1.8	Chopping wood	4.9
cello	2.3	Climbing hills (no load)	6.9
flute	2.0	Climbing hills (with 5-kg load)	7.4
horn	1.7	Cycling (moderately)	5.7
piano	2.3	Dancing (aerobic or ballet)	6.0
trumpet	1.8	Dancing (ballroom or square)	5.5
violin	2.6	Field hockey	7.7
woodwind	1.8	Ice skating	5.5
Volleyball (non-competitive)	2.9	Jogging (10-minute mile)	10.2
Walking (2 m.p.h.)	2.5	Karate or judo	6.5
Writing	1.7	Roller-skating	6.5
		Rope-skipping	12.0
Moderate intensity		Skiing (water or downhill)	6.8
Callisthenics (no weights)	4.0	Squash	12.1
Croquet	3.0	Surfing	6.0
Cycling (leisurely)	3.5	Swimming (fast)	7.0
Gardening (no lifting)	4.4	Tennis (doubles)	6.0
Golf (without cart)	4.9		

NB These activities can often be done at variable intensities, assume that the intensity in each case is not excessive and that the courses are flat (no hills) unless otherwise specified.

select from activities corresponding to 6–7 METs (e.g. badminton, water-skiing and fast swimming).

A disadvantage of the MET system is that it does not make any allowance for environmental factors or differing skill levels.

Time

The conditioning period (exclusive of a warm-up and a cool-down) should progress up to 20 minutes.

Sedentary individuals and those with known pathologies should be guided towards lower intensity, longer duration exercise. To begin with, they will be unable to exercise for long (e.g. 10 minutes) at the desired intensity. The emphasis should then be on increasing the exercise duration as opposed to increasing the exercise intensity. In other words, as fitness improves, the duration of the conditioning part of the exercise should be increased in 5-minute increments, with the duration of the warm-up and cool-down remaining constant.

An exercise training session which lasts longer than an hour is more likely to provoke musculoskeletal overuse injury.

Warm-up The warm-up is the preparatory phase of an exercise session and has an important role in reducing the risks of musculoskeletal injury and cardiovascular complications. In its simplest form, a warm-up would involve performing the prescribed exercise at a much lower intensity (e.g. slow walking, pedalling without any resistance, etc.).

A typical warm-up for a cardiac population lasts 15 minutes (dependent on the intensity of the exercise to follow) and should include the following elements:

- range of movement/mobilizing exercises for the main joints
- low-intensity aerobic exercise to allow the cardiovascular system to accommodate the increased demands being placed upon it
- static muscle stretches
- skill rehearsal (practice of any co-ordinated patterns of movement used during conditioning period).

One of the major purposes of the warm-up is to prepare the cardiovascular system for the physical exertion ahead. If individuals attempt strenuous exercise without having warmed up, then their heart rate will rise rapidly in response to the sudden increase in demand. This in turn causes a sudden and large increase in the myocardial oxygen demands, predisposing the individual to arrhythmias and/or ischaemia.

A warm-up allows more time for the selective redistribution of the body's cardiac output (see p. 190). Without this, the muscles are forced to work anaerobically, leading to a build-up of lactic acid. This then causes the muscles to fatigue at a workload or level that they might otherwise have been capable of sustaining.

As the name suggests, a warm-up slowly elevates the temperature of the body as a whole and in particular the temperature of the muscles. This increase in temperature reduces the viscosity of the muscles so that they contract more efficiently. Warm muscles, ligaments and tendons are able to lengthen more readily when stretched. This greatly reduces the likelihood of sprained muscles and other musculoskeletal injuries.

Cool-down When the training portion of the exercise session ends, it is important not to stop abruptly but to gradually reduce the level of activity before stopping. A cool-down is therefore described as the period of lower intensity exercise at the end of an exercise session. The structure of a cool-down is essentially the reverse of the warm-up. There are several reasons why a cool-down is important.

• During exercise, venous blood is assisted in its return to the heart by the action of the skeletal muscles wrapped around the veins. If a person suddenly stops exercising (particularly if the body is in an upright posture), then without the muscle pump to maintain venous return, blood begins to pool in the extremities. This can lead to postexercise hypotension, resulting in fainting or the unpleasant symptoms of light-headedness and dizziness.

- Even though the exercise is over, the active skeletal muscles still need a large supply of oxygenated blood to replenish their energy reserves. If the heart's stroke volume is less because of the smaller venous return, then the heart rate has to remain elevated in order to maintain the cardiac output (cardiac output = stroke volume × heart rate). This means that myocardial oxygen consumption continues to rise even though the person has stopped exercising.

- Maintaining an adequate blood flow to the skeletal muscles into the recovery period enhances the removal of the waste products of metabolism (e.g. lactic acid) which may have accumulated during exercise. These waste products have been blamed for much of the muscle soreness that develops following exercise.

Continuous versus interval training methods As the name suggests, during continuous exercise, after a warm-up, the level of exercise is maintained at a steady intensity for the duration of the training period. The session is completed by a cool-down period before stopping.

However, untrained individuals are usually unable to sustain such an intensity for the desired period of time. During interval training, there is the usual warm-up and cool-down but the training period is interspersed with short periods of lower intensity exercise (active recovery). Thus interval training allows unfit individuals to complete the desired duration at their prescribed intensity.

Type of exercise

When recommending the type of exercise a person should do to improve his or her fitness and stamina, the following factors need to be considered.

- The activity should involve isotonic rhythmic movement of as large a number of different muscle groups as possible. This then utilizes aerobic pathways and places a demand on the oxygen transport system.
- The activity should be of sufficient intensity to cause the heart and respiratory rate to rise.
- The activity should be one that the person is capable of continuing for 10–30 minutes at a time.
- The activity should require minimal skill levels to reduce the person's likelihood of injury.
- The participant should find the activity enjoyable. This makes the exercise programme easier to comply with.
- If special facilities/equipment are needed, then these should be readily accessible and affordable.

Exercise progression

Progression should be made by adjusting the frequency and the duration. It is usual to build up tolerance by increasing the frequency of the exercise sessions, then the duration. For safety reasons, the exercise intensity should

Table 7.2 Suggested guidelines for exercise prescription – unsupervised exercise

	Frequency	Intensity		Time (minutes)
		%HRmax	RPE	
Healthy, active adults	2–4/week	75–85%	14–16	30–40
Healthy, sedentary adults	3–5/week	65–80%	12–14	20–30
Asymptomatic adults with two or more risk factors	3–5/week	60–75%	12–13	20–30
Chronic stable angina pectoris	Twice daily	10 beats below ischaemic threshold	10–11	5–10
Within first 2 months after uncomplicated MI or CABG	Once daily	40–55%	10–11	15–20
2 months following uncomplicated MI or CABG	4–6/week	60–75%	12–13	20–30

remain constant. Table 7.2 shows the recommended exercise prescription for differing patient populations. If the exercise intensity is controlled using the METs system already discussed, then as the person's fitness improves, the same exercise may no longer be equivalent to a 'moderate' intensity.

For example, people with a functional capacity of 5 METs would initially select an activity equal to around 3 METs, e.g. walking at 3 mph. As they became fitter, their functional capacity would improve, say to 7 METs. If, however, they continued to choose walking at 3 mph as their training method, then instead of exercising at 60% of their maximum, they would only be exercising at 40% of their functional capacity. If, however, exercise intensity is guided by heart rate or perceived exertion levels, then individuals would be automatically adjusting the amount of exercise they were doing in order to stay within their training zone.

Exercise safety

Contraindications to exercise Contraindications to exercise listed by the ACSM (2000) include:

- unstable angina
- resting systolic blood pressure >200 mmHg
- resting diastolic blood pressure >110 mmHg
- symptomatic orthostatic blood pressure drop of >20 mmHg
- critical aortic stenosis
- acute systemic illness or fever
- uncontrolled atrial or ventricular arrhythmias
- resting sinus tachycardia >120 bpm
- uncompensated congestive heart failure
- third-degree AV heart block
- active pericarditis or myocarditis

- recent embolism
- thrombophlebitis
- resting ST segment displacement (>2 mm)
- uncontrolled diabetes.

Injuries (both musculoskeletal and cardiovascular) resulting from exercise are generally avoidable. Exercise participants must be made aware of and understand the risks associated with non-compliance with their individual exercise prescription. It is important to recognize and address any exercise misconceptions (e.g. 'no pain – no gain') which may place an individual at unnecessary risk.

The incidence of serious adverse events during supervised outpatient cardiac rehabilitation exercise training has been estimated to be 1 in 60 000 participant-hours (Fletcher et al 2001).

Exercise testing should be used to screen out high-risk individuals. Such individuals usually require further medical or surgical intervention and should therefore be guided to a supervised low-intensity, low-duration, high-frequency exercise plan.

During an exercise test, specific indicators of a poor clinical status are:

- decrease in systolic blood pressure during exercise testing or failure of systolic blood pressure to rise despite increasing workload
- exercise test terminated at a low workload because of myocardial ischaemia (>2 mm ST depression)
- appearance of serious ventricular arrhythmias.

Other clinical markers of high-risk status include:

- a myocardial infarction complicated by congestive heart failure, cardiogenic shock and/or complex ventricular arrhythmias
- multiple myocardial infarctions
- impaired ventricular function (i.e. ejection fraction <25%)
- angiographic evidence of significant (>75%) occlusions in the left main or left anterior descending coronary arteries
- an unpredictable pattern of angina.

Cardiovascular complications are more prevalent during vigorous or competitive exercise when warning symptoms such as feeling unwell, dizziness, chest pain and breathlessness are ignored. Patients should therefore be encouraged to report any change in their typical cardiac symptoms (e.g. increasing frequency of angina during activities of daily living or failure of quick-acting nitrates to relieve angina once it has developed) and should be reminded not to exercise if they have forgotten to take their usual medications. Isometric exercise or activities that involve a large isometric component should be discouraged for the reasons previously discussed.

Participants should not exercise within 2 hours of eating a meal, otherwise blood flow is diverted away from the gut and the digestive process is hindered. Cardiac patients should be advised on how to gradually warm up prior to exercise (at least 15 minutes) and then how to cool down prior to stopping, thus reducing the risk of serious cardiovascular complications.

Orthopaedic problems may be either chronic overuse injuries such as shin splints, caused by repetitive trauma, or acute injuries such as sprained ligaments caused by sudden excessive overloading of the soft tissues. Most are the result of inadequate warm-up, unaccustomed vigorous exercise or poor technique. Patients with known orthopaedic problems should be guided towards lower impact exercise which causes less stress on the bones and joints.

Resistance training Most household, recreational and occupational activities require equal, if not greater, upper body strength than cardiovascular fitness. Increasing evidence now points to the value of light upper body resistance training to complement an aerobic training programme for cardiac patients. It is important to point out that these strengthening programmes emphasize isotonic muscle work using high repetitions of light weights. Isometric muscle work should be minimized. There is a risk that patients with evidence of myocardial ischaemia and/or poor ventricular function could develop wall motion abnormalities or ventricular arrhythmias during resistance training (ACSM 2000).

METHODS OF MEASURING EXERCISE TOLERANCE

An accurate knowledge of a person's aerobic exercise capacity is needed in order to give appropriate exercise advice. This can be obtained subjectively by using a questionnaire such as those shown in Boxes 7.2 and 7.3.

To obtain a 'gold standard' measurement of a person's aerobic capacity, a graded exercise test should be done with ECG and blood pressure monitoring. The most commonly used treadmill test is the Bruce Protocol that involves an increase in both treadmill speed and gradient every 3 minutes. This test is often criticized because the first stage is often too hard for unfit patients (starting speed 1.7 mph and an uphill gradient of 10%) and there is a relatively large increase in workload from one stage to the next. For cardiac patients, a modified Bruce Protocol is used. This has two preliminary stages and therefore starts at a lower intensity. Detailed description of this and various other protocols for exercise testing can be found elsewhere (Fletcher et al 2001).

Clinically, it is usually not feasible for all patients to undergo such a test in which case, for uncomplicated low-risk patients (providing there are no contraindications), 'field' tests can be used without the need for ECG monitoring and direct medical supervision.

The 6-minute walking test is the simplest type of maximal exercise test which does not necessitate the use of laboratory equipment. For this test patients are instructed to walk up and down a 10-metre course, aiming to cover as much ground as possible in the time permitted. The examiner then records the distance covered. A criticism of this test is that because it is self-paced, it is subject to patients' motivation and as such is open to bias.

■ **BOX 7.2   Duke activity scale index (DASI) (Hlaty et al 1989)**

Can you?

1. Take care of yourself, i.e. eating, dressing, bathing or using the toilet.	2.75
2. Walk indoors, such as around your house.	1.75
3. Walk a block or two on level ground.	2.75
4. Climb a flight of stairs or walk up a slope.	5.50
5. Run a short distance.	8.00
6. Do light work around the house – dusting, washing dishes.	2.70
7. Do moderate work around the house – vacuuming, sweeping floors, carrying in groceries.	3.50
8. Do heavy work around the house – scrubbing floors, lifting/moving furniture.	8.00
9. Do yard work – raking leaves, weeding, pushing a power mower.	4.50
10. Have sexual relations.	5.20
11. Participate in moderate recreational activities – golf, bowling, dancing, doubles tennis.	6.00
12. Participate in strenuous sports – swimming, singles tennis, football, basketball, skipping.	7.50

DASI = sum of weights for 'yes' replies

$VO_2max = DASI + 9.6 \times 0.43$

On the other hand, the 12-minute shuttle-walking test is a reproducible test that is easy to implement (Singh et al 1992).

For some health professionals, it may not be possible to carry out an objective measurement of physical fitness. In this case patient questionnaires such as the Duke Activity Status Index (Hlaty et al 1989) can be used to estimate functional capacity.

BARRIERS TO THE UPTAKE OF REGULAR EXERCISE

Iliffe et al (1994) remind us that exercise initiatives seem to influence those who would have taken up exercise anyway, the so-called 'worried well'. One of the problems of leading a sedentary lifestyle is that such people rarely place significant demands on their cardiovascular system. Consequently, they have little idea of their true level of fitness and as such have no incentive to improve it. Fitness assessments are one way of motivating individuals to take part in regular aerobic exercise, particularly if they know subsequent retesting is to be carried out. If the person is being expected

■ BOX 7.3   Physical activity index

I avoid walking if I can and prefer to drive/get a lift/use public transport.	0
I occasionally walk instead of driving/getting a lift/using public transport.	1
I go for short easy walks (<15 min) at least three to four times a week.	2
I go for short easy walks (<15 min) at least five to six times a week.	3
I go for 10- to 15-minute brisk walks at least three to four times a week.	3
I use the stairs every day for exercise.	4
I go for 10- to 15-minute brisk walks at least five or more times a week.	4
I go for 15- to 30-minute brisk walks at least three to four times a week.	5
I go for 15- to 30-minute brisk walks at least five or more times a week.	6
I participate in recreational activities of moderate intensity*	
− once or twice a week	6
− three to four times a week	7
− five or more times a week	8
I participate in recreational activities of vigorous intensiy[†]	
− once or twice a week	8
− three to four times a week	9
− five or more times a week	10

*Moderate intensity = within individual's exercise capacity − breathing faster than normal but able to sustain comfortably

[†]Vigorous intensity = intense enough to represent a substantial challenge to the person's cardiovascular system

to carry out an exercise programme unsupervised, regular contact with the health-care professional is essential. This can vary from regular telephone contact to getting the person to complete a weekly exercise diary. Feedback and encouragement are essential for giving patients confidence that they can change. Pollock & Schmidt (1995) remind us that drop-out from supervised rehabilitation does not automatically mean that the desired behavioural changes are not being maintained. All too often the reason for non-attendance is unknown (Horgan et al 1992). Finding out the reasons for drop-out is crucial.

Membership of health clubs and sports facilities can be outwith the budgets of many patients. Local authorities often have a discount scheme for those who are retired, unemployed, disabled or on a low income. Another reason people give up an exercise programme is that the goals and expectations they were given were unrealistic. Patients who expect sudden, major changes in their health will become discouraged when they fail to see an immediate improvement. In fact, the benefits of secondary prevention may not be evident until 3 or more years after MI (Pollock & Schmidt 1995). Unrealistic goals should be discouraged (for example, a previously inactive 50-year-old taking up rock climbing as a hobby).

It is essential to obtain accurate baseline measures of a person's current physical capacity, so that the intensity can be set at the right level.

The ideal situation is initially to have the patient undergo a graded exercise test, the results of which can be used to set exercise intensity. Relying on subjective information can be misleading. If open questioning is used, most people tend to overestimate their physical abilities. Exercise scales such as those shown in Boxes 7.2 and 7.3 will give more objective data.

Exercise adherence is highest amongst those who have an individualized exercise programme. This means taking time to find out factors such as the person's likes and dislikes and his or her ease of access to facilities. Information about the existence and location of various organized exercise groups should be prominently displayed. Consideration should be given not only to the mode of exercise, but to the duration and frequency expected. Despite the fact that swimming is known to be a good aerobic exercise, if the swimming pool is not within easy travelling distance then compliance will be much lower. Campbell et al (1994), on examining the attitudes of postmyocardial infarction patients to cardiac rehabilitation, found that the greatest influence foreseen on attendance was the travelling distance involved. Another reason may be that the exercise is perceived as boring or unexciting.

One example of a highly successful strategy is that employed by general practitioners in Hailsham (Jelley 1993). Here, GPs can prescribe exercise in much the same way as medication. Patients then take their prescription to their local leisure centre and can then attend for a 10-week supervised programme of exercise.

The more complex the behavioural change needed, the harder it is to achieve long-term compliance. Most cardiac patients need to alter several habits. It is essential to introduce change gradually in a positive and realistic manner.

Cardiac patients are often presented with a list of don'ts. It is helpful to reinforce the idea that exercise is a positive step as opposed to being told to refrain from a behaviour perceived as enjoyable. Newton et al (1991) found that exercisers showed much better psychosocial adjustment after MI, confirming the benefits of exercise in restoring self-esteem.

Increasing exercise may not be the first priority in which case, it is better to try to encourage exercise as part of the normal way of life. Simple changes such as taking the stairs rather than waiting for the lift or elevator or getting off the bus one or two stops early and walking the rest of the way soon have a cumulative effect. Equally as important is enlisting the active support of spouses, partners and families. Age should not be a barrier to exercise, since it has the potential not only to enhance a person's well-being but also to decrease the morbidity and mortality of those over 65 (Pescatello & DiPietro 1993).

The link between inactivity and heart disease needs to be clearly established in the patient's mind. Otherwise their exercise habits are very difficult to change. The health professional's role lies not only in providing education on the health-related benefits of regular exercise and how to realize these safely and effectively but in being a source of example and motivation.

■ KEY POINTS

- Numerous studies indicate that regular physical activity reduces cardiovascular morbidity and mortality.
- The health-related benefits of regular exercise make it an important strategy in the primary and secondary prevention of CHD.
- Seventy percent of the adult population in the UK do not take enough exercise. If exercise is to maintain its beneficial effects it must be habitual. Fitness cannot be stored. What counts most is current exercise. Athleticism in youth does not confer any additional protection against coronary heart disease in later life.
- Moderate exercise is just as cardioprotective as vigorous exercise.
- The incidence of musculoskeletal and cardiovascular complications is greatest during vigorous activity and competitive exercise.
- Before embarking on an exercise programme, medical clearance should be obtained from the person's GP.
- The exercise prescription should be individualized. Parameters such as type, intensity, duration and frequency should be specified.
- Set realistic exercise objectives.
- To improve cardiovascular fitness an exercise session should be composed of a warm-up, cardiovascular endurance training then a cool-down.
- With all forms of exercise, it is advisable to begin at a relatively easy level and gradually progress as able.

■ PRACTICAL EXERCISE

Identify the cardiac rehabilitation programmes running in your area. How are patients encouraged to keep physically active once they are discharged from the programme? What can you do to promote a physical, activity lifestyle for your patients?

REFERENCES

Allied Dunbar, Health Education Authority, Sports Council 1992 Allied Dunbar National Fitness Survey: a report on activity patterns and fitness levels. Main findings and summary document. Sports Council, Health Education Authority, London

American College of Sports Medicine (ACSM) 1998 The recommended quantity and quality of exercise for developing and maintaining cardiorespiratory and muscular fitness, and flexibility in healthy adults. Medicine and Science in Sports and Exercise 30(6): 975–991

American College of Sports Medicine (ACSM) 2000 Guidelines for exercise testing and prescription, 5th edn. Lea & Febiger, Philadelphia

Balady GJ 1993 Types of exercise. Arm–leg and static–dynamic. Cardiology Clinics 11(2): 297–308

Bhopal R, Unwin N 1995 Cycling, physical exercise and the Millennium Fund. British Medical Journal 311(7001): 344

Birk TJ, Birk C 1987 Use of ratings of perceived exertion for exercise prescription. Sports Medicine 4: 1–8

Blair SN, Kampert JB, Kohl HW 3rd et al 1996 Influences of cardiorespiratory fitness and other precursors on cardiovascular disease and all cause mortality in men and women. Journal of the American Medical Association 276: 205–210

Blamey A, Mutrie N, Aitchison T 1995 Health promotion by encouraged use of stairs. British Medical Journal 311(7000): 289–290

British Heart Foundation 2002 Coronary heart disease statistics. www.dphpc.ox.ac.uk/bhfhprg/stats/2000/2002/physicalactivity.html

Brodie D, Liu X, Bundred P et al 1998 Age-related heart rate thresholds to optimize aerobic training in cardiac rehabilitation. Coronary Health Care 2(1): 11–16

Campbell RM, Grimshaw J, Rawles J et al 1994 Cardiac rehabilitation: the agenda set by post myocardial infarction patients. Health Education Journal 53: 409–420

DeBusk RF 1990 Training effects of long versus short bouts of exercise in healthy subjects. American Journal of Cardiology 65: 1010–1013

Department of Health 1999 Health survey for England 1998. Stationery Office, London

Department of Health 2001 Exercise referral systems: a national quality assurance framework. www.doh.gov.uk/exercisereferrals/

Fletcher G, Balady G, Amsterdam E et al 2001 Exercise standards for testing and training: a statement for healthcare professionals from the American Heart Association. Circulation 104(14): 1694–1740

Hall LK 1993 Developing and managing cardiac rehabilitation programs. Human Kinetics, Champaign, IL

Health Education Board for Scotland (HEBS) 1997 Strategic statement on promotion of physical activity in Scotland. Health Education Board for Scotland, Edinburgh

Hlaty M, Boineau R, Higginbotham M et al 1989 A brief, self administered questionnaire to determine functional capacity. The Duke Activity Index. American Journal of Cardiology 64: 651–654

Horgan J, Bethen H, Carson P et al 1992 Working party report on cardiac rehabilitation. British Heart Journal 67: 412–418

Iliffe S, Tai S, Gould M et al 1994 Prescribing exercise in general practice. Look before you leap. British Medical Journal 309: 494–495

Jelley S 1993 Prescription for health. Healthline 1: 18–19

Joliffe JA, Rees K, Taylor R et al 2000 Exercise based rehabilitation for coronary heart disease (Cochrane Review). Cochrane Library, Issue 4. Update Software

Lee IM, Paffenburger RS 2000 Associations of light, moderate and vigorous intensity physical activity with longevity: the Harvard Alumni Health Study. American Journal of Epidemiology 151: 293–299

Leon AS 1997 Physical activity and cardiovascular health. Human Kinetics, Champaign, IL

Murphy M, Hardman A 1998 Training effects of short and long bouts of brisk walking in sedentary women. Medicine and Science in Sports and Exercise 30(1): 152–157

Murphy M, Nevill A, Hardman A 2000 Different patterns of brisk walking are equally effective in decreasing postprandial lipaemia. International Journal of Obesity and Related Metabolic Disorders 24(10): 1303–1309

Newton M, Mutrie N, McArthur J 1991 The effects of exercise in a coronary rehabilitation programme. Scottish Medical Journal 36: 38–41

O'Connor GT, Buring JE, Yusuf S et al 1989 An overview of randomized trials of rehabilitation with exercise after myocardial infarction. Circulation 80: 234–244

Oldridge NB, Guyatt GH, Fischer ME et al 1988 Cardiac rehabilitation after myocardial infarction. Combined experience of randomized clinical trials. Journal of the American Medical Association 260(7): 945–950

Pate RR, Pratt M, Blair SN 1995 Physical activity and public health: a recommendation from the Centers for Disease Control and Prevention and the American College of Sports Medicine. Journal of the American Medical Association 273(5): 402–407

Pescatello LS, DiPietro L 1993 Physical activity in older adults. An overview of health benefits. Sports Medicine 15(6): 353–364

Pollock ML, Schmidt DH 1995 Heart disease and rehabilitation, 3rd edn. Human Kinetics, Champaign, IL

Singh SJ, Morgan M, Scott S et al 1992 Development of a shuttle walking test of disability in patients with chronic airways obstruction. Thorax 47: 1019–1024

Uren NG, Lipkin DP 1992 Exercise training as therapy for chronic heart failure. British Heart Journal 67: 430–433

FURTHER READING

British Heart Foundation and the National Primary Care Facilitation Programme 2001
 Physical activity toolkit. A training pack for healthcare teams. Details on how to obtain a
 copy are available on: www.bhf.org.uk/publications

Booklets and leaflets – a full range should be available from the health promotion
 department of your local health board.

USEFUL ADDRESSES

Association of Chartered Physiotherapists in Cardiac Rehabilitation
Chartered Society of Physiotherapy
14 Bedford Row
London WC1R 4ED
Tel: 020 7306 6666

British Association for Cardiac Rehabilitation
c/o British Cardiac Society
9 Fitzroy Square
London W1T 5HW
Tel: 020 7692 5413

Chest, Heart and Stroke Northern Ireland
21 Dublin Road
Belfast BT2 7HB
Tel: 028 9032 0184

Chest, Heart and Stroke Scotland
5 North Castle Street
Edinburgh EH2 3LT
Tel: 0131 225 6963

Health Development Agency
Holborn Gate
330 High Holborn
London WC1V 7BA
Tel: 020 7430 0850

Health Education Board for Scotland
Woodburn House
Canaan Lane
Edinburgh EH10 4SG
Tel: 0131 536 5500

Health Promotion Agency for Northern Ireland
18 Ormeau Avenue
Belfast BT2 8HS
Tel: 028 9031 1611

Health Promotion and Public Health Strategy Divisions
National Assembly for Wales
Cathays Park
Cardiff CF10 3NQ
Tel: 029 2068 1245

Lifestyle management: facilitating behavioural change

Paul Bennett

8

INTRODUCTION

Coronary heart disease (CHD) is dependent, to a large extent, on our behaviour and our psychological circumstances. Cigarette smoking, dietary behaviour, exercise levels and the prevalence and impact of psychological stress are considered key behavioural risks. Major health promotion initiatives have attempted to bring about appropriate behavioural change through programmes targeted at large populations. Increasingly common, however, are programmes targeted at changing the behaviour of individuals identified through screening as being at risk (e.g. OXCHECK Study Group 1994).

This chapter will provide a brief overview of some of the processes thought to determine health-related behaviours. It will then examine how these, and a few relatively simple counselling methods, may help promote behavioural change. Space limitations mean that the issues and methods introduced here cannot be considered in great depth. A list of suggested reading, in which they are described in greater detail, is provided at the end of the chapter.

MODELS OF HEALTH BEHAVIOUR

Human behaviour is complex and difficult to predict. Decisions are frequently a response to chance events and apparently random thought processes. Nevertheless, a number of models of behavioural decision making have been developed. None pretends to be all encompassing. Rather, they try to provide a basic understanding of at least some of the processes underlying our behaviour. Some of these models are described below. More complex models exist, but this section does not aspire to providing a text on psychology and human decision making. Rather, it seeks to identify the basic processes to be considered when counselling behavioural change, particularly in relation to behaviours implicated in CHD.

Health Belief Model

The Health Belief Model (Becker 1974) suggests that the likelihood of individuals engaging in a particular health-related behaviour is a function of their perceptions of the relationship between that behaviour and an illness, their perceived susceptibility to that illness, its seriousness and the particular costs and benefits involved in engaging in any behaviour. The costs may be social, financial, physical, and so on. Factors influencing adherence to antihypertensive medication, for example, may include the perceived health benefits (often not immediately obvious), the hassle of remembering to take medication and concerns about side-effects and the long-term use of medication. A final influence on the uptake of any behaviour is the presence of cues to action. These may take the form of a reminder to engage in some form of action, including such things as health checks, reminders from doctors on routine visits, and so on.

Although we may ultimately wish to optimize our health, whether or not we engage in health-promoting behaviours is as much, if not more, governed by short-term costs and benefits than by longer term possible health outcomes. An individual may consider adopting a low-fat diet to reduce his or her risk of CHD, but be beset by more immediate problems. Their family may not wish to change their diet, they may have to learn new cooking methods, eat less favoured foods, perhaps even increase the cost of their shopping. These short-term costs may override the benefits of potential long-term health gains and prevent appropriate behavioural change. Research conducted with working-class mothers who smoke affords a further example (e.g. Jacobson 1981). Many such women chose to smoke cigarettes in the full knowledge of the associated health risks. Those that did frequently reported that smoking helped them cope with adverse life conditions and that they would be less able to cope with their responsibilities towards their family if they stopped smoking. To promote change in this group of women would clearly involve more than simple advice on the health risks of smoking.

Stage of change

A frequent assumption made in counselling is that the person receiving advice or counselling is willing and able to make use of any information given. This, clearly, is not always the case: people differ over time in their willingness to consider or adopt change. One of the first models to appreciate this was developed by Prochaska & DiClemente (1984). Their model was particularly useful as it identified both the process of change and the counselling strategies most likely to move people toward behavioural change.

Prochaska & DiClemente identified five stages of change. The first stage is known as precontemplation. Here, little or no thought is given to adopting a new behaviour: most smokers, for example, at any one time are not actively considering stopping smoking. The next stage is known as contemplation, in which the individual begins to consider changing his or her behaviour. The movement from precontemplation to contemplation may result from an individual developing a chest infection, hearing of the illness of a fellow smoker, and so on. Reaching this stage does not, however, guarantee behavioural change and people can still slip back to the precontemplation stage (for example, when they recover from illness), and frequently do. However, some may move to a more active consideration of change even achieving behavioural change. The stages of active consideration and achievement of change are referred to as the 'planning' and 'action' stages. The final stage is one of consolidation and maintenance of any behavioural change. However, a frequent risk at this stage is that the person relapses to the contemplation or even precontemplation stage.

In any counselling process it is important that the counsellor be aware of what stage the client is at. Providing strategies for smoking cessation to a smoker at the precontemplation stage is likely to be ineffective. Rather, strategies should seek to shift the smoker into the contemplation or even planning stage. There is good evidence that such a shift is rarely achieved through direct attempts at persuasion, which often harden attitudes rather than change them (whatever the person may say at the time of interview). However, a technique known as motivational interviewing, described later in the chapter, may be of use here.

Social cognitive theory

A basic tenet of social cognitive theory (Bandura 1986) is that behaviour is guided by its expected consequences. The more positive these are, the more likely one is to engage in any particular behaviour. That said, many behaviours persist when what may seem to be negative health consequences are likely to follow. One reason for this is that in general, short-term rewards are more salient than long-term probabilistic health gains: the individual on a diet may all too frequently give in to the immediate gratification of a cream bun rather than achieving the more distant goal of losing weight.

A second important aspect of social cognitive theory is known as self-efficacy. This refers to a person's confidence in his or her ability to carry out an action or achieve a particular goal. People are unlikely to attempt change if they do not think they will succeed in doing so. This has powerful implications for counselling. First of all, it suggests that any suggested behavioural change must lie within the perceived capabilities of the individual: change may sometimes need to be made in gradual stages if necessary. Secondly, it cautions against decisions concerning behavioural change being determined by epidemiological considerations alone. For example, if an individual carries several risk factors for CHD, including smoking, poor diet and lack of exercise, it may be tempting to first try to address the most 'risky' behaviour, in this case probably smoking. However, if the person does not believe he can quit smoking, his consequent lack of success may make him reluctant to try to change other 'risky' behaviours.

Theory of planned behaviour

Throughout much of the 1950s and 1960s psychologists and others assumed that individuals' attitudes were the primary determinants of their behaviour and that to change behaviour simply required changing attitudes. Smokers, for example, were assumed to smoke because they had a positive attitude towards smoking rather than because of addictive processes or social pressure. Unfortunately, attitudes rarely predict behaviour and a number of models have added further factors in attempts to be more predictive of behaviour. One of the most important of these is known as the theory of planned behaviour (Ajzen 1985). This assumes that the key determinant of behaviour is one's intention to behave in a certain way. Behavioural intentions are, in turn, derived from three broad influences: the individuals' attitudes to the behaviour, the attitudes they perceive others important to them as having (so-called social norms), and the 'availability' of the behaviour to them. Availability refers to whether or not individuals have access to a given behaviour, recognizing the economic, social and personal constraints that may exist. This model explains, at least in part, why people do not always behave in accordance with their attitudes. Some ex-smokers, for example, may have a number of negative attitudes towards smoking but smoke when with friends who smoke, as the social pressure they encounter may compete with their personal attitudes.

What the model does not address are findings that although attitudes, social norms and availability strongly predict intentions to behave in certain ways, intentions frequently do not predict behaviour. So marked is this failure of intentions that the phenomenon has become known as the behaviour–intention gap. What seems to predict behaviour is firstly an intention to behave, then the number and complexity of plans the individual makes in order to put that intention into practice (e.g. Gollwitzer 1999). Smokers are much more likely to quit smoking if they have thought through *how* they will quit smoking, deal with the difficulties of withdrawal, cravings to smoke, and so on, than if they try to quit without this forethought.

Comment

These models provide some understanding of the decision-making process related to health behaviours. None provides a complete account. Between them, however, they offer some insight into the processes which govern health-related decisions. However, they identify some key insights that should be borne in mind when helping people change. People are most likely to consider change when:

- the advantages of change outweigh the disadvantages
- they hold a positive attitude towards change
- they believe themselves capable of achieving any necessary change
- the social group of the individual is supportive of change.

Actually achieving change is most likely when:

- there is a strong intention to attempt change
- individuals believe they have the ability to put the plans into action
- they have developed plans of *how* to change
- the social support continues.

CHANGING BEHAVIOUR

The process of helping people change their behaviour can vary in complexity from simple provision of information to dealing with complex issues and adverse emotional responses to new health risk information. The approach that needs to be followed will be determined by, amongst other things, the length of time available for counselling, the characteristics of the individual being screened and the 'depth' to which the counsellor is prepared to explore issues relevant to the patient. The following section will examine three issues: motivating behavioural change; facilitating behavioural change through information giving; and helping people cope with the adverse emotional effects of receiving risk information.

Some basic skills

Whatever approach is adopted, some basic skills are necessary to involve people in the counselling process. A key predictor of adherence to recommended therapeutic regimens is an individual's level of satisfaction with his or her care. This in turn is strongly influenced by the quality of communication with professional staff. Good counselling depends on an appropriate relationship between therapist and client. At its most basic, this involves the therapist showing warmth towards the client, being able to understand the difficulties the client is facing from his perspective and reflecting this back to him (empathy) and being honest in their relationship (see Rogers 1961). Sufficient time should also be allocated to the consultation process and additional time identified if necessary. On a more pragmatic note, participants should sit at approximately right angles with no obstacles such as a desk in the way. This arrangement allows each person to see the other fully and to make and break eye contact as necessary. Direct face-to-face contact makes it difficult to look away and can be seen as confrontational. An open posture, sitting very slightly forward, emphasizes interest and listening.

Motivating behavioural change

There is a clear goal to screening: to identify and, where possible, change risk factors for CHD. However, it should not be assumed that all those attending screening are motivated and willing to do so. As the most appropriate intervention will differ according to the individual's level of motivation to change, it is useful to identify at what stage of change the person is in relation to each risk behaviour.

Where individuals are motivated to change risk behaviours, the counselling process should focus on developing strategies for change. If, however, the individual is in the precontemplation stage, the most appropriate intervention is to try and increase his motivation to change: to shift him through the stages of change. As previously noted, this is usually not best achieved through direct attempts at persuasion; this may only lead to increased resistance to change. An alternative approach to motivating change is known as motivational interviewing (Miller & Rollnick 2002).

The primary goal of the motivational interview is to encourage individuals to explore their own, perhaps conflicting, beliefs about and attitudes towards a particular behaviour and behavioural change. This process is thought to result in a state of cognitive dissonance: an aversive state that may result in individuals reconsidering their attitudes towards behavioural change. The process is deliberately non-confrontational and at its most basic provides the individual with the space to actively consider the benefits or disadvantages of his present behaviour or behavioural change.

A key strategy is to focus people's attention on both the 'good' and 'less good' aspects of the behaviour they may benefit from changing. By inviting people to consider both 'good' and 'less good' aspects of their behaviour, they may experience dissonance and begin to consider change, without the pressure resulting from more direct attempts at persuasion. In addition, the initial focus on the 'good things' about the individual's behaviour reduces threat or confrontation. Individuals can then be asked to identify the 'less good'. Open questioning techniques may facilitate exploration of these issues. Finally, the counsellor can summarize both good and less good aspects of the behaviour, so they are starkly identified.

- What are the good things about your (lack of exercise)?
- What are the less good things about your (lack of exercise)?
  - How does it affect you?
  - What don't you like about it?
- Summary of the information given, in 'your' language: e.g. 'So, not exercising gives you time to .... On the other hand, you ...'

Following this phase, it may be useful to ask whether the individual would like information about the issues raised in this discussion. The decision whether to offer information or not must depend on the individual's response to this enquiry. Some will make it clear that they are not interested: others may be neutral or willing to consider change.

Information exchange

To maximize the effectiveness of any information given, it is important that it is presented in a manner which makes it easy to understand and remember. Unfortunately, this is not always the case. When dealing with a variety of behaviours, advice is often presented piecemeal. Issues related to smoking are dealt with after taking a smoking history, dietary advice is given following discussion of eating habits, and so on. Such an approach necessarily interrupts the acquisition of information with discussion of new issues, interfering with memory and consideration of any information given. Accordingly, advice on behavioural change should generally be presented at the end of any screening interview. Some simple guidelines can ensure maximal impact of any information given. These are described by Nichols (1984), who identified three stages in the process of giving information:

- Initial check on the person's present level of knowledge
- Information provision
- Accuracy check: ensuring any information has been remembered and understood.

Information check

Before giving information it is important to find out what the person knows and what he or she wants to know. Unnecessary reiteration can thus be avoided and information pitched at a level consistent with the individual's present knowledge. It will also allow the counsellor to identify any misconceptions the person has about his or her risk or risk behaviours.

Information provision

The language used should be appropriate to the person to whom the information is being given. Jargon should be avoided: words and phrases that are routine to health-care workers may be totally alien to others. Equally, vague phrases, such as 'Your blood pressure is a little high', are best avoided. These frequently confuse and can lead to a misunderstanding of the nature of the problem.

Where a number of risk factors are identified, it may be best to focus on only one of them and to suggest that the person returns to discuss the others. In addition, it is important to identify which of any risk or preventive behaviours the person would like to know about. Basing the choice of information solely on epidemiological risk ('Your smoking is probably causing you the most risk for heart disease. Perhaps I could give you some advice on how to cut down …') is likely to be of little benefit. Asking people what they wish to know about is more likely to identify behaviours amenable to change. Once the areas of information have been chosen, a few rules of thumb may help effective information exchange.

- Do not overload people with information; if necessary, they can come back for more.
- Information should be given clearly in short and simple sentences.
- The language used should mirror that of the person.
- Information should be given issue by issue, not as a jumble of related and unrelated information.
- Repetition increases memory – in the words of a famous researcher in interpersonal interaction: 'Tell 'em what you're going to tell 'em, tell 'em, tell 'em what you've told 'em'.

Some of these points are exemplified in the following dialogue between a practice nurse and a smoker with a high serum cholesterol level.

Nurse: As you know, we've found some things which increase your risk of having a heart attack. It's no news to you that you smoke, and you know this raises your risk. But you didn't know that your cholesterol levels were high. If you would like to reduce your risk of heart attack, it would be helpful to cut out your smoking and reduce your cholesterol levels. I wonder how you feel about doing either of these …

Mr J: Well, I've tried to stop smoking so many times. I know it's bad for me, but it's really difficult to stop. My cholesterol reading was a bit of a shock, though – perhaps I could have a go at changing that.

Nurse: OK; let's talk about how to reduce your cholesterol now. If you would like to look at some ways of cutting down smoking, perhaps we could do that another time. What do you think that you are eating or doing that is making your cholesterol levels high?

Later:

Nurse: From what you've told me, I think there are a number of things you could do to reduce your cholesterol levels. Firstly, you could cut down the amount of fatty meat you eat and eat more vegetables. Secondly, you could change how you cook some of your food. Finally, you could reduce the amount of crisps and chocolate you eat, perhaps by replacing them with a lower fat snack. Let's look at each of those in turn …

In this condensed and brief dialogue the nurse has gone through some of the key stages in appropriate advice giving. First of all, he identified what Mr J wanted advice on at present, while making it clear that advice on other issues could be given another time should Mr J wish it. He then explored Mr J's understanding of the causes of high cholesterol levels. Finally, at the end of this process, the nurse broke down the type of information to be given into three clear categories: cutting down fatty meat; changing cooking methods; changing snacks. This explicit categorization, followed by more detailed information on each issue, increases the likelihood that the information will be remembered.

Accuracy check

It is important to check explicitly that participants in the screening and advice process have understood any information given. If nothing else, such a check will serve to strengthen memory. It will also reduce the risk of inappropriate action arising from misunderstanding. Care must be taken not to patronize, but an accuracy check can be achieved with some subtlety by, for example, asking patients whether they have any questions, whether explanations were clear or which of any suggestions made they would find useful to try out.

The impact of adverse information

Although for the professionals involved, the identification of risk factors for CHD and facilitating appropriate change are routine procedures, some individuals will inevitably respond to information with alarm and anxiety. Indeed, one study found that over one third of people who had their cholesterol measured and were found to have 'safe' levels still reported significantly increased health anxieties many months after the screening procedure. Not surprisingly, then, the impact of receiving adverse health information can, in vulnerable individuals, result in significant anxiety.

The most immediate effect of this is that people may take little notice of information they are given. High levels of anxiety interfere with concentration and memory. In the longer term, anxiety may result in the individual feeling overwhelmed and not being able to make use of any advice given. Conversely, it may result in excessive and inappropriate behavioural change (see Case Study 8.1). Accordingly, it is important to reassure individuals that their risk may be reduced by appropriate behavioural or pharmacological change and to ensure that risk reduction information is given at a time when the individual is receptive to this, either later in a screening session or at a later appointment.

Having informed an individual of his or her risk, some pause in the counselling process may be advisable. To find out how the person feels, a simple question may suffice. If any factual concerns are expressed, these may be allayed by provision of information. If the person indicates more serious upset, time may be required to permit expression of any fears or anxieties. It is important at this stage that the person is made to feel that it is acceptable to express upset or concern.

Tempting as it may be, the goal of the counsellor is not to try to reassure inappropriately, but to allow the individual to talk about his or her feelings and emotions. Listening quietly may be the counsellor's only response at this stage. If concerns are felt, but not expressed, individuals may be too distracted by their own thoughts to process any information given. Only after a period in which anxieties are expressed may the individual be receptive to information concerning how they may reduce their risk for CHD.

■ CASE STUDY 8.1

Mr F was screened for CHD risk as part of a local screening programme. He was advised to cut down his saturated fat intake and to take more exercise in order to reduce his risk. Three months later he was seen by a dietitian in order to monitor his progress. Despite not being overweight at the time of initial counselling, in the 3 months following screening he had lost over 2 stones in weight. He looked haggard and his clothes were, almost literally, hanging off him. He told the dietitian that he had cut his fat intake drastically, through eating vegetables, salad and very little else. He was frightened to eat anything which he thought contained fat. His family were experiencing problems as they could not cope with the diet he had imposed on himself, and his wife was preparing his food separately from that for the rest of the family. He was exercising constantly and spent up to 2 hours a day exercising by riding his bicycle. He was also very anxious about his cholesterol and fretted about it on a daily basis. The changes he had made, while apparently complying with the advice given, were excessive and had resulted in his and his family's misery.

A PROBLEM-SOLVING APPROACH

While many individuals will require relatively simple advice, and act upon it appropriately, the advice necessary and how this may be implemented may not always be obvious. Consider the case of Mrs T (Case Study 8.2). The case history, while being perhaps somewhat unusual in its specifics, highlights a common problem resulting from inappropriate or casual advice giving.

The counselling process of Gerard Egan (1990) emphasizes the importance of appropriate analysis of the problem the individual is facing. Only when this has been achieved can an appropriate solution to the problem be identified. A further element of Egan's approach is that the job of the counsellor is not to act as an expert solving the person's problems once identified. Instead, their role is to mobilize the individual's own resources both to identify problems accurately and to arrive at strategies of solution. Counselling is problem oriented. It is focused specifically on the issues at hand and in the 'here and now'. Egan's model of counselling involves three phases:

- problem exploration and clarification
- goal setting
- facilitating action.

■ CASE STUDY 8.2

Mrs T, a 43-year-old obese woman, attended a screening programme for CHD risks conducted in her local GP's surgery. She was found not only to be significantly overweight, but also to have raised serum cholesterol levels. As a consequence she attended a clinic where she was seen by a dietitian. She was given advice on 'healthy eating' and a diet sheet and asked to come back in 1 month. When her weight and cholesterol levels were measured at this time, they were found to be unchanged: if anything, they had increased.

At this point the dietitian explored in depth some of the issues preventing change. Mrs T had a good understanding of what comprised a 'healthy' and 'unhealthy' diet and had been placed on similar diets to the one prescribed a number of times previously without any benefit. Further discussion revealed that the main reason for her eating excessively and consuming high-fat food was lack of support within her family. Her two sons, who had flats of their own but who used the family home much as a hotel, would frequently arrive home from the pub late at night and demand a 'fry-up'. She, reluctantly, accepted the role of provider and cooked their food, but found it difficult not to nibble while she did so. As a result, although she may have eaten carefully during the day, she frequently finished the day eating high-fat foods. Not only did this increase her calorific intake, it also reduced her motivation to diet the following day, as she saw herself as having 'ruined' her diet. This recurring process significantly eroded her motivation to diet over the long term. As a result of this problem exploration, Mrs T identified that the problem she was facing was not learning how to diet but how to stop cooking for her sons late at night. This then became the focus of future discussions.

Some people may not need to work through each stage of the counselling process. Others may be able to work through all the phases in one session. Yet others may require more than one session. However, it is important to deal with each stage sequentially and thoroughly. Flitting from stage to stage will serve only to confuse both the counsellor and the individual, while thoroughness will reduce the risk of identifying incorrect problems or solutions, as in the case of Mrs T.

Problem exploration and clarification

The goal of the first stage of counselling is to help the person identify the problems he or she is facing (or may face) in achieving change. The problem can be lack of information, in which case provision of information may be all that is required. However, individuals can face other problems. Some of these may surface immediately on receiving initial health information ('I'm not sure how I'm going to sort these dietary changes with my family') or later ('I don't know – I tried to carry out your advice on cutting down fat, but my weight still seems to be going up'). Responses of this sort should prompt further probing. The goal is to clarify *exactly* what problems the individual is facing: only then can appropriate problem-solving strategies be applied.

Some skills or strategies that are particularly pertinent to this stage of counselling are:

- direct questioning and prompts
- silence and minimal prompts
- empathic feedback.

The most obvious way of eliciting information is to ask direct questions. These should be open ended, in order to discourage one-word answers. Questions such as 'What do your family eat on a typical weekend?' are likely to elicit much more information than 'How often do your family eat green vegetables?'. A second approach similar to direct questioning is known as prompting. Here, requests for information take the form of prompts and probes: 'Tell me about …', 'Describe …'.

It is important to mix direct questioning with other techniques of encouraging the person to explore relevant issues. One such method involves the use of silence or minimal prompts ('uh-huh'). By its very nature, problem exploration leads individuals to consider matters they have not previously addressed. The process cannot be rushed and filling silences with new questions may interrupt their thoughts and impede the proper exploration of problems.

A further method of encouraging problem exploration is through the use of empathic feedback. Reflecting back to people an understanding of their situation or feelings through a simple phrase can be highly effective. Such feedback also serves to verify the counsellor's understanding.

Take the example of Mrs T.

Mrs T: Well it's disappointing that my cholesterol levels haven't changed, but I really have no willpower. As soon as I just look at food I seem to put on weight.

Counsellor:	That seems nothing short of miraculous! It may help us to find out what you are eating that's causing the problem. What do *you* think is keeping your weight on?
Mrs T:	I don't know (pause). Well I know what to eat, and when to eat. It seems so difficult to stick to a diet sometimes, though. Sometimes I stick to the diet, but often the whole things seem to collapse. I don't know – nothing seems to work with me.
Counsellor:	You seem quite despondent. But, you can eat appropriately at times. Tell me about the things that help you diet.
Mrs T:	Oh, I'm not sure … I think …
Counsellor:	Tell me about some of the things that get in the way of dieting.
Mrs T:	I suppose one thing that really gets me down is the way my boys treat the house like a hotel and expect me to cook for them all the time. And they always want fry-ups!

Here, the counsellor has managed through direct questioning to move from a situation where everything and nothing seems to be contributing to Mrs T's failure to lose weight to identification of a key factor. She also highlighted the success Mrs T did report, in an attempt to focus on her success and to increase her confidence that change is achievable, before once more identifying things that prevented her dieting appropriately.

Goal setting

Once particular problems have been identified, some people may feel they have the resources to deal with them and need no further help in making appropriate changes. Others, however, may need further support in determining what they want to change and how to change it. The first stage in this process is to help the individual to decide the goals he or she wishes to achieve and to frame his or her goals in specific rather than general terms (e.g. 'I will go to the gym on Tuesday and Thursday evenings' versus 'I must do more exercise').

If the final goal seems too difficult to achieve in one step, the elaboration of subgoals working towards the final goal should be encouraged. Short-term success in achieving modest, short-term goals is more likely to motivate further change than pursuing difficult-to-attain, long-term goals. It is easier to lose 2 pounds of weight per week than to strive for a 3-stone weight loss over an ill-defined time period.

Goals must pay heed to people's resources and their social and environmental circumstances. Even a short walk lasting 10 minutes two or three times a week may be a sufficient initial goal for a 'couch potato'. Goals which are too adventurous may prove impossible to achieve and the resultant failure fosters a general unwillingness to attempt future change: 'I knew it would happen; I tried and I failed'. In the case of Mrs T, the aim at this stage of counselling would be to identify goals both in terms of weight loss and not cooking 'fry-ups' for her sons. How she sets about achieving these can then be explored in detail in the third stage of counselling.

Some goals may be apparent following the problem exploration phase. However, should this not be the case, Egan identified a series of strategies designed to help the client identify and set goals:

- summarizing
- providing relevant information
- challenging to provide new perspectives.

A good summary provides a concise and structured means for focusing on the changes required.

Counsellor: Let's look at what we've got now. You've identified a number of things which are contributing to your weight problem. You find it difficult to keep long-term targets, such as losing 2 stones of weight before Christmas, you don't exercise as much as you used to, and you've developed a liking for ice cream …

Mrs F: Yes, that about sums it up. I guess I do need to do something about these things. I suppose I could set about doing more exercise …

Challenge involves inviting the person to explore new perspectives. It is particularly useful when the person appears locked into old ways of thinking or feels little can be done. As noted in the section on motivational interviewing, direct challenges, however well phrased ('Well, why don't you try to lose 2 pounds of weight a week?'), are likely to result in resistance to change or feelings of defeat. Accordingly, challenge in this context involves inviting the individual to explore new solutions, using phrases such as:

- 'Perhaps it would be useful to consider some different ways of looking at solutions to this problem.'
- 'I wonder if there are any other things you could do to deal with this problem.'

Facilitating action

Once goals have been established in the second phase of counselling, some individuals may feel they need no further support in achieving them. Others, who by this stage may have a good idea of what they want to achieve, can remain unsure of how to achieve them. Discussion between the counsellor and the person may still be necessary. One useful strategy at this stage is to brainstorm. This involves thinking through as many possibilities as possible, forsaking quality for quantity. Once a list has been generated, these possibilities can then be sifted and focused strategies developed.

Counsellor: Be as adventurous as you like – just think of as many solutions as you can. We can weed out the good ideas in a few minutes. You never know, some of the 'crazy' solutions may turn out to be the answer to the problem.

Consider the possibilities simply for establishing a new 'fitness plan':

- Join a local gymnasium.
- Attend aerobic classes at a leisure centre.

- Walk or cycle to work.
- Join up with friends to form an exercise group.
- Set up a crèche with friends to take it in turns to look after children while you exercise.
- Go for a brisk walk during the lunch hour.
- Buy a bicycle.
- Attend a course of lessons in a new sport.
- Buy an aerobics videotape.
- Walk to the local shops instead of taking the car.

Exercises

To practise listening skills

Sit with a friend for a period of 10 minutes and use the various strategies to explore an interest they have or an issue they wish to explore. Try not to interrupt or interject your own ideas or things you wish to say, and to keep them focused on the issue at hand. The goal is simply to listen and allow the other person to talk about *one* issue. It sounds simple but this exercise can be extremely difficult.

More advanced practice

To practise more skills, it may be helpful to role play with a colleague a problem presented by a client you have seen recently. Explicitly stage the process through the three phases of counselling and stop after each phase to discuss how the experience of being counselled felt from the client's perspective. The goal is not to provide expert feedback, but that of the client. This, after all, is the most important aspect of counselling and can provide important insights into your own skills and methods.

STRESS AND STRESS MANAGEMENT TRAINING

As noted previously, helping people cope with the stress of receiving 'bad news' can involve listening to them express their anxieties and concerns so these can be dealt with constructively. However, many people report having to cope with long-term stress resulting from their life situation. Although there are a number of stress management techniques that may help people cope with stress, these should not be seen as distinct from the approach developed by Egan, who noted that achieving some goals may necessitate learning new skills. Stress management skills may be seen as falling into this category.

Most stress management strategies are based on the model of stress developed by Lazarus & Folkman (1984). This model suggests that stress is a process and can be described as a series of stages. The first stage of the stress process is usually (but not exclusively) an environmental event. The model suggests we do not all respond to such events in the same way. Some may respond to a high-stress work situation with enthusiasm and enjoyment; others may feel overwhelmed and distressed. The trigger event, therefore, forms the beginning of a complex chain of internal events and cannot be seen simply as the 'stress' in itself. The next stage in the process involves an appraisal of the environmental stimulus. If regarded as something the person feels confident he or she can cope with, an event is likely to have minimal impact. A stress response will occur when the event is viewed as demanding or having potential harm to the individual *and* the individual feels he or she will have difficulty coping. The response may involve increased autonomic arousal, increased muscular tension, feeling 'stressed' or anxious and some degree of 'stressed' behaviour.

Stress management involves dealing with each of the stages in the stress process. Stress may be obviated by changing environmental circumstances. It may be reduced by modifying the individual's various responses to these circumstances. However, relaxation is the stress management skill most frequently taught. It can be useful for a number of reasons. First, it can reduce unpleasant physical sensations and chronic tiredness. Second, it provides individuals with a means of gaining some control over their response to stress. Finally, relaxation is relatively easy to teach and use. This section will concentrate on teaching these skills. Other techniques involved in stress management are discussed in Meichenbaum (1985) and, in the context of CHD, by Bennett (1993).

Relaxation training

The goal of relaxation training is to help people be as relaxed as possible throughout the day and, in particular, at times of stress. Although learning relaxation involves lying or sitting quietly for some minutes away from the hustle and bustle of everyday life, its ultimate value is in its application at times of stress. There is little to be gained by becoming increasingly tense during the day and only unwinding at night in a comfy chair. However expert someone may become in this sort of relaxation, it will do little to ameliorate the effects of daily stress. Learning to use relaxation skills appropriately involves developing awareness of stress evidenced through physical tension throughout the day, and learning to minimize this tension. It is best achieved using three interacting stages:

• learning relaxation skills
• learning to monitor tension in daily life
• learning to use relaxation skills at times of stress.

Learning relaxation skills

The first stage involves learning to relax under optimal conditions. Ideally, the individual should be talked through a series of relaxation instructions by the counsellor before practising at home. Time, and other considerations, often preclude this and home practice with a tape often has to suffice. The most effective tapes promote gradual relaxation throughout the body, by means of tensing and relaxing specific muscle groups systematically. The order in which the muscles are relaxed varies but a typical exercise may involve the following stages (the tensing procedure is described in brackets).

• Hands and forearms (making a fist)
• Upper arms (touching fingers to shoulder)

- Shoulders and lower neck (hunching shoulders)
- Back of neck (pushing back against support)
- Lips (pushing them together)
- Forehead (frowning)
- Abdomen/chest (holding deep breath)
- Abdomen (tensing stomach muscles)
- Lower legs and feet (pointing foot up and toward head, not lifting leg).

Each muscle group should be tensed just sufficiently to feel the effects, affording practice at recognizing and relaxing away 'normal' levels of tension. In order to apply relaxation at times of actual stress, regular daily practice is essential. Individuals need to overlearn the skill, so that it becomes a habitual response and can be performed 'to order'. As they become more practised, they can cut down the tensing component, focusing instead on the immediate relaxation of the muscle groups. The regularity of practice can be reduced with developing expertise.

Monitoring physical tension

While learning relaxation skills, individuals can begin to monitor their levels of physical tension. As they learn to relax, most people become increasingly aware of periods during the day when they are particularly tense or incidents in the day which may trigger tension. Formal stress management programmes often ask people to record their tension at regular intervals during the day or when they are feeling particularly tense, as this helps to identify likely triggers and any pattern of stress that may occur (see Table 8.1). This may feel too formal for many counsellors, but can be a useful exercise. Note in the example that the stressors identified are those of everyday life, the stressors most people have to deal with using stress management techniques.

Using relaxation skills

To be useful, relaxation needs to be integrated into daily life. After one or two weeks of monitoring tension and learning relaxation, patients can begin to gradually incorporate relaxation into their daily lives. This can be done by using tension as a cue to an attempt to relax as much as is possible in the circumstances in which the person finds herself. Use can be made of coffee and other breaks during the day to relax fully. However, the goal of

Table 8.1 A typical 'tension diary'

Time	Level of tension (0–10)	Trigger
08.00	9	Rushing to get kids to child minder
09.00	6	Driving and arriving at work still feeling rushed
10.00	4	General tension at work
11.00	2	Coffee break – bliss!
12.00	3	General work
13.00	7	Annoyed – had to work over lunch

relaxation training is to help people relax as fully as is appropriate while maintaining their daily routine or when dealing with particular stressors. This level of relaxation takes practice and time to achieve. Accordingly, relaxation is best used to reduce even relatively low levels of excess tension. Accumulated minor stresses during the day can be more wearing than occasional larger stresses. In addition, the consistent use of relaxation techniques can prepare the person to cope with times of greater stress. Without practice, use of relaxation skills at such times may be difficult if not impossible.

CONCLUSION

Appropriate behavioural change in those at risk for CHD can reduce risk of disease. However, while optimizing health is a goal of screening, individuals' motivation and ability to change are frequently more rooted in the 'here and now'. Some people may not place a high value on possible future health gain some years hence and be unwilling or unready to change. Others may be motivated and able to act on information provided during the screening process. Yet others may wish to change but lack the confidence or problem-solving skills to enable this.

The goal of the counsellor is to identify where in this continuum of change people lie and to tailor any intervention accordingly. Those who are unmotivated may benefit from the opportunity simply to consider the pros and cons of change, with the goal of counselling being no more than to facilitate this process. Those in the second group will benefit from clear and structured information provision. The final group will benefit most from a problem-solving approach such as that developed by Egan.

Use of the strategies for facilitating behavioural change suggested here may mean that the screening process takes longer than many of the original models of screening and counselling (e.g. Fullard et al 1983). It is difficult to conduct the form of information giving or counselling described here within the 20 minutes per person time constraints initially considered to be about the optimum. However, the probability of achieving lasting behavioural change in any but the most motivated and self-confident individual is significantly greater than that likely to be achieved by the simple educational techniques. Accordingly, while they may appear time consuming, their 'cost effectiveness' is likely to be high.

■ KEY POINTS

- Decisions concerning health-related behaviours are not simply based on their health consequences. Other factors involved include the immediate costs and benefits of engaging in any behaviour and the availability of the behaviour to the individual.
- At any one time an individual may be more or less motivated to change his or her behaviour. A key aspect of counselling is to identify what 'stage of change' the individual is at and to tailor any intervention accordingly.

- The quality of communication in the counselling process is central to facilitating appropriate behavioural change.

- Even where any behavioural change required is relatively simple, time should be given to exploring motivational factors and enhancing motivation to change.

- Facilitating some behavioural change may simply require the provision of appropriate information. This process involves: an initial check on present knowledge; the provision of information; and an accuracy check.

- Information given should be structured and relevant to the individual's level of knowledge and the individual's own desired behavioural change.

- Care should be taken to detect and pre-empt inappropriate levels of anxiety following the provision of adverse health information.

- Facilitating behavioural change may require more complex counselling. This may involve three stages: problem exploration and clarification; goal setting; facilitating action.

- Skills and strategies primarily involved in the problem exploration stage are: direct questioning and prompts; silence and minimal prompt; and empathic feedback.

- Goals must be concrete and within the resources of the individual. Some strategies which help individuals define their goals are: summarizing; providing relevant information; challenge.

- One useful way of facilitating plans for achieving goals is the use of 'brainstorm' techniques.

- Stress is a process, with identifiable, interacting 'stages': a 'trigger event'; cognitive appraisal; and a stress response including stressed behaviour and physical tension.

- Relaxation focuses on one part of this process, reducing physical tension. Learning relaxation involves three stages: learning relaxation skills; learning to monitor tension in daily life; learning to use relaxation skills at times of stress.

REFERENCES

Ajzen I 1985 From intentions to action: a theory of planned behaviour. In: Kuhl J, Beckham J (eds) Action control: from cognitions to behaviours. Springer, New York

Bandura A 1986 Social foundations of thought and action: a social cognitive theory. Prentice Hall, Englewood Cliffs, NJ

Becker MH 1974 The health belief model and personal health behaviour. Health Education Monographs 2: 324–508

Bennett P 1993 Counselling for heart disease. British Psychological Society, Leicester

Egan G 1990 The skilled helper: models, skills, and methods for effective helping. Brooks/Cole Publishing, Monterey, CA

Fullard E, Fowler A, Gray JAM 1983 Facilitating prevention in primary care. British Medical Journal 289: 1585–1587

Gollwitzer PM 1999 Implementation intentions – strong effects of simple plans. American Psychologist 54: 493–503

Jacobson B 1981 The ladykillers: why smoking is a feminist issue. Pluto, London

Lazarus RS, Folkman S 1984 Stress, appraisal and coping. Springer, New York

Meichenbaum D 1985 Stress inoculation training. Pergamon Press, Oxford

Miller WR, Rollnick S 2002 Motivational interviewing, 2nd edn. Guilford, New York

Nichols KA 1984 Psychological care in physical illness. Croom Helm, London

OXCHECK Study Group 1994 Effectiveness of heart checks conducted by nurses in primary care: results of the OXCHECK Study after one year. British Medical Journal 308: 3008–3012

Prochaska JO, DiClemente CC 1984 The transtheoretical approach: crossing traditional foundations of change. Don Jones, Homewood, IL

Rogers CR 1961 On becoming a person. Houghton Mifflin, Boston

FURTHER READING

Bennett P 1993 Counselling for heart disease. British Psychology Society, Leicester

Egan G 1998 The skilled helper: a problem-management approach to helping. Brooks/Cole Publishing, Monterey, CA

Meichenbaum D 1985 Stress inoculation training. Pergamon Press, Oxford

Rollnick S, Mason P, Butler C 1999 Health behaviour change. A guide for practitioners. Churchill Livingstone, Edinburgh

Medical management of coronary heart disease

Kanarath P. Balachandran   Keith G. Oldroyd

9

■ CONTENTS

STABLE CORONARY HEART DISEASE

Angina has three cardinal features – retrosternal chest discomfort, provocation by exertion or stress and prompt relief by rest or nitrates. Patients with two out of three of these characteristics are considered to have atypical chest pain and patients with only one out of three should be described as having non-cardiac chest pain. Thus angina is a clinical diagnosis and the typical history is easy to recognize. The majority of patients with angina have CHD but it is important to remember that a significant minority have other forms of cardiovascular disease, including aortic stenosis and cardiomyopathy.

Medical therapy for angina

Nitrates

Nitrates in their various forms are an essential component of the drug therapy of angina. Their main mode of action is venous dilatation with consequent reductions in preload and myocardial oxygen demand. At higher doses direct arterial dilatation can be produced. The vascular effects of nitrates are not dependent on the presence of an intact endothelium. Sublingual glyceryl trinitrate spray is used for rapid relief of acute anginal attacks. Isosorbide dinitrate or mononitrate can be used for prophylaxis of angina. An asymmetric regimen (8 am, 2 pm and 6 pm for dinitrate and 8 am and 2 pm for mononitrate) is recommended to avoid tolerance. Transdermal nitrate patches are available, as are once-daily modified-release oral nitrate preparations. The latter are designed to prevent the development of tolerance but they are expensive and some authorities recommend their use only for individual patients unable to comply with asymmetric regimens. Buccal administration of nitrates avoids the problem of variable absorption and is a viable alternative to intravenous therapy in patients with unstable angina or heart failure. The main adverse effects of nitrates are headache, flushing and postural hypotension which can be particularly troublesome in the elderly.

β-Adrenoceptor blockers (Table 9.1)

β-Blockers reduce myocardial oxygen consumption by slowing the heart rate both at rest and on exercise and by reducing the force of contraction of the myocardium. Cardioselective β-blockers have less activity at β_2-receptors but they are not cardiospecific and will still provoke bronchoconstriction in patients with reversible airways obstruction. β-blockers are the agents of first choice for the treatment of angina. They are effective and have additional cardioprotective effects although this has only been demonstrated in patients with a prior history of myocardial infarction (MI). The main adverse effects are bradycardia, fatigue, impotence and bronchoconstriction. Some β-blockers such as labetalol and carvedilol have additional vasodilatory effects. Sotalol in high doses has additional class III antiarrhythmic activity. Although there is no clear correlation between lipid solubility and central nervous system side-effects, if these are a problem switching to a drug with low lipophilicity, such as atenolol, may help. β-Blockers with partial agonist activity (intrinsic sympathetic activity, ISA) should be avoided, as they have not been shown to have any cardioprotective effects. In the past, β-blockers have been said to be contraindicated in patients with congestive heart failure (CHF) but this is no longer the case and, indeed, β-blockade is now the optimal therapy for the treatment of angina in patients with CHF.

Calcium channel blockers (Table 9.2)

There are three distinct types of calcium antagonist in common use: the dihydropyridines (e.g. nifedipine, amlodipine), diltiazem and verapamil. The dihydropyridines act mainly on vascular smooth muscle, producing

Table 9.1 Selected properties and maintenance doses of a variety of β-blockers

	Cardioselective	Vasodilatation	Usual daily dose in angina (mg)
Atenolol	+	−	50–100
Metoprolol	+	−	100–200
Bisoprolol	+	−	5–10
Timolol	−	−	20–40
Propranolol	−	−	120–240
Sotalol	−	−	160–240
Carvedilol	−	+	25–50

Table 9.2 Cardiovascular effects of the three different classes of calcium channel blocker

	Vasodilatation	Heart rate	Contractility
Nifedipine	+ +	↑	−
Diltiazem	+	↓	↓
Verapamil	−	↓↓	↓↓

coronary and systemic arterial vasodilatation. Verapamil has its main effects on the myocardium, including the atrioventricular node, but unlike β-blockers has no propensity to cause bronchoconstriction. Although diltiazem is often thought of as a half-way house between the two, it shares more of the properties of verapamil than nifedipine. All of these drugs are available in a range of different delivery systems. The pharmacokinetic profiles of the available sustained-release preparations differ slightly and it is recommended that they should be prescribed by brand name.

Potassium channel openers

These agents are a chemically diverse group, which share the ability to relax vascular smooth muscle. Nicorandil is the only example available for use clinically. Although considered by many to be a relatively new drug it was in fact licensed for the treatment of angina in Japan in 1983. Despite this, it is still not available in the USA. Its predominant effect is systemic and coronary vasodilatation without any change in contractility. This makes it particularly attractive in patients with impaired ventricular function. Interestingly, even in diseased segments of coronary artery, nicorandil appears able to produce some dilatation. Potassium channels are also involved in preconditioning, the phenomenon whereby myocardium exposed to a brief episode of ischaemia is rendered relatively resistant to subsequent ischaemia. Some evidence exists to suggest that nicorandil may pharmacologically precondition the myocardium. In an attempt to demonstrate whether this is of clinical significance, nicorandil has been subjected to a placebo-controlled randomized trial to assess its ability to modify clinical outcomes in patients with stable angina. The IONA Study (2002) indicated that when added to standard antianginal therapy, nicorandil reduced hospital readmissions but did not reduce death or non-fatal myocardial infarction. This result has been interpreted to confirm its efficacy as an antianginal drug but to provide no evidence of any preconditioning.

Appropriate selection of drug therapy in angina

The choice of therapy should be based on the pattern of angina experienced by the patient and on any concomitant medical conditions.

1. Effort angina with consistent ischaemic threshold usually reflects increased oxygen demand – use a β-blocker if possible. If not tolerated or the patient has contraindications, use either diltiazem or verapamil.

2. Variable ischaemic threshold may reflect variable coronary vasomotor tone/oxygen supply – use either diltiazem or verapamil.

3. Variant angina – pain at rest, particularly with ST segment elevation during ischaemic episodes – use either diltiazem or verapamil with nitrates and/or nicorandil. High doses of the calcium channel blocker are often required in this condition.

4. Co-existent ventricular dysfunction/CHF – use β-blockade starting at low dose with slow titration. Nitrates, nicorandil and dihydropyridine calcium channel blockers are all alternatives if β-blockade is poorly tolerated.

5. Asthma/chronic obstructive airways disease (COAD) – patients with genuine asthma will not tolerate β-blockade – use diltiazem or verapamil with nicorandil and/or nitrates. However, many patients with COAD have no reversible airways obstruction and will tolerate β-blockade. This is important as the two conditions commonly co-exist. Often a supervised trial of β-blockade is necessary to confirm tolerance.

6. Co-existent aortic stenosis – use β-blockade or rate-limiting calcium antagonists or low doses of nitrates; avoid potent vasodilators which may have the effect of increasing the degree of left ventricular outflow obstruction.

If a single drug fails to control symptoms adequately, a second and if necessary a third drug from different antianginal groups may be added (triple therapy). Some general guidelines are outlined below:

1. Maximize the dose of the initially selected drug before adding a second agent.
2. The addition of a β-blocker to either diltiazem or verapamil does not usually improve antianginal efficacy and is associated with an increased risk of bradycardia.
3. Dihydropyridines are unattractive as monotherapy but work well in conjunction with β-blockers.

Common questions patients ask about antianginal therapy

Question. The GTN spray makes me dizzy and gives me a headache. What can I do?

Answer. Switch to sublingual tablets and as soon as you feel the angina resolving, spit the tablet out.

Question. How should I use my GTN tablets/spray?
Answer. Take GTN before any activities which regularly provoke angina. Do not worry about the GTN losing its effect – this is rarely a problem.

Question. I am on regular nitrate tablets – when should I take them?
Answer. Take the tablets on waking and after lunch with no evening dose. If you get frequent symptoms at night, take the tablets before bed and on waking with no dose in between.

Question. The tablets have helped my angina but I have swollen legs by nighttime (nifedipine, amlodipine, etc.). Should I continue with them? Should I be on a water tablet?
Answer. Unless your doctor feels the swollen legs are a sign of heart failure there is no need to take diuretics. Usually elevating the legs above waist level when resting or if necessary a reduction in dose controls this problem. If the swelling persists and is very troublesome you may have to change tablets. Only if this is not felt to be an option should you use a diuretic and then only in low dosage.

Question. The tablets have helped my angina but I feel very tired (β-blockers). Will this get better?
Answer. It may do. Some β-blockers cause sleep disturbance and if this is the case, withdrawal of therapy is usually required. Some patients with CHD have sleep disturbance as part of a depressive mood disorder and this may require specific therapy. Other causes of fatigue should be considered, e.g. heart failure, anaemia or hypothyroidism. If all of these have been excluded and the fatigue continues to be very troublesome, then dose reduction or withdrawal should be considered.

Who needs coronary angiography?

A case can be made for performing coronary angiography in all patients with angina on the grounds that this is the best method of risk stratification. However, there is no evidence base to support this strategy and in most health-care systems an initial attempt to risk stratify patients is performed non-invasively using an exercise test, stress echo or myocardial perfusion imaging. The results of such testing are considered in conjunction with the patient's symptoms when making a decision to proceed or not to coronary angiography. In general, angiography is a prelude to revascularization and should certainly be offered to the patient in the following circumstances:

- continuing angina despite adequate medical therapy – usually at least two antianginal drugs plus aspirin and a statin if appropriate
- continuing angina and a positive stress test
- asymptomatic patients but with a previous MI and a positive exercise test
- unstable angina or non-ST elevation MI, particularly if there are high-risk features such as elevated troponin or dynamic ECG changes.

Percutaneous coronary intervention (Figs 9.1, 9.2)

Percutaneous coronary intervention (PCI) using an inflatable balloon was the original technique of non-surgical revascularization. This has now largely been replaced by coronary stent implantation. PCI success and complication rates vary according to the type of lesion being dilated but most centres now report overall success rates in excess of 90% for all lesions treated. The success rate for chronic total occlusions has always been lower, averaging around 70%. A number of non-balloon devices have a limited role in particular situations.

- *Directional atherectomy (DCA)* – a combined balloon and rotating blade device which removes plaque and allows it to be retrieved for analysis; good in certain anatomical locations. Combined DCA/stenting is associated with very low restenosis rates.
- *Rotational atherectomy* – a very high-speed rotating burr, which ablates plaque into microparticles; good for calcified lesions.

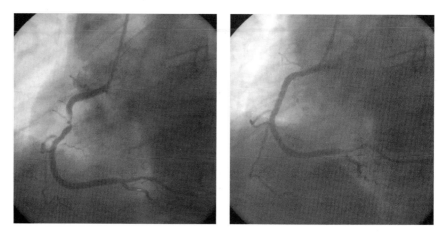

Figure 9.1 Direct stenting of a focal mid-right coronary artery stenosis.

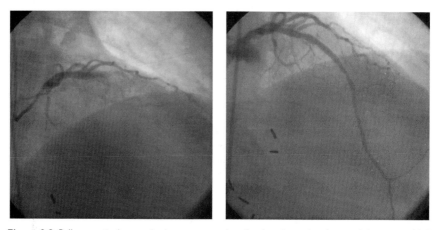

Figure 9.2 Balloon angioplasty and subsequent stenting of a chronic total occlusion of the proximal left anterior descending artery.

- *Extraction atherectomy* – a variety of devices exist using various techniques to 'hoover' out material from the vessel lumen; good for thrombus.

None of these techniques has been convincingly demonstrated to be any better than conventional balloon angioplasty/stenting in any given situation.

Coronary stents

Stents are implanted percutaneously in coronary and other arteries to create a scaffold and maintain the patency of the vessel lumen. Dotter implanted the first vascular stents in canine popliteal arteries in 1969 (Dotter 1969). Currently there are a large number of metallic vascular stents suitable for implantation in the coronary arteries, and many more in the pipeline. Stenting has been successful because it addresses the two main problems of conventional balloon angioplasty – abrupt vessel closure (AVC) and restenosis.

AVC is the phenomenon whereby a vessel subjected to balloon angioplasty occludes during or in the first few hours after the procedure. It is to a certain extent an unpredictable adverse event, occurs in up to 5% of patients and previously often led to myocardial infarction or a need for urgent coronary bypass surgery. Placement of a stent into a vessel that has acutely occluded or has the features of threatened acute closure usually stabilizes the situation and often no other therapy is required.

Restenosis following balloon angioplasty is due to a combination of inadequate initial dilatation, elastic recoil of the artery, negative remodelling (vessel shrinkage post dilatation) and neointimal proliferation. The individual contribution of each of these phenomena varies from lesion to lesion and patient to patient but stenting reduces restenosis by essentially abolishing recoil and remodelling. Two large randomized multicentre trials conducted in parallel in the USA (STRESS: Fischman et al 1994) and Europe (BENESTENT I: Serruys et al 1994) showed conclusively that elective implantation of the Palmaz–Schatz stent reduced restenosis compared to conventional balloon angioplasty (Table 9.3). Of even greater importance was the demonstration that there were parallel highly significant reductions in adverse clinical endpoints and the need for reintervention.

In the stent group of BENESTENT there was a 10% incidence of bleeding compared to 1.6% in the balloon angioplasty group. This was related to the particularly intensive antithrombotic regimen employed in an attempt to

Table 9.3 Effect of elective implantation of the Palmaz–Schatz stent on restenosis (defined as a diameter stenosis of $>50\%$ at 6 months) in two randomized clinical trials of stenting versus conventional PTCA

	n	PTCA	Stent	% reduction in restenosis	p value
STRESS	410	43	29	33	0.01
BENESTENT	520	33	22	33	< 0.03

prevent stent thrombosis. This regime also required the patient to stay in hospital for 5–7 days post procedure. In 1995, Colombo et al published data on a large series of patients undergoing stent implantation guided by intravascular ultrasound. They showed that in around 70% of cases, the apposition between the stent and the vessel wall was suboptimal when the stent was deployed using conventional balloon pressures. High-pressure (17–18 atmospheres) dilatations following stent implantation optimized deployment and abolished the need for anticoagulation. This study heralded the first revolution in the practice of interventional cardiology. Patients were now able to go home on the same day or at most one day after their procedure on antiplatelet therapy alone (aspirin and/or ticlopidine, later clopidogrel) with the risk of bleeding and stent thrombosis both below 1%. Since then coronary stenting has become the routine method of PCI, being performed in 80–90% of all cases.

Drug-eluting stents

Although stenting reduces restenosis, it by no means abolishes the problem. Restenosis following stent implantation is almost entirely due to neointimal proliferation and, depending on a number of patient- and lesion-specific characteristics, restenosis rates may vary from <10% to 50%. Known predictors of instent restenosis include diabetes, lesions in the proximal left anterior descending artery or saphenous vein grafts, long lesions, small vessels and chronic total occlusions.

A huge amount of research has been conducted in an attempt to find some means of controlling neointimal growth in the stented artery and very recently significant progress has been achieved. A number of drugs have been coated on to a variety of stents and been shown to almost completely inhibit neointimal proliferation in humans and abolish clinical restenosis. These include rapamycin, a cytostatic drug used orally in renal transplant patients, and paclitaxel, a cytotoxic drug used in the treatment of a variety of cancers. The obvious attraction of using the stent itself for local drug delivery is that only very low doses are required to achieve efficacy, with no resultant systemic toxicity. At the time of writing none of these devices is available for clinical use but it is likely that at least one drug-eluting stent will be in routine use in the near future and that their introduction will herald a second revolution in the practice of interventional cardiology.

Surgical revascularization

Current techniques of coronary artery bypass surgery (CABG) usually involve the placement of one or more arterial conduits. This is based on data showing that the long-term patency of arterial grafts is superior to that of saphenous veins. The left internal mammary artery (LIMA) is used in most cases to bypass the left anterior descending (LAD) coronary artery. The LIMA is almost always left attached to the subclavian artery (pedicled graft) so that only a single surgical anastomosis is required. Some surgeons may also use the right internal mammary artery to bypass either the circumflex or right coronary arteries. In this case, the graft may be pedicled or it may be detached and used as a free graft. There is some evidence that the latter technique produces better results. Other arterial conduits which can be used include the radial, gastroepiploic and inferior gastric arteries. Complete arterial revascularization, even for three-vessel coronary disease, is becoming more common. Nonetheless, most patients receive one or more venous conduits and a common approach is to use the LIMA for the LAD and two vein grafts for the circumflex and right coronary arteries.

Just as PCI has improved technically in the past decade, so there have been parallel advances in cardiac surgery. Devices have been developed which can temporarily stabilize segments of the myocardium, allowing the surgeon to anastomose selected grafts to a beating heart. This avoids the need for cardiopulmonary bypass and may reduce the mortality and morbidity, especially stroke, associated with CABG. So far, however, only a limited number of surgeons are practising 'off-pump' surgery and no randomized trials have confirmed superiority over the conventional technique.

Indications for revascularization

Patients are offered revascularization either to relieve symptoms refractory to medical therapy or in the belief that revascularization will improve prognosis (secondary prevention); often both indications apply in the same patient.

Selection of patients for PCI

Historically the ideal patient for PCI had single-vessel, single-lesion disease and these were the only patients treated in the early days of the technique. Now, because of improvements in operator experience, catheter design and imaging quality, and particularly stents, many patients with multivessel disease are treated by PCI. If it is considered that complete revascularization of every stenosed artery is not necessary, some of these patients may be treated by single-vessel PCI to the most severe or 'culprit' lesion and this will usually substantially relieve angina. In others, multivessel PCI may be performed. Comparisons between the effects of different treatment strategies have been undertaken but as this is such a rapidly evolving field the results are often of historical interest only.

Medical therapy versus surgery

The 10-year results of the randomized trials comparing CABG and medical therapy in CHD were the subject of a meta-analysis (Yusuf et al 1994). These trials recruited patients with either stable angina not severe enough to warrant surgery or a previous MI. In reality, they compared a strategy of immediate surgery versus one of medical therapy with surgery later if symptoms worsened. After 10 years, 41% of patients randomized to initial medical therapy had actually undergone CABG compared to 93% of those randomized to CABG. The CABG group had significantly lower total mortality than the medical treatment group at all time points though the absolute benefit decreased as time progressed (Table 9.4 and Fig. 9.3). This waning of the initial effects of surgery mirrors the natural history of graft occlusion.

Subgroup analysis suggested that the benefits of surgery were greatest in those with left main stem stenosis or proximal three-vessel disease. In two-vessel disease with involvement of the LAD artery, the odds ratio for reduction in mortality with surgery was of borderline significance (0.34–1.01); without LAD involvement there was no significant mortality benefit with surgery. In univariate analysis, the relative benefits of surgery over medical therapy were not significantly affected by other risk factors such as left ventricular dysfunction, previous MI, abnormal exercise test and age. However, when these factors are considered together the absolute survival benefit did increase with increasing risk. In other words, if a patient with left main stem stenosis or proximal three-vessel disease also has one or more of the above risk factors, this increases the likelihood that the patient's

Table 9.4 Summary of results of a meta-analysis of randomized trials comparing CABG and medical therapy in stable coronary heart disease

Follow-up	Reduction in mortality with CABG (%)	95% confidence intervals
5 years	39	23–52
7 years	32	17–44
10 years	17	2–30

Adapted from Yusuf et al 1994.

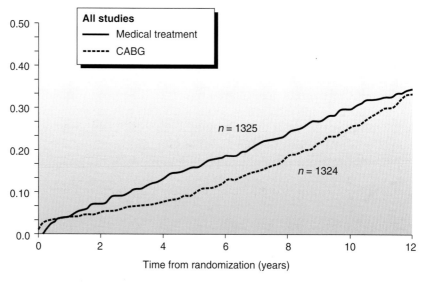

Figure 9.3 Survival curve over time. Long-term survival in all the randomized studies of medical therapy versus CABG for patients with coronary heart disease and angina is not in itself severe enough to warrant surgery (adapted from Yusuf et al 1994).

survival will be improved by surgery rather than medical therapy. None-theless, the mean extension of survival with CABG over 10 years was only 4.3 months. Even in the highest risk groups as assessed by standard risk scoring, the mean extension of survival was only 8–10 months. The current results of CABG may be better, due to a number of factors including:

- higher frequency of arterial revascularization
- greater use of aspirin with consequently lower early graft occlusion
- improvements in the techniques of cardiopulmonary bypass and myocardial preservation
- off-pump surgery
- improved control of risk factors following CABG.

However, there have also been substantial improvements in medical ther-apy since the time of these trials and at least three interventions not widely used at the time have been shown to reduce mortality in CHD – aspirin, angiotensin-converting enzyme inhibitors and lipid lowering with statins or fibrates. In addition, the CABG trials were almost exclusively men only and none recruited patients aged more than 65. Further trials are required to compare modern medical and surgical therapy in women, the elderly and in the subgroups in which no clear advantage of surgery was demonstrated. However, it is unlikely that these will ever be performed.

Medical therapy versus PCI

Some comparisons have been made between these two strategies but again they are of little relevance to contemporary practice as the PCI groups were not routinely stented and did not receive optimal adjunctive pharmaco-logical therapy.

The ACME trial did suggest that over a 6-month follow-up period PCI resulted in better relief of angina and a greater improvement in exercise capacity compared to medical therapy in patients with initially mild symp-toms and single-vessel disease (Parisi et al 1992). In clinical practice, how-ever, PCI is not generally used in patients with stable angina as an alternative to medical therapy. Rather, it is reserved for suitable patients who have poorly controlled angina despite medical therapy.

The RITA-2 trial directly compared medical therapy with PCI in 1018 ran-domized patients. Of these, 53% had angina class $\geqslant 2$ and 40% had two or more vessel disease. Median follow-up was 2.7 years. The PCI arm had sig-nificantly better symptomatic relief and improved exercise times but there were more deaths and non-fatal myocardial infarctions in the intervention arm (6.3% versus 3%, $p = 0.02$). However, there was significant crossover with 23% of the initially medically treated patients undergoing revascular-ization (RITA-2 Trial Participants 1997).

PCI versus CABG

The follow-up data from several trials comparing PCI and CABG have been reported. Most have excluded single-vessel disease as there is general agreement that if possible this should be dealt with non-surgically with the option of CABG being reserved for the future development of more diffuse disease. Some of the trials demanded that the operators attempt complete revascularization of all target vessels, whilst others were less stringent. The largest of these was the Bypass Angioplasty Revascularization Investigation (BARI 2000) that recently reported 7-year follow-up outcomes. Overall there was no difference in mortality or non-fatal myocardial infarction rates. Mortality in diabetics was significantly less in the CABG arm (23.6% versus 44.7%, $p < 0.001$) but diabetes was not a prespecified subgroup and this finding requires verification. Generally patients randomized to PCI have consistently lower event-free survival, primarily because approximately 30% of such patients require at least one repeat procedure for restenosis. Nevertheless, in the RITA-1 trial conducted in the UK (Schulpher et al 1994), the initial average cost of treating a patient randomized to PCI was about 52% of that for CABG. Despite reinterventions, total costs in the PCI group were still 20% less than with CABG at 2 years.

Both RITA-1 and BARI were performed prior to the introduction of coronary stenting. The ARTS Study was a randomized comparison of CABG and stenting in patients with multivessel disease. An attempt was made to achieve equivalent revascularization in both groups although this was not entirely successful. As anticipated, there was no difference in rates of death or non-fatal myocardial infarction over the first 12 months of follow-up. Stenting reduced restenosis so that the need for reintervention in patients randomized to PCI fell from around 30% in the balloon angioplasty studies described above to around 15% (Serruys et al 2001). At 12 months the costs associated with an initial strategy of PCI were around 3000 euros less than with CABG.

Studies are planned to compare CABG with multivessel stenting using drug-eluting stents. If in these studies the need for repeat procedures in the PCI group is less than 5% then multivessel stenting will become the treatment of choice for all patients in whom it is technically feasible.

ACUTE CORONARY SYNDROMES

ST elevation myocardial infarction (STEMI)

The most effective means of preventing the late consequences of MI is to attempt to limit the initial injury by restoring normal myocardial perfusion as rapidly as possible. The vast majority of MI is due to thrombus formation in a coronary artery, usually at the site of a pre-existing atheromatous plaque. There are two main methods of dealing quickly with this occlusive coronary thrombus: intravenous administration of a variety of fibrinolytic, antithrombotic and antiplatelet drugs or PCI.

Thrombolytic therapy

Thrombolytic therapy vs placebo A series of large randomized placebo-controlled clinical trials clearly showed the benefits of thrombolytic therapy with significant reductions in mortality in the ISIS-2 trial using streptokinase (SK; ISIS-2 Collaborative Group 1988), the AIMS trial using anistreplase (AIMS Trial Study Group 1988) and the ASSET trial using recombinant tissue plasminogen activator (rt-PA) (Wilcox et al 1988).

Thrombolytic comparisons The ISIS-3 and GISSI-2 trials that directly compared SK, anistreplase and rt-PA showed no differences between these three agents in 30-day mortality (GISSI-2 1990, ISIS-3 Collaborative Group 1993). Anistreplase was never commercially available. SK is far less expensive than rt-PA and in many countries became the drug of choice. However, these results surprised many investigators as previous small studies employing angiography to determine infarct-related artery patency had shown that more arteries were open 90 minutes post therapy with rt-PA than with SK. These studies had also indicated the need to follow up the administration of rt-PA with intravenous heparin rather than the subcutaneous heparin employed in ISIS-3.

Primarily because of this criticism the GUSTO-I trial was conducted (GUSTO Investigators 1993). The rt-PA arm of this study employed an accelerated or 'front-loaded' regimen in which a bolus dose was given and the remaining dose was administered in 90 minutes. It was then followed up with intravenous heparin for at least 24 hours. GUSTO-I showed an overall reduction in absolute mortality of 1% with accelerated rt-PA and intravenous heparin at the expense of three additional major intracerebral haemorrhages per 1000 patients treated (GUSTO Investigators 1993). Following the demonstration of this modest but statistically significant effect, the use of rt-PA increased, particularly in patients presenting early (<4 hours) with extensive anterolateral infarctions in which subgroup analysis suggested the greatest differential benefit.

Bolus thrombolytic therapy rt-PA and SK are given as infusions. It was thought that drugs designed for bolus administration might result in earlier reperfusion with improved outcomes. GUSTO-III compared reteplase given as a double bolus 30 minutes apart with front-loaded rt-PA (Topol et al 2000). ASSENT-2 compared tenecteplase given as a single bolus with rt-PA (ASSENT-2 Investigators 1999). These two trials demonstrated equivalence but not superiority. Subsequently in ASSENT-3 full-dose tenecteplase with enoxaparin was shown to be significantly better than full-dose tenecteplase with UFH (ASSENT-3 Investigators 2001). Bolus administration is clearly ideal for use in the community by paramedics and even in hospital, when there is no time wasted preparing the double dummy infusions required in the trials, a few crucial minutes may be saved.

Thrombolytic therapy vs reduced-dose thrombolysis combined with platelet glycoprotein IIb/IIIa (GP IIb/IIIa) receptor inhibitors In pilot studies employing coronary angiography to assess infarct artery patency, combined administration of reduced-dose thrombolytic therapy together with a platelet GP IIb/IIIa inhibitor was associated with earlier and more complete reperfusion compared with full-dose thrombolytic therapy alone. Of course, this had also been shown for rt-PA compared to SK but it was subsequently difficult to show a mortality advantage. Similarly the large mortality trials comparing these two strategies failed to confirm a mortality advantage. GUSTO-V used half-dose reteplase with abciximab (Topol 2001). One of the three arms of ASSENT-3 used half-dose tenecteplase and abciximab. Both showed minor but significant reductions in reinfarction with the combination therapy at the expense of more bleeding.

In ASSENT-3 the full-dose tenecteplase/enoxaparin combination produced similar results to the half-dose tenecteplase/abciximab combination but is significantly cheaper and simpler to administer, with lower bleeding complications. It may become the gold standard for pharmacological reperfusion but it should be noted that the trial regimen required the enoxaparin to be given for 7 days which is rather longer than most patients with acute MI now stay in hospital. The tenecteplase/abciximab combination does have the potential advantage of providing an optimal pharmacological background for patients who fail to reperfuse and proceed to rescue PCI.

PCI in acute STEMI

Some patients have relative or absolute contraindications to thrombolytic therapy and should be referred for PCI as the only means of achieving reperfusion. In certain subgroups such as those presenting late or with cardiogenic shock, thrombolytic therapy is ineffective. In the latter group early revascularization is of proven benefit (Hochman et al 2001). Direct comparisons of thrombolytic therapy with plain old balloon angioplasty in randomized trials have shown higher rates of reperfusion with PCI and a meta-analysis confirmed a significantly higher event-free survival at short-term follow-up (Michels & Yusuf 1995). This emphasizes the secondary preventive effect of rapid, complete and sustained restoration of normal flow in the infarct-related artery. The initial results of stent implantation in MI were less clear as there was a suggestion that antegrade flow declined in some patients following deployment of the stent possibly as a result of distal embolization of plaque material and/or thrombus. More recently, coronary stenting with adjunctive GP IIb/IIIa blockers has been associated with excellent outcomes in acute MI (Montalescot et al 2001; Table 9.5).

Logistically very few hospitals can provide round-the-clock primary PCI for acute myocardial infarction. In most units PCI is used in patients who fail to reperfuse with thrombolytic therapy (rescue PCI). However,

Table 9.5 Clinical outcomes in the ADMIRAL study showing the benefit of administering abciximab prior to stent implantation in patients with acute MI (Montalescot et al 2001)

	Abciximab + stenting ($n = 149$)	Placebo + stenting ($n = 150$)	RR (95% CI)
30-day death, reinfarction, urgent TVR	6.0%	14.6%	0.41 (0.18–0.93)
6-month death, reinfarction, urgent TVR	7.4%	15.9%	0.46 (0.22–0.93)

conventional ECG criteria to diagnose failed reperfusion are only 70–80% sensitive and specific. Considering this and the fact that stents and GP IIb/IIIa receptor blockers have improved the results of PCI in AMI, there is a trend towards early angiography and PCI if appropriate, even in patients who appear to have reperfused (adjunctive PCI).

PCI in non-ST elevation acute coronary syndromes (ACS)

The first series of trials assessing the role of early routine angiography and revascularization in this patient subgroup were negative. However, in FRISC-II (Wallentin et al 2000) and TACTICS-TIMI 18 (Cannon et al 2001), performed following the introduction of routine stenting and platelet glycoprotein IIb/IIIa blockers, the early revascularization strategy was clearly superior to the alternative of medical therapy with revascularization only for recurrent or inducible ischaemia. Most of the benefit was seen in high-risk patients characterized by ECG evidence of ischaemia, elevated troponin levels and diabetes.

Unfractionated heparin
STEMI

In the acute therapy of MI intravenous unfractionated heparin (UFH) is routinely administered for 24–48 hours after the use of rt-PA. At the moment none of the low molecular weight heparins (LMWH) are approved for use with either thrombolytic drugs or GP IIb/IIIa inhibitors. However, it is anticipated that co-administration will be approved over the next 2–3 years (see above). There is no clear evidence of any additional benefit with either intravenous or high-dose (12 500 units twice daily) subcutaneous UFH after the use of SK.

Non-ST elevation ACS

When there is electrocardiographic evidence of ischaemia, intravenous UFH significantly reduces the frequency of ischaemic episodes compared to aspirin with bolus heparin or thrombolytic therapy (Serneri et al 1990). However, it has largely been replaced with LMWH (see below).

Low molecular weight heparin

The various LMWHs have several advantages over UFH. They directly inhibit factor Xa (Xa:IIa inhibitory activity ratio >2:1), thereby producing a greater anticoagulant effect. They have predictable bio-availability and can be given as once- or twice-daily subcutaneous injections without the need for any monitoring.

STEMI

ASSENT-3 has suggested that enoxaparin combined with full-dose tenecteplase is superior to the same thrombolytic drug with UFH.

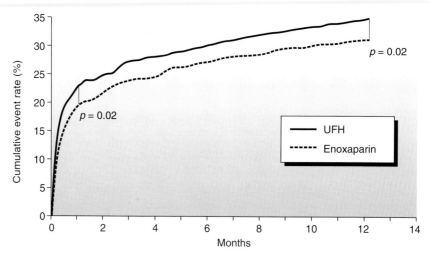

Figure 9.4 Cumulative event rate (death, MI, refractory angina) in the ESSENCE trial showing the superiority of LMWH (enoxaparin) over unfractionated heparin (UFH).

Non-ST elevation ACS

The ESSENCE and TIMI-IIB trials have demonstrated the superiority of enoxaparin over UFH in preventing death, MI and recurrent ischaemia in non ST-elevation ACS (Antmann et al 1999; Fig. 9.4). Dalteparin was found to be equivalent to UFH in the same clinical setting (Klein et al 1997), emphasizing that different LMWHs may have different biological effects.

Warfarin
STEMI

A number of clinical trials in the prethrombolytic era established the beneficial effects of oral anticoagulation with warfarin following MI. In a population of MI patients who have received thrombolytic therapy, warfarin and aspirin is superior to aspirin alone (WARIS-II, presented at ESC 2001). In practice, however, all patients receive aspirin unless contraindicated and warfarin is added for specific indications such as atrial fibrillation or the demonstration of mural thrombus on echocardiography.

Non-ST elevation ACS

Combination therapy with aspirin and moderate-intensity anticoagulation has so far not shown any clear superiority over aspirin alone in preventing recurrent events in patients with unstable angina (OASIS Investigators 2001). As a therapeutic option this has in any event been superseded by combined aspirin/clopidogrel therapy and in future, this may also apply to MI patients.

Direct thrombin inhibitors

These agents bind to thrombin and inhibit all its major actions, including fibrin generation and platelet activation. The prototype is hirudin derived from the leech *Hirudo medicinalis*. Several hirudin preparations have been produced by recombinant DNA technology. They have been compared to UFH in several clinical settings including MI, ACS and PCI. The safety profile of the direct thrombin inhibitors appears to be better than UFH but to date none has been shown to be conclusively superior in clinical trials (HERO-2 Investigators 2001). Of greater relevance, there are no data comparing thrombin inhibitors and LMWHs.

Glycoprotein IIb/IIIa receptor blockers

The binding of fibrinogen to the platelet GP IIb/IIIa receptor is the final common pathway of platelet aggregation. Several drugs (oral and intravenous) have been developed which block this receptor and thereby induce potent antiplatelet effects. The oral GP IIb/IIIa blockers have not shown any benefit in the clinical trials conducted so far. However, the story with intravenous agents is different.

Abciximab

This is a chimeric (half-human, half-mouse) monoclonal antibody directed against the GP IIb/IIIa receptor. It exhibits tight irreversible binding with a long biological half-life. This means that bleeding complications are difficult to deal with and usually require platelet transfusions. On the other hand, it has actions against a range of other cellular receptors in addition to the GP IIb/IIIa and this may confer additional long-term effects. It has proved to be of unequivocal benefit when used in the setting of PCI, reducing short- and long-term mortality, non-fatal MI and reintervention rates. This has been observed in all settings in which PCI is employed:

- non-ST elevation ACS (CAPTURE Investigators 1997)
- high-risk PCI (EPIC Investigators 1994)
- elective PCI (EPILOG Investigators 1997)
- coronary stenting (EPISTENT Investigators 1998)
- stenting in acute MI (ADMIRAL; Montalescot et al 2001).

Interestingly, however, two large multicentre trials evaluating the effect of abciximab outwith the setting of PCI have both been negative:

- non-ST elevation ACS (GUSTO-IV; Simoons 2001)
- MI (abciximab plus half-dose reteplase vs full-dose reteplase; GUSTO-V; Topol 2001).

Eptifibatide/tirofiban

These are both short-acting small molecule GP IIb/IIIa blockers. Their effect is lost 3–4 hours after administration is discontinued which makes bleeding complications easier to treat. On the other hand, they are very specific for the GP IIb/IIIa receptor, a property that may in theory be a disadvantage in comparison to abciximab. In the placebo-controlled studies in the setting of PCI, initial results with both eptifibatide (IMPACT-II Investigators 1997) and tirofiban (RESTORE Investigators 1997) were disappointing, probably because of underdosing. In a second study (ESPRIT Investigators 2000), a double-bolus regimen of eptifibatide was used prior to stent implantation. This produces levels of platelet inhibition approaching those achieved with abciximab and was shown to be of significant benefit. In the non-interventional treatment of ACS, both eptifibatide (PURSUIT Trial Investigators 1998) and tirofiban (PRISM-PLUS Trial Investigators 1998) are of proven efficacy in terms of reducing death and non-fatal MI.

Comparisons of GP IIb/IIIa blockers

So far there has only been one head-to-head study (Stone et al 2002) in which patients were randomized to receive either abciximab or tirofiban prior to elective PCI. At 30 days clinical outcomes were superior in the abciximab group but this difference had disappeared at 1 year. Nevertheless, the only drug with a proven long-term effect on mortality following PCI is abciximab (Fig. 9.5).

Who should receive a GP IIb/IIIa blocker?

In the UK the National Institute for Clinical Excellence (NICE 2002) has recommended that all patients undergoing PCI should receive abciximab as at the moment neither of the other two drugs is licensed for use in this setting. Cost restraints have precluded any unit following this advice and in fact, most of the benefit can be achieved by targeting patients at high risk of periprocedural adverse events, including diabetics, patients with angiographic evidence of intraluminal thrombus, those with an elevated troponin and those undergoing multivessel intervention. The NICE also recommend administration of one of the small-molecule drugs in the coronary care unit prior to PCI in high-risk patients. This is the so-called upstream regimen as

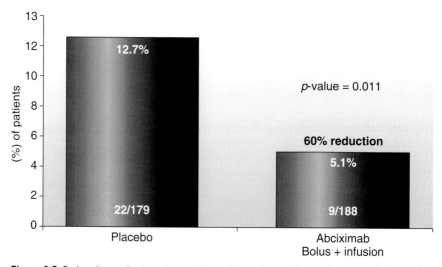

Figure 9.5 Reduced mortality in patients with unstable angina or MI at study entry with abciximab therapy at 3 years follow-up in the EPIC study.

employed in TACTICS-TIMI 18 (Cannon et al 2001) but currently it is not commonly utilized, largely because of cost considerations.

Aspirin

Aspirin is a critical component of the immediate treatment of all acute coronary syndromes and in MI produces the same magnitude of mortality reduction as streptokinase given alone (ISIS-2 Collaborative Group 1988).

Clopidogrel

Clopidogrel is an inactive drug in vitro that has potent platelet antiaggregatory effects in vivo. It acts by non-competitive but selective antagonism of ADP-induced platelet aggregation, thereby blocking platelet GP IIb/IIIa activation. Active metabolites generated in the liver are responsible for the effects as the presence of a portojugular shunt renders it inactive. It is effective in preventing in-stent thrombosis and has taken over from ticlopidine in this clinical setting (Bertrand et al 2000).

The recently published CURE study (2001) indicates that the combination of clopidogrel and aspirin is superior to aspirin alone in the non-interventional treatment of non-ST elevation ACS. Significant reductions were observed in the incidence of stroke and non-fatal myocardial infarction although there was no reduction in overall mortality (CURE 2001). It should be emphasized that very few patients in this study were revascularized or received GP IIb/IIIa inhibitors. However, in those who did go on to PCI, there was some evidence of an additional benefit in patients receiving pretreatment with clopidogrel.

Clopidogrel has been compared with aspirin in the CAPRIE trial (1996). This enrolled 19 185 patients with an equal proportion having suffered an MI, an ischaemic stroke or having documented peripheral vascular disease. Overall clopidogrel was associated with an 8.7% relative reduction in the combined endpoints of ischaemic stroke, MI or vascular death (5.32% versus 5.83% per year; $p = 0.042$). Certain high-risk groups like diabetics and those with prior CABG appeared to derive the maximum benefit. The incidence of gastrointestinal bleeding was also less in the clopidogrel group.

In general, our current practice is to reserve the use of clopidogrel to the following patients:

- intolerant of aspirin
- in combination with aspirin in patients who continue to experience ischaemic events despite aspirin therapy
- for 2–4 weeks following coronary stent implantation
- in patients with ACS who are not scheduled for revascularization or in whom revascularization is not possible.

SECONDARY PREVENTION IN CORONARY HEART DISEASE

Strategies for secondary prevention in patients with CHD have almost exclusively involved studies of various drug interventions in patients with a prior MI. There are virtually no data on the effects of most current thera-pies on the outcome of patients with stable angina pectoris but without any history of prior MI. Extrapolation of the data from post-MI studies to this latter group of patients is difficult as the two groups have different natural histories and event rates. In addition, epidemiological studies suggest that up to one third of such patients in the community are unrecognized, i.e. they have had silent infarctions (Sugurdsson et al 1995).

Aspirin

Primary prevention

Two major studies have been conducted. In the United States, more than 22 000 male physicians aged 40–84 were randomized to either aspirin 325 mg every other day or placebo for 5 years. Though the incidence of cardiovas-cular death was not reduced, there was a 44% relative reduction in MI in the aspirin-treated group. This effect was limited to those older than 50 years (Steering Committee of Physicians' Health Study 1989). A similar study in the UK involving more than 5000 physicians followed up for 6 years failed to show any reduction in MI in the aspirin-treated arm. However, a number of protocol crossovers diluted the power of this study (Peto et al 1988).

Secondary prevention

In this setting the benefits of aspirin are more clearly established. The data from the Antiplatelet Trialists' Collaboration confirm that antiplatelet ther-apy, mainly aspirin, significantly reduces vascular events (vascular death, non-fatal stroke and myocardial infarction) in patients at high risk, i.e. those with a prior history of vascular disease or other conditions associated with an increased risk of occlusive vascular disease such as atrial fibrillation and valvular heart disease (Table 9.6; Antiplatelet Trialists' Collaboration 1994a). These reductions were significant in middle and old age, in men and women, in hypertensive and normotensive patients and in diabetic and

Table 9.6 Summary of secondary preventive effects of antiplatelet therapy (mainly aspirin) from the Antiplatelet Trialists' Collaboration

	n	Vascular events prevented per 1000 patients treated	2p value
Acute MI	~20 000	40 at 1 month	<0.0001
Previous MI	~20 000	40 at 2 years	<0.0001
Previous stroke/TIA	~10 000	40 at 3 years	<0.0001
Unstable angina	~4000	50 at 6 months	<0.0001
Other cardiovascular disease*	~14 000	20 at 1 year	<0.0001

*Stable angina, vascular surgery, angioplasty, atrial fibrillation, valvular heart disease, peripheral vascular disease.
MI myocardial infarction.
TIA transient ischaemic attack.

non-diabetic patients. The optimal duration of treatment in each patient category remains undetermined but is at least 2–3 years. Similar meta-analysis has confirmed the beneficial effects of aspirin on graft or arterial patency following vascular surgery/angioplasty and the ability of aspirin to reduce the incidence of venous thrombosis and pulmonary embolism in both medical and surgical patients (Antiplatelet Trialists' Collaboration 1994b,c).

Angiotensin-converting enzyme inhibitors (ACEI)

The original hypothesis that ACEI would favourably influence the outcome after MI was based on animal studies that showed ACEI could favourably modify ventricular remodelling. This is the term used to describe the complex changes in ventricular size and shape involving expansion of both the infarcted and non-infarcted regions of the myocardium which follow MI. Around one third of patients demonstrate significant remodelling after MI, the best predictors of this being the presence of a large transmural anteroapical infarction and also the presence of heart failure. Although the initial few weeks of ventricular remodelling may help to maintain cardiac function, mortality at 8 weeks is higher in patients experiencing infarct expansion (Eaton et al 1979). The magnitude of the increase in left ventricular volume may be the single best predictor of an adverse prognosis following MI.

Mortality trials with ACEI in MI

All the randomized placebo-controlled trials showed a significant reduction in mortality at a variety of follow-up times, except the CONSENSUS II trial which was halted prematurely because of a non-significant excess mortality in the enalapril group. The study authors themselves believed that this was due to the early administration of intravenous enalaprilat, which may have provoked an excess incidence of harmful hypotension (Swedberg et al 1992). The pattern of results in all the trials is similar to that seen in the β-blocker trials, i.e. the relative risk reduction is greatest in the AIRE trial which selected the highest risk group of patients (Fig. 9.6; AIRE Investigators 1993). These patients were also identified without the need for any sophisticated measurements of ejection fraction.

In the GISSI-3 (1994) and ISIS-4 (ISIS-4 Collaborative Group 1995) trials, which recruited essentially all patients with MI and so avoided the issue of patient selection, smaller risk reductions were seen. This may in fact represent a similar magnitude of effect in patients similar to those recruited in AIRE and little or no effect in patients at low risk. The SAVE trial, which recruited patients at intermediate risk, produced an intermediate risk reduction (Pfeffer et al 1988). In the HOPE study (2000) treatment with ramipril reduced mortality and non-fatal myocardial infarction in a range of patients with vascular disease. It is not clear whether this effect was mediated by blood pressure reduction alone or by specific inhibition of the renin–angiotensin axis.

β-Adrenoceptor blockade

Several studies have confirmed the ability of β-blockers to improve the prognosis of patients with MI. Both cardioselective and non-cardioselective

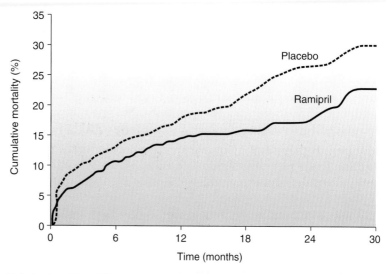

Relative hazard 0.73 (95% CI 0.60 to 0.89) $p = 0.0002$

Figure 9.6 Reduction in the risk of death from all causes in the AIRE study (AIRE Study Investigators 1993).

drugs appear to work, though agents with partial agonist activity such as oxprenolol are much less effective (Yusuf et al 1985). More recently and in parallel with studies in congestive heart failure, carvedilol has been shown to reduce mortality and recurrent infarction in post-MI patients with left ventricular ejection fractions <40% (CAPRICORN Investigators 2001).

Calcium channel blockade
Nifedipine
Several trials have confirmed that nifedipine has no beneficial effects on survival when used routinely in patients with prior myocardial infarction (Held et al 1989). In fact, the trend is for mortality to be increased.

Diltiazem
In the Multicentre Diltiazem Postinfarction Trial (MDPIT) no benefits of treatment with diltiazem were seen. On the contrary, there was evidence of a harmful effect in patients with significant left ventricular dysfunction (MDPIT Research Group 1988). In a randomized trial restricted to patients with non-Q wave infarction, diltiazem in a high dosage of 360 mg daily produced a significant reduction in reinfarction (Gibson et al 1986).

Verapamil
In the second Danish Verapamil Infarction Trial a modest benefit was observed but only in patients with well-preserved ventricular function (DAVIT-II 1990). An important feature of the protocol in these two trials

was that patients requiring β-blocker therapy because of angina, arrhythmias or hypertension were excluded and elective use of β-blockade for secondary prevention was not allowed.

Nitrates

Despite the theoretical attractions of nitrate therapy two mega-trials have failed to show any mortality reductions in patients treated with intravenous followed by transdermal nitrates (GISSI-3 1994) or oral nitrates (ISIS-4 Collaborative Group 1995) for 4–6 weeks after MI. However, nitrates are still widely used in acute MI for specific indications such as persistent myocardial ischaemia, heart failure and control of hypertension both before and after thrombolytic therapy.

Lipid-lowering drugs

The critical role of lipid-lowering drug therapy in the primary and secondary prevention of CHD has been clarified over the past 10 years and is addressed elsewhere in this book (see Chapter 3).

CONGESTIVE HEART FAILURE

Coronary heart disease and particularly MI is now the major cause of congestive heart failure (CHF) in the developed world. As such, the primary prevention of CHD by risk factor modification should ultimately feed through into a reduction in the incidence of CHF. In similar fashion, more rapid and complete restoration of adequate myocardial perfusion in patients who have sustained an acute MI, with early administration of thrombolytic therapy and/or PCI, should also reduce the subsequent development of CHF. Meanwhile, the incidence of CHF is rising and by the time it has developed the coronary artery disease process is usually so advanced that there is very little scope left for secondary prevention.

Digoxin

Digoxin has been used for 200 years and yet its role in CHF has only been defined recently. It is clearly helpful in patients with CHF and atrial fibrillation where its rate-limiting properties result in improved haemodynamic status. It is now clear that there are also some benefits in patients in sinus rhythm. Both the RADIANCE (Packer et al 1993) and PROVED (Uretsky et al 1993) trials demonstrated that withdrawal of digoxin in patients with mild to moderate CHF stabilized on diuretics, ACE inhibitors and digoxin resulted in significant and rapid deterioration. These trials were not powered to show a reduction in mortality but the larger Digitalis Investigation Group study (1997) demonstrated that, despite being associated with improved quality of life and reduced hospital admission rates, no overall survival advantage was demonstrated.

Digoxin acts by blocking the myocardial NaK-ATPase, thereby increasing intracellular calcium and thus exerting a positive inotropic effect. It also increases baroreceptor sensitivity, thereby reducing sympathetic and enhancing parasympathetic output leading to peripheral vasodilatation. These effects lead to reduction in the myocardial oxygen consumption and improved cardiac function. Digoxin should be avoided in the early stages following a myocardial infarction as its arrhythmogenic potential can increase mortality. It is generally reserved for the later stages of chronic CHF and in patients with atrial fibrillation.

Diuretics

No clinical trials have addressed the question of whether diuretics have any effect on disease progression or survival in patients with CHF. There is no doubt that diuretic therapy improves symptoms and thereby quality of life in patients with CHF. Even in mild CHF, trials attempting to use ACEI alone have not been successful. As such, they are an essential part of the treatment and will probably never be the subject of survival studies. There are, however, a number of adverse features associated with diuretic therapy, which may unfavourably influence disease progression and survival. These include electrolyte disturbances and activation of the renin–angiotensin system. Some of these may be offset in part by the concomitant use of ACEI. Generally, it is good practice to maximize ACEI dosages in the hope that this will allow the use of the minimum dosage of diuretics commensurate with keeping the patient's clinical condition stable.

Spironolactone

Although spironolactone is conventionally considered as a diuretic, its benefit in CHF relates to specific antagonism of the deleterious effects of aldosterone. Aldosterone levels are increased in CHF and this causes sodium retention, potassium and magnesium depletion, loss of baroreceptor sensitivity and promotion of myocardial fibrosis. The RALES study confirmed that low doses of spironolactone (25–50 mg od) added to otherwise optimal therapy for CHF (including ACEI, digoxin and β-blockers) produce a 27% reduction in mortality (Pitt et al 1999b). However, when adding spironolactone to a patient's therapy, it is important to closely monitor renal function and serum potassium levels.

Angiotensin-converting enzyme inhibitors

There is no doubt that ACEI improve symptoms and effort capacity in patients with CHF and as such they are an essential part of therapy. In terms of CHD prevention, there is also ample evidence to support their use.

Co-operative North Scandinavian Enalapril Survival Study (CONSENSUS I)

This trial of the use of enalapril in severe class IV heart failure showed, for the first time, that a therapy for heart failure could improve the prognosis. Indeed, the effect was so marked that the trial was stopped prematurely (CONSENSUS Trial Group 1987).

Studies of Left Ventricular Dysfunction (SOLVD)

In the treatment arm of this study, patients with mild to moderate class II–III CHF and an ejection fraction <35% were randomized to enalapril or placebo in addition to their previous therapy, usually digoxin and diuretics. Patients with an ejection fraction <35% but no symptoms of CHF, i.e. asymptomatic left ventricular dysfunction or functional class I, were recruited into the prevention arm. This study differs from the postinfarction trials described above in that patients with recent (<1 month) myocardial infarction were excluded. However, around 70% of the patients did have ischaemic heart disease. In the treatment arm, over an average follow-up period of 41 months there was a 16% (95% CI: 5–26%) reduction in mortality with the bulk of this effect being due to a reduction in death from progressive heart failure as opposed to any reduction in sudden death (SOLVD Investigators 1991). In the prevention arm with a lower risk group of patients, enalapril produced no significant reduction in either total or cardiovascular mortality. The combined endpoint of death and the development of CHF was significantly reduced (SOLVD Investigators 1992).

Heart Outcomes Prevention Evaluation Study (HOPE)

The earlier trials of ACEI have always used the presence of significant LV systolic dysfunction (EF <40%) as a prerequisite for commencing therapy. The results of the HOPE study argue for its initiation in the pre-LV dysfunction stage. In this large randomized multicentre trial, treatment with ramipril in patients with vascular disease or diabetes and one cardiovascular risk factor without any evidence of systolic dysfunction resulted in improved life expectancy. This study emphasizes the beneficial vascular effects of ACE inhibition and has lead to more widespread and earlier use of this unique class of drugs (HOPE Investigators 2000).

Assessment of Treatment with Lisinopril and Survival Trial (ATLAS)

The importance of achieving maximum inhibition of the angiotensin-converting enzyme and blocking formation of angiotensin II is reflected in the ATLAS trial (ATLAS Study Group 1999), which showed greater haemodynamic and clinical benefits with high-dose lisinopril (32.5–35 mg), compared to low dose (2.5–5 mg). In practice it is important that patients receive maximum tolerated doses of the prescribed drug.

Angiotensin II blockers

These novel drugs act by inhibition of the angiotensin II receptor and several drugs in this class have been approved for use in systemic hypertension.

Losartan and valsartan have been studied in the setting of CHF. The ELITE-II study which compared losartan with captopril showed that fewer patients randomized to captopril died or were hospitalized due to heart failure and failed to confirm the hypothesis that AII blockers are superior to ACEI (Pitt et al 1999a). Addition of the AII blocker valsartan to captopril in the Val-HEFT trial did not improve outcomes in the combination arm compared to captopril alone (presented at AHA 2000). Unlike ACEI, AII blockers do not stimulate the kinin pathway, which may have beneficial effects, and this may be responsible for the trial results. Currently AII blockers are used in patients intolerant of ACEI, due to intolerable cough or angio-oedema.

β-Blockers

Waagstein et al (1975) advocated the use of β-blockers in CHF nearly 25 years ago but as in the case of ACEI, this did not become accepted practice until the demonstration of dramatic beneficial effects in randomized trials. So far two highly β_1-selective blockers, bisoprolol and metoprolol, and two non-selective β-blockers, carvedilol and bucindilol, have been evaluated. In the CIBIS-II trial (CIBIS-II Investigators 1999), patients with mild to moderate heart failure randomized to bisoprolol (target dose 10 mg daily) achieved marked reductions in mortality, sudden death and hospitalizations. Similarly treatment with metoprolol (target dose 200 mg slow release daily) in the MERIT-HF study (1999) resulted in impressive reductions in mortality and morbidity. Carvedilol is a non-selective β-blocker with additional antioxidant and α-blocking properties. It is the only β-blocker so far to demonstrate benefit in severe heart failure (Packer et al 2001). Interestingly, bucindilol, another non-selective β-blocker with additional vasodilating properties, was not associated with mortality benefit (BEST Investigators 2001).

It appears that there are subtle differences in the effects of various β-blockers in CHF and only drugs for which an evidence base exists should be prescribed. It is important to realize that β-blockers may initially cause both haemodynamic and clinical deterioration. It is current practice to initiate these drugs in small doses with slow increments in 2–3-week intervals to the maximum tolerated dose. Studies have shown that following a reduction in the LV ejection fraction in the first few weeks of treatment, the ejection fraction steadily improves and often exceeds the baseline values with prolonged treatment. This phenomenon of reversed remodelling has only been demonstrated with β-blockers.

ARRHYTHMIAS

Many patients with CHD have arrhythmias, some of which are clinically silent. It is crucially important to establish the correct electrocardiographic diagnosis. Frequent ambulatory recordings may be required and if doubt remains it may be necessary to implant a long-term recording device or proceed to electrophysiological study. Co-existent ventricular dysfunction or heart failure that can be worsened by the negative inotropic effect of many antiarrhythmic drugs often complicates drug therapy of arrhythmias in patients with CHD. It is beyond the scope of this chapter to discuss details of the management of specific arrhythmias but some generally applicable comments relevant to patients with CHD are made below.

Symptomatic arrhythmias requiring therapy

Atrial fibrillation (AF)

In an elderly asymptomatic patient this may not require specific therapy. If it is chronic and the ventricular rate is rapid, it can be slowed by any drug that slows conduction through the atrioventricular (AV) node, i.e. digoxin, β-blocker or verapamil. The choice is often determined by co-existing disease. Consideration should be given to attempting to restore sinus rhythm in most symptomatic patients. Amiodarone is the best drug for both facilitating electrical cardioversion and maintaining sinus rhythm. If external cardioversion fails internal cardioversion may be successful and can be performed with the appropriate equipment under local anaesthesia. In patients who remain in AF, lifelong therapy with warfarin is required to reduce the risk of cardiac thromboembolism. Paroxysmal atrial fibrillation is often treated with sotalol or amiodarone. Class 1 drugs (flecainide, propafenone) should be avoided in patients with CHD and/or CHF.

Supraventricular tachycardia

Most narrow complex regular tachycardias are due to re-entry circuits involving the AV node. As such they are not caused by CHD but they may co-exist. Drugs which modify AV node conduction are effective but it is sometimes necessary to use other agents such as amiodarone. A permanent cure can often be provided by radiofrequency ablation. Atrial flutter can be more difficult to deal with and is often associated with CHD. Again the main role of drug therapy is to slow the ventricular rate. Pharmacological or more often electrical cardioversion to sinus rhythm is usually successful.

Ventricular fibrillation/tachycardia

Patients with a history of a prior MI and ventricular tachycardia occurring beyond the first 48 hours after MI are a high-risk group for sudden death. Late ventricular tachycardia is usually due to electrical instability in and around the scar tissue of the original infarct. If acute ischaemia and other provoking factors are excluded then therapy will be required.

Several trials have compared the implantable cardioverter-defibrillator (ICD) with various antiarrhythmic drugs (amiodarone, sotalol, metoprolol) in patients who have survived an out-of-hospital cardiac arrest or have experienced haemodynamically unstable ventricular tachycardia (secondary prevention). These trials (AVID Investigators 1997, Connolly 1998) demonstrated the superiority of ICD therapy.

Patients with poor LV function (EF <35%) and inducible ventricular tachycardia on programmed ventricular stimulation also have a high risk of sudden death. The MADIT (Moss et al 1996, 2002) and MUSTT (Buxton et al 1999) trials randomized patients in this subgroup to ICD or anti-arrhythmic therapy and again demonstrated an improved outcome with the ICD option.

In the UK, the NICE has advised that ICD therapy should be routinely considered in all patients in the above categories.

Postmyocardial infarction/CHF

The Cardiac Arrhythmia Suppression Trial showed that the use of class I antiarrhythmic therapy in patients with prior MI and asymptomatic complex ventricular ectopy caused rather than prevented sudden death (CAST Investigators 1989). This finding is probably related to the ability of all antiarrhythmic drugs to also exert proarrhythmic effects. Empirically amiodarone significantly reduces sudden cardiac death rates following myocardial infarction but its effect on total mortality is unclear. Total mortality was reduced in the BASIS (Burkart et al 1990) trial but was not in the larger CAMIAT (Cairns et al 1997) trial despite a 50% reduction in arrhythmic mortality.

There is increasing evidence that high-risk post-MI patients with or without CHF benefit from ICD therapy. A recent trial in post-MI patients with low ejection fraction randomized patients to amiodarone or ICD therapy (Moss et al 2002). It was not a requirement of this study that the patient had experienced either symptomatic ventricular tachycardia or that ventricular arrhythmias had been demonstrated either by Holter recording or by programmed ventricular stimulation. Despite this, the trial was terminated prematurely because of a significant reduction in mortality in patients randomized to ICD. The recent implantation of an ICD in the Vice-President of the USA, Dick Cheney, is a reflection of the growing enthusiasm for this approach in high-risk (or high-profile) patients.

Drug eluting stents

Although stenting reduces restenosis, it by no means abolishes the problem. Restenosis following stent implantation is almost entirely due to neo-intimal proliferation and depending on a number of patient and lesion-specific characteristics, restenosis rates may vary from <10% to 50%. Known predictors of instent restenosis include diabetes, lesions in the proximal left anterior descending artery or saphenous vein grafts, long lesions, small vessels and chronic total occlusions. A huge amount of research has been conducted in an attempt to find some means of controlling neo-intimal growth in the stented artery and significant progress has been achieved. A number of drugs have been coated on to a variety of stents and have been shown to almost completely inhibit neointimal proliferation in humans and to abolish clinical restenosis. These include rapamycin, a cytostatic drug used orally in renal transplant patients and paclitaxel, a cytotoxic drug used in the treatment of a variety of cancers. The obvious attraction of using the stent itself for local drug delivery is that only very low doses are required to achieve efficacy with no resultant systemic toxicity. The RAVEL study (2002) was a randomized trial that compared both angiographic and clinical endpoints in patients with chronic stable angina and single vessel coronary artery disease who were randomized to either stenting with a bare metal stent or a sirolimus coated stent. At 6 months, angiographic restenosis rates were significantly lower in the coated stent group (0% vs 26%). This reduction in restenosis was reflected in improved clinical outcomes at 1 year, which was entirely due to a reduction in the rate of revascularization.

Drug eluting stents are now commercially available but are about three times more expensive than the bare metal stents. However if the improved outcomes are established in larger currently ongoing trials, this will offset the initial higher costs.

■ KEY POINTS

- β-Blockers, calcium channel blockers, nitrates and nicorandil all relieve angina but there is no evidence that any of these therapies can improve the survival of patients with angina and no history of myocardial infarction.
- All patients with CHD should be assessed by a cardiologist with a view to coronary angiography to assess the extent of their disease. The historical threshold for referral is too high.
- A strategy of early revascularization in all high-risk patients with non-ST elevation ACS has been shown to be superior to the 'watch and wait' option of intervention only for recurrent symptoms or inducible ischaemia.
- Randomized studies performed in the late 1970s showed that compared to medical therapy, CABG improves the survival of patients with significant stenosis of the left main coronary artery or significant proximal stenosis of all three coronary arteries, particularly if there is also ventricular dysfunction or CHF.
- Randomized studies performed in the 1990s have shown that for many categories of CHD, there is no difference in survival or subsequent rates of myocardial infarction between patients treated by PCI and those treated by CABG.
- Restenosis following PCI results in a much higher incidence of repeat procedures compared to CABG but restenosis can be reduced by stenting and may be further reduced by drug-eluting stents.
- In acute MI, aspirin and prompt reperfusion of the occluded coronary artery by either thrombolytic drugs or PCI improve survival.
- Following MI, all patients should continue on aspirin, β-blockers, ACEI and a statin. Amiodarone and warfarin may be of benefit in specific subgroups.
- Digoxin, diuretics, ACEI and β-blockers all improve the symptoms of CHF.
- ACEI reduce mortality in all categories of CHF. If ACEI cannot be tolerated because of cough switch to an AII receptor blocker. If ACEI induce renal failure consider renal angiography.
- β-Blockers also improve mortality in all categories of CHF but should be initiated cautiously.
- Spironolactone improves mortality in moderate to severe heart failure.
- Implantable cardioverter-defibrillators are superior to antiarrhythmic drug therapy in the primary and secondary prevention of sudden cardiac death.

REFERENCES

AIMS Trial Study Group 1988 Effect of intravenous APSAC on mortality after acute myocardial infarction: preliminary report of a placebo-controlled clinical trial. Lancet I: 547

AIRE (Acute Infarction Ramipril Efficacy) Study Investigators 1993 Effect of ramipril on mortality and morbidity of survivors of acute myocardial infarction with clinical evidence of heart failure. Lancet 342: 821–828

Antiplatelet Trialists' Collaboration 1994a Collaborative overview of randomised trials of antiplatelet therapy – I: prevention of death, myocardial infarction, and stroke by prolonged antiplatelet therapy in various categories of patients. British Medical Journal 308: 81–106

Antiplatelet Trialists' Collaboration 1994b Collaborative overview of randomised trials of antiplatelet therapy – II: maintenance of vascular graft or arterial patency by antiplatelet therapy. British Medical Journal 308: 159–168

Antiplatelet Trialists' Collaboration 1994c Collaborative overview of randomised trials of antiplatelet therapy – III: reduction in venous thrombosis and pulmonary embolism by antiplatelet prophylaxis among surgical and medical patients. British Medical Journal 308: 235–246

Antmann EM, Cohen M, Radley D et al 1999 Assessment of the treatment effects of enoxaparin for unstable angina/non Q wave myocardial infarction: TIMI 11B-ESSENCE meta-analysis. Circulation 100: 1602–1608

ASSENT-2 (Assessment of the Safety and Efficacy of a New Thrombolytic) Investigators 1999 Single-bolus tenecteplase compared with front-loaded alteplase in acute myocardial infarction: the ASSENT-2 double-blind randomised trial. Lancet 354: 716–722

ASSENT-3 Investigators 2001 Efficacy and safety of tenecteplase in combination with enoxaparin, abciximab, or unfractionated heparin: the ASSENT-3 randomised trial in acute myocardial infarction. Lancet 358: 605–613

ATLAS Study Group 1999 Comparative effects of low and high doses of the angiotensin converting enzyme inhibitor lisinopril on morbidity and mortality in chronic heart failure. Circulation 100: 2312–2318

AVID (Antiarrhythmics Versus Implantable Defibrillators) Investigators 1997 A comparison of antiarrhythmic drug therapy with implantable defibrillators in patients resuscitated from near fatal ventricular arrhythmias. New England Journal of Medicine 337: 1576–1583

BARI 2000 Seven year outcome in the Bypass Angioplasty Revascularisation Investigation (BARI) trial by treatment and diabetic status. Journal of the American College of Cardiology 35: 1130–1133

Bertrand ME, Rupprecht H-J, Urban P et al 2000 Double-blind study of the safety of clopidogrel with and without a loading dose in combination with aspirin compared with ticlopidine in combination with aspirin after coronary stenting. Circulation 102: 624–629

BEST Investigators 2001 A trial of the beta-blocker bucindilol in patients with advanced chronic heart failure. New England Journal of Medicine 344: 1659–1667

Burkart F, Pfisterer M, Kioski W et al 1990 Effect of antiarrhythmic therapy on mortality in survivors of myocardial infarction with asymptomatic complex ventricular arrhythmias. Basel Antiarrhythmic Study of Infarct Survival (BASIS). Journal of the American College of Cardiology 16: 1711–1718

Buxton AE, Lee KL, Fisher JD et al 1999 A randomised study for the prevention of sudden death in patients with coronary artery disease. Multicentre Unsustained Tachycardia Trial (MUSTT) Investigators. New England Journal of Medicine 341: 1882–1890

Cairns JA, Connolly SJ, Roberts R et al 1997 Randomised trial of outcome after myocardial infarction in patients with frequent or repetitive ventricular premature depolarisations. Canadian Amiodarone Myocardial Infarction Arrhythmia (CAMIAT) Trial. Lancet 349: 675–682

Cannon CP, Weintraub WS, Demopoulos LA et al 2001 Comparison of early invasive and conservative strategies in patients with unstable coronary syndromes treated with the glycoprotein IIb/IIIa inhibitor tirofiban. New England Journal of Medicine 344(25): 1879–1887

CAPRICORN Investigators 2001 Effects of carvedilol on outcome after myocardial infarction in patients with left-ventricular dysfunction: the CAPRICORN randomised trial. Lancet 357: 1385–1390

CAPRIE Steering Committee 1996 A randomised trial of clopidogrel versus aspirin in patients at risk of ischaemic events. Lancet 348: 1329–1339

CAPTURE Investigators 1997 Randomised placebo-controlled trial of abciximab before and during coronary intervention in refractory unstable angina. Lancet 349: 1429–1435

CAST (Cardiac Arrhythmia Suppression Trial) Investigators 1989 Preliminary report: effect of encainide and flecainide on mortality in a randomised trial of arrhythmia suppression after myocardial infarction. New England Journal of Medicine 321: 406–412

CIBIS-II Investigators 1999 The Cardiac Insufficiency Bisoprolol Study II (CIBIS II). A randomised trial. Lancet 353: 9–13

Colombo A, Hall P, Nakamura S et al 1995 Intracoronary stenting without anticoagulation accomplished with intravascular ultrasound guidance. Circulation 91: 1676–1688

Connolly SJ, on behalf of the CIDS Investigators 1998 The CIDS study: final results. Oral presentation at the annual session of the American College of Cardiology, Atlanta, March 29

CONSENSUS Trial Group 1987 Effects of enalapril on mortality in severe congestive heart failure. Results of the Cooperative North Scandinavian Enalapril Survival Study. New England Journal of Medicine 316: 1429–1435

CURE Investigators 2001 Effects of clopidogrel in addition to aspirin in patients with ACS without ST-segment elevation. New England Journal of Medicine 345: 494–502

DAVIT-II (Danish Study Group on Verapamil in Myocardial Infarction) 1990 Effect of verapamil on mortality and major events after acute myocardial infarction. American Journal of Cardiology 66: 779–785

Digitalis Investigation Group 1997 The effect of digoxin on mortality and morbidity in patients with heart failure. New England Journal of Medicine 336: 525–533

Dotter CT 1969 Transluminally placed coilspring endarteria tubegrafts. Long-term patency in canine popliteal. Invest Radiol 4: 329–32

Eaton LW, Weiss JL, Berkley BH et al 1979 Regional cardiac dilatation after acute myocardial infarction. New England Journal of Medicine 350: 57–62

EPIC Investigators 1994 Use of a monoclonal antibody directed against the platelet glycoprotein IIb/IIIa receptor in high-risk coronary angioplasty. The EPIC Investigation. New England Journal of Medicine 330: 956-961

EPILOG Investigators 1997 Platelet glycoprotein IIb/IIIa receptor blockade and low dose heparin during percutaneous coronary revascularisation. New England Journal of Medicine 336: 1689–1696

EPISTENT Investigators 1998 Randomised placebo-controlled and balloon-angioplasty controlled trial to assess the safety of coronary stenting with use of platelet glycoprotein IIb/IIIa receptor blockade. Lancet 352: 87–92

ESPRIT Investigators 2000 Novel dosing regimen of eptifibatide in planned coronary stent implantation (ESPRIT): a randomised placebo-controlled trial. Lancet 356: 2037–2044

Fischman DL, Leon MB, Baim DS et al 1994 A randomised comparison of coronary-stent placement and balloon angioplasty in the treatment of coronary artery disease. New England Journal of Medicine 331: 496–501

Gibson RS, Boden WE, Theroux P et al 1986 Diltiazem and reinfarction in patients with non-Q-wave infarction. New England Journal of Medicine 315: 423–429

GISSI-2 (Gruppo Italiano per lo Studio della Sopravivenza nell'Infarto Miocardico) 1990 A factorial randomised trial of alteplase versus streptokinase and heparin versus no heparin among 12 490 patients with acute myocardial infarction. Lancet 336: 65–71

GISSI-3 (Gruppo Italiano per lo Studio della Sopravivenza nell'Infarto Miocardico) 1994 Effects of lisinopril and transdermal glyceryl trinitrate singly and together on 6 week mortality and ventricular function after acute myocardial infarction. Lancet 343: 1115–1122

GUSTO Investigators 1993 An international randomised trial comparing four thrombolytic strategies for acute myocardial infarction. New England Journal of Medicine 329: 673–682

Held PH, Yusuf S, Furberg CD 1989 Calcium channel blockers in acute myocardial infarction and unstable angina: an overview. British Medical Journal 229: 1187–1192

HERO-2 (Hirulog and Early Reperfusion or Occlusion) Trial Investigators 2001 Thrombin-specific anticoagulation with bivalirudin versus heparin in patients receiving fibrinolytic therapy for acute myocardial infarction: the HERO-2 randomized trial. Lancet 358: 1855–1863

Hochman JS, Sleeper LA, White HD et al 2001 One-year survival following early revascularization for cardiogenic shock. Journal of the American Medical Association 285: 190–192

HOPE (Heart Outcomes Prevention Evaluation) Study Investigators 2000 Effects of angiotensin converting enzyme inhibitor, ramipril on cardiovascular events in high-risk patients. New England Journal of Medicine 342: 145–153

IMPACT II Investigators 1997 Randomised placebo-controlled trial effect of eptifibatide on complications of percutaneous coronary intervention: IMPACT-II. Lancet 349: 1422–1428

IONA Trial Investigators 2002 Effect of nicorandil on coronary events in patients with stable angina. The Impact of Nicorandil in Angina (IONA) randomised trial. Lancet 359: 1269–1275

ISIS-2 (Second International Study of Infarct Survival) Collaborative Group 1988 Randomised trial of intravenous streptokinase, oral aspirin, both, or neither among 17,187 cases of suspected acute myocardial infarction. Lancet 2: 349–360

ISIS-3 (Third International Study of Infarct Survival) Collaborative Group 1993 ISIS-3: a randomised comparison of streptokinase vs tissue plasminogen activator vs anistreplase and of aspirin plus heparin vs aspirin alone among 41 229 cases of suspected acute myocardial infarction. Lancet 339: 753–770

ISIS-4 (Fourth International Study of Infarct Survival) Collaborative Group 1995 ISIS-4: a randomised factorial trial assessing early oral captopril, oral mononitrate, and intravenous magnesium sulphate in 58,050 patients with suspected acute myocardial infarction. Lancet 345: 669–681

Klein W, Buchwald A, Hillis SE et al 1997 Comparison of low molecular weight heparin with unfractionated heparin acutely and with placebo for 6 weeks in the management of unstable coronary artery disease. Fragmin in Unstable Coronary Artery Disease (FRIC) study. Circulation 96: 61–68

MDPIT (Multicenter Diltiazem Postinfarction Trial) Research Group 1988 The effect of diltiazem on mortality and reinfarction after myocardial infarction. New England Journal of Medicine 319: 385–392

MERIT-HF Study Group 1999 Effect of metoprolol CR/XL in chronic heart failure: Metoprolol CR/XL Randomised Intervention Trial in Congestive Heart Failure (MERIT-HF). Lancet 353: 2001–2007

Michels KB, Yusuf S 1995 Does PTCA in acute myocardial infarction affect mortality and reinfarction rates? Circulation 91: 476–485

Montalescot G, Barragan P, Wittenberg O et al 2001 Platelet glycoprotein IIb/IIIa inhibition with coronary stenting for acute myocardial infarction. New England Journal of Medicine 344(25): 1895–1903

Moss AJ, Zareba W, Hall J et al 2002 Prophylactic implantation of a defibrillator in patients with a myocardial infarction and reduced ejection fraction. MADIT II trial. New England Journal of Medicine 346: 877–883

Moss AM, Hall WJ, Cannom DS et al 1996 Improved survival with an implanted defibrillator in patients with coronary disease at high-risk for ventricular arrhythmia. New England Journal of Medicine 335: 1933–1940

NICE 2002 Glycoprotein 2a/3b inhibitor guidance for acute coronary syndromes. NICE 2002/046

OASIS Investigators 2001 Effects of long-term, moderate-intensity oral anticoagulation in addition to aspirin in unstable angina. The Organization to Assess Strategies for Ischemic Syndromes (OASIS) Investigators. Journal of the American College of Cardiology 37: 475–484

Packer M, Georghiade M, Young J et al 1993 Withdrawal of digoxin from patients with chronic heart failure treated with angiotensin converting enzyme inhibitors. New England Journal of Medicine 329: 1–7

Packer M, Coats AJS, Fowler MB et al for the Carvidilol Prospective Randomised Cumulative Survival Study Group (COPERNICUS) 2001 Effect of carvidilol on survival in severe chronic heart failure. New England Journal of Medicine 344: 1651–1658

Parisi AF, Folland ED, Hartigan P 1992 A comparison of angioplasty with medical therapy in the treatment of single-vessel coronary artery disease. New England Journal of Medicine 326: 10–16

Peto R, Gray R, Collins R et al 1988 Randomised trial of prophylactic daily aspirin in British male doctors. British Medical Journal 296: 313–316

Pfeffer MA, Lamas GA, Vaughan DE, Parisi AF, Braunwald E 1988 Effect of captopril on progressive ventricular dilatation after anterior myocardial infarction. New England Journal of Medicine 319: 80–86

Pitt B, Poole-Wilson B, Segal R et al 1999a Effects of losartan versus captopril on mortality in patients with symptomatic heart failure. ELITE-II. Journal of Cardiac Failure 5: 146–155

Pitt B, Zannad F, Remme WJ et al 1999b The effect of spironolactone on morbidity and mortality in patients with severe heart failure. New England Journal of Medicine 341: 709–717

PRISM-PLUS Trial Investigators 1998 Inhibition of platelet glycoprotein IIb/IIIa receptor with tirofiban in unstable angina and non-Q-wave myocardial infarction. New England Journal of Medicine 338: 1488–1497

PURSUIT Trial Investigators 1998 Inhibition of platelet glycoprotein IIb/IIIa with eptifibatide in patients with acute coronary syndromes. New England Journal of Medicine 339: 436–443

RAVEL study group 2002 New England Journal of Medicine 346: 1773–1780

RESTORE Investigators 1997 Effects of platelet glycoprotein IIb/IIIa blockade with tirofiban on adverse cardiac events in patients with unstable angina or acute myocardial infarction undergoing coronary angioplasty. Circulation 96: 1445–1453

RITA-2 Trial Participants 1997 Coronary angioplasty versus medical therapy for angina: the second Randomised Intervention Treatment for Angina (RITA-2) trial. Lancet 350: 461–468

Schulpher MJ, Seed P, Henderson RA et al 1994 Health service costs of coronary angioplasty and coronary artery bypass surgery: the Randomised Intervention Treatment of Angina (RITA) trial. Lancet 344: 927–930

Serneri GGN, Gensini GF, Poggesi L et al 1990 Effect of heparin, aspirin or alteplase in reduction of myocardial ischaemia in refractory unstable angina. Lancet 335: 615–618

Serruys PW, de Jaegere P, Kiemeneij F et al 1994 A comparison of balloon-expandable-stent implantation with balloon angioplasty in patients with coronary artery disease. New England Journal of Medicine 331: 489–495

Serruys PW, Unger F, Sousa JE et al 2001 Comparison of coronary artery bypass surgery and stenting for the treatment of multivessel disease. New England Journal of Medicine 344: 1117–1124

Simoons ML 2001 Effect of glycoprotein IIb/IIIa receptor blocker abciximab on outcome in patients with acute coronary syndromes without early coronary revascularisation: the GUSTO IV-ACS randomised trial. Lancet 357: 1915–1924

SOLVD Investigators 1991 Effect of enalapril on survival in patients with reduced ejection fractions and congestive heart failure. New England Journal of Medicine 316: 293–302

SOLVD Investigators 1992 Effect of enalapril on mortality and the development of heart failure in asymptomatic patients with reduced left ventricular ejection fractions. New England Journal of Medicine 327: 685–691

Steering Committee of the Physicians' Health Study Research Group 1989 Final report of the aspirin component of the ongoing Physicians' Health Study. New England Journal of Medicine 321: 129–135

Stone GW, Moliterno DJ, Bertrand M et al 2002 Impact of clinical syndrome acuity on the differential response to two glycoprotein IIbIIIa receptor inhibitors in patients undergoing coronary stenting. Circulation 105: 2347–2354

Sugurdsson E, Thorgeirsson G, Sigvaldason H, Sigfusson N 1995 Unrecognized myocardial infarction: epidemiology, clinical characteristics, and the prognostic role of angina pectoris. The Reykjavik Study. Annals of Internal Medicine 122: 96–102

Swedberg K, Held P, Kjekshus J et al on behalf of the CONSENSUS II Study Group 1992 Effects of early administration of enalapril on mortality in patients with acute myocardial infarction. Results of the Cooperative North Scandinavian Enalapril Survival Study II (CONSENSUS II). New England Journal of Medicine 327: 678–684

Topol EJ 2001 Reperfusion therapy for acute myocardial infarction with fibrinolytic therapy or combination reduced fibrinolytic therapy and platelet glycoprotein IIb/IIIa inhibition: the GUSTO V randomised trial. Lancet 357: 1905–1914

Topol EJ, Ohman EM, Armstrong PW et al 2000 Survival outcomes 1 year after reperfusion therapy with either alteplase or reteplase for acute myocardial infarction: results from the Global Utilization of Streptokinase and t-PA for Occluded Coronary Arteries (GUSTO) III trial. Circulation 102: 1761–1765

Uretsky BF, Young JB, Shahidi FE et al 1993 Randomised study assessing the effect of digoxin withdrawal in patients with mild to moderate chronic congestive heart failure: results of the PROVED trial. Journal of the American College of Cardiology 22: 955–962

Waagstein F, Hjalmarson A, Varnauskas E, Wallentin I 1975 Effect of chronic beta-adrenergic blockade in congestive cardiomyopathy. British Heart Journal 37: 1022–1036

Wallentin L, Lagerqvist B, Husted S et al 2000 Outcome at 1 year after an invasive compared with a non-invasive strategy in unstable coronary-artery disease: the FRISC II invasive randomised trial. Lancet 356: 9–16

Wilcox RG, Olsson CG, Skene AM et al 1988 Trial of tissue plasminogen activator for mortality reduction in acute myocardial infarction. Anglo-Scandinavian Study of Early Thrombolysis (ASSET). Lancet ii: 525–529

Yusuf S, Peto R, Lewis J et al 1985 Beta blockade during and after myocardial infarction: an overview of the randomised trials. Progress in Cardiovascular Disease 27: 335

Yusuf S, Zucker D, Peduzzi P et al 1994 Effect of coronary artery bypass graft surgery on survival: overview of 10 year results from randomised trials by the Coronary Artery Bypass Graft Surgery Trialists Collaboration. Lancet 344: 563–570

FURTHER READING

Journals

- General cardiology: *New England Journal of Medicine; Lancet; British Medical Journal*
- Specialist cardiology: *Circulation; American Journal of Cardiology; Journal of American College of Cardiology; American Heart Journal; Heart*

Books

Braunwald E 2001 Heart disease. A textbook of cardiovascular disease, 6th edn. WB Saunders, Philadelphia

Hurst R 2001 The heart, 10th edn. McGraw-Hill, New York

Julian DG, Camm AJ, Fox K, Hall RJC, Poole-Wilson PA 1996 Diseases of the heart. Baillière Tindall, London

Swanton RH 2000 Cardiology. Blackwell Science, Oxford

Websites

Important clinical trial results are often posted on www.theheart.org within hours of being presented.

Cardiac rehabilitation

10

Laura McIntosh

■ **CONTENTS**

INTRODUCTION

Cardiac rehabilitation has progressed from an exercise-based treatment for angina pectoris to a complex and comprehensive service that serves as an integral part in the prevention and rehabilitation of coronary heart disease (CHD).

The National Service Framework (NSF) for CHD, standard 12 (DoH 2000), states that:

> 'NHS trusts should put in place agreed protocols and systems of care so that, prior to leaving hospital, people admitted to hospital suffering from CHD have been invited to participate in a multidisciplinary programme of secondary prevention and cardiac rehabilitation'.

This view is mirrored in the CHD Task Force report for National Health Service Scotland (CHD/Stroke Task Force 2001) which recommends that:

> 'NHS boards should, as part of their CHD strategy, plan to commission services to deliver cardiac rehabilitation (CR) in accordance with the forthcoming SIGN guideline, and integrated with the local managed clinical network for cardiac services'.

People with CHD are at increased risk of premature death, heart attack and other vascular events. However, there is much that can be done to reduce these risks. This process of risk reduction and secondary prevention involves a range of interventions and preventive strategies. These include prophylactic medications, therapeutic and behavioural interventions to promote the adoption of a healthy lifestyle and reduce CHD risk factors.

People with CHD are faced with the challenge to make significant changes to the way that they behave and live and some will also have chronic psychological problems following the diagnosis of CHD. Thus cardiac rehabilitation and secondary prevention measures aim not only to reduce the risk of subsequent cardiac problems and death but also to promote return to a full and normal life.

DEFINITION OF CARDIAC REHABILITATION

Cardiac rehabilitation has been defined by the World Health Organization (1993) as the:

'Sum of activities required to influence favourably the underlying cause of the disease as well as the best possible physical, mental and social conditions, so that they (people) may by their own efforts preserve or resume when lost, as normal a place as possible in the community. Rehabilitation cannot be regarded as an isolated form or stage of therapy but must be integrated within secondary prevention services of which it forms only one facet'.

The SIGN guideline (SIGN 2002) for cardiac rehabilitation quotes an excellent definition.

'Cardiac rehabilitation is the process by which patients with cardiac disease, in partnership with a multidisciplinary team of health care professionals, are encouraged and supported to achieve and maintain optimal physical and psychological health'.

Both the above definitions demonstrate that cardiac rehabilitation is a complex intervention with numerous desired outcomes and goals.

Unfortunately the development of cardiac rehabilitation over the last 20–30 years has taken place in an ad hoc and sometimes random manner. Many groups started through British Heart Foundation start-up grants or with support from the medical charity Chest, Heart and Stroke. Staff ran many of the programmes as a goodwill gesture and the content and quality of programmes across the UK were and are, to a certain extent, very different. In an effort to standardize care and provide services that reflect best practice, the British Association of Cardiac Rehabilitation (BACR) produced national guidelines for the rehabilitation of the cardiac patient in 1995; these guidelines also included an overview of research findings as well as information on exercise testing and motivating adults to exercise (Coats et al 1995).

In a review of cardiac rehabilitation services in England and Wales in 1997 (Thompson et al 1997), wide variations in resources and focus of programmes were still documented despite the BACR guidelines. Following this review in England and Wales, recommendations were made for the introduction of guidelines both to provide a framework for, and to determine minimum service provision for, cardiac rehabilitation programmes. This review formed the basis of the recommendations outlined in the NSF Chapter 7 (DoH 2001). In Scotland a SIGN guideline (SIGN 2002) for cardiac rehabilitation was also published.

Production of these national guidelines in England, Wales and Scotland should take cardiac rehabilitation forwards. They have been produced to ensure that there is equity and quality in the services provided across the UK. In an effort to ensure such equity and quality of NHS services, the Clinical Standards Board for Scotland (CSBS) (CSBS 2001) has been developed to run a system of quality assurance and accreditation of clinical services. The CSBS produced standards for secondary prevention following acute myocardial infarction in December 2000. Peer review visits were made to all health board areas in Scotland between November 2000 and August 2001 to assess performance against the standards. Cardiac rehabilitation was assessed as part of this review. Following the review it was noted that cardiac rehabilitation, with an identified co-ordinator, exists in most hospitals and is available to all patients regardless of age or gender. There has therefore been some progress. However, the CSBS noted that there was still some overreliance on staff goodwill and short-term/project-based finance for cardiac rehabilitation programmes (CSBS 2001).

EVIDENCE FOR BENEFIT

The recent systematic review (Jolliffe et al 2001) of exercise-based rehabilitation for coronary heart disease reported on outcome in over 8000 CHD patients. The pooled effect estimates that for mortality from all causes, the exercise-only intervention showed a 27% reduction. Similarly, comprehensive cardiac rehabilitation reduced mortality from all causes compared to usual care, but to a lesser (13%) and non-significant degree.

There were no significant differences, however, in the rate of non-fatal MIs between the intervention and control groups, which may mean that although the number of MIs was not reduced, there was a significant reduction in the severity of the MI, which is obviously an important effect as it would lead to reduced morbidity and, of course, mortality.

It should also be noted that the majority of the patients included were male. Programmes might need to be adapted to meet the needs of women with CHD (Jolliffe et al 2001). In addition, many studies included in the Cochrane review were based on work undertaken in the early 1980s and much has changed since then in terms of improved medical and lifestyle management of cardiac patients. However, this systematic review remains a core component of the evidence base for cardiac rehabilitation because there have been few large randomized trials examining mortality in the intervening years.

An important objective of cardiac rehabilitation is to improve quality of life but evidence supporting improvement in this dimension of health is limited (Pell 1997). This is not surprising. There is an inherent difficulty in both defining and measuring quality of life. The current literature supports the value of quality of life improvement as a treatment goal for patients with cardiac disease, but recommends that further research is needed to determine the optimal test instrument and method of interpreting scores (Shepherd & Franklin 2001).

AIMS AND CONTENT OF CARDIAC REHABILITATION

The aims of cardiac rehabilitation are to return patients to optimum health within the confines of their disease, to highlight individual risk factors and encourage patients to initiate long-term changes where indicated. Cardiac rehabilitation also provides the opportunity to educate relatives. For this reason family and friends should be encouraged to participate in the education process. Cardiac rehabilitation also provides the environment where patients and family acknowledge their role in accepting responsibility for their health and emphasizes the necessity of dealing with a progressive disease. There has to be a balance between preventing recurrence of coronary events (secondary prevention) and helping patients to come to terms with their diagnosis and to overcome any memories, misconceptions and fears which may be impeding their recovery. The BACR guidelines suggest that when setting up a cardiac rehabilitation programme, 'it is useful to consider a structure which will cater for the needs of patients at the different stages of their disease and recovery process' (Coats et al 1995). This structure traditionally consists of four phases, each phase representing a different component of the patient's journey of care.

Phase one

Occurs during an inpatient stay or after a stepwise change in the patient's condition, e.g. acute MI, admission for revascularization, admission with unstable angina.

Phase two

This is usually defined as the early postdischarge period. Often this is a time when patients feel isolated and insecure.

Phase three

This has historically taken the form of a structured outpatient cardiac rehabilitation programme.

Phase four

This is where long-term maintenance of lifestyle changes occurs once the formal rehabilitation programme has finished.

Phase one

During this phase there will be many issues that are important for the patient and the team of health-care professionals involved with care. Issues to consider at this time are: medical evaluation, reassurance and education, risk factor assessment, correction of cardiac/other misconceptions, risk stratification, mobilization and discharge planning. Most rehabilitation teams are multidisciplinary and advice and education may be given by the most relevant health-care professional. For example, the physiotherapist will give advice about exercise or the pharmacist about pharmaceutical agents. However, it is important for each team member to be aware of the information that their colleagues give so that patients do not receive misleading or incongruent messages.

The key elements of care above were identified by Thompson (1989) in his randomized controlled trial of in-hospital nursing support for first-time MI patients and the BACR has adopted them into its guidelines.

This is a time when involvement and support of partner and family are crucial. Studies have shown that some partners of those with heart disease may stay awake to make sure that their loved one is still alive (Thompson & Coldie 1988). Overprotection is also common. Thus advice and reassurance to family and friends will be of paramount importance.

Reassurance

There needs to be discussion of immediate medical concerns and issues but also vocational and financial matters. Sometimes these are at the forefront of patients' minds and the quicker they are reassured that the event need not necessarily have a negative effect on their life, the better. One study showed that a nurse counsellor can improve the patient's and the partner's knowledge of heart disease and reduce anxiety and depression compared with those receiving usual care (Johnston et al 1999).

Misconceptions

Misconceptions may affect the patient's potential recovery and it is thus important to establish what misconceptions the patients may have about CHD and deal with them in a realistic way (Lewin et al 1992).

Risk factor assessment

This will include an assessment of overall needs and, more specifically, an assessment of the coronary risk factors involved. Identifying risk factors is an integral part of the rehabilitation process and it is carried out throughout the four phases of rehabilitation. The main modifiable risk factors of smoking, hypertension and hyperlipidaemia are considered below and in the preceding chapters.

At this point in phase one discussions should be initiated about preventive strategies and necessary lifestyle changes. Information should be collected about risk factors, including: family history of CHD, personal history of CHD, smoking history, dietary habits and blood lipid profile, body mass index, blood pressure and history of hypertension, diabetes, physical activity levels and functional capacity, emotional status/stress, anxiety and depression, socio-economic status, vocational status and leisure activities.

Advice at this stage must be tailored to patients' needs and willingness to make changes to their life. It is important that the cardiac rehabilitation professional is seen as a supporter of patients in their efforts to make lifestyle change, rather than as a disciplinarian. For every risk factor and lifestyle factor where behaviour change is required, the patient's readiness to change should be recorded in their rehabilitation notes to facilitate effective interventions in the later stages of rehabilitation. It also keeps all members of the multidisciplinary team aware of the patient's stage of change, thus reducing the risk of hostility and wasted time giving information that the patient is not ready to receive.

Smoking Smoking cessation advice is given if applicable. The positive aspects of stopping should be emphasized, i.e. the fact that stopping smoking halves the likelihood of further MI (WHO 1993). Encouraging a belief in the patient's own ability to succeed is crucial. Use of a range of strategies, including alternative therapies and nicotine replacement therapy (not recommended until a minimum of 4 weeks post cardiac event), should also be considered.

Cholesterol and diet Lipid profile will be discussed with the patient and recommended levels will be advised. Advice about diet in terms of weight reduction, if applicable, and reduction in dietary fat, improved intake of fruit and vegetables and safe alcohol levels will be offered. An explanation of the benefits and use of cholesterol-lowering medications will also be offered.

Hypertension Advice on managing hypertension should be offered, including the use of antihypertensive medication, reasons for prophylactic medication, namely aspirin and β-blockers, benefits, contraindications and possible side-effects.

Exercise Physical activity should be encouraged within limitations of general well-being and ongoing cardiac symptoms, taking into account previous level of fitness. A personalized home programme/prescription for exercise should be given, with written information about exercise progression over the weeks when the patient is at home prior to attending the rehabilitation classes.

Stress, anxiety and depression Anxiety and depression can be common and this has been shown to affect recovery adversely (Williams et al 1986) so identification and interventions to treat these conditions are an important part of the overall management of the patient following an acute cardiac event.

In terms of dealing with relatives, it should be remembered that they might experience the hospital admission in a more alarming way than the patient, who may be too ill to be aware of the surroundings and the severity of their condition. Listening to, and dealing with, their fears and anxieties is essential because the patient's recovery process may be hindered by their terror. Providing information on medications, investigations, the patient's progress and what they can expect when the patient gets home is good practice to reduce unnecessary worry, uncertainty and anxiety. The initial time at home can be particularly stressful for relatives and clear guidelines on what the patient should and should not be undertaking are useful, together with contact details for information and support. Relaxation techniques can be offered and taught, for example simple relaxation tapes to use in a personal stereo whilst in the ward.

Despite general health warnings and health education, some patients are more likely to blame stress for their heart condition rather than their use of tobacco or poor diet whereas others will refuse to acknowledge stress despite very difficult social and personal issues that surround them. Being given time to express their anxieties and fears and indeed openly voice feelings which they have previously denied is crucial for some patients. Allowing themselves to admit anger, fear and sadness may be something patients have never experienced and they will need to be reassured that such feelings are normal for all of us. Allowing patients to express their feelings without judgement can provide a long overdue release. Privacy is paramount in these situations and the issue of confidentiality is important. You should inform patients that if you felt they were a danger to themselves or others, you would reserve the right to inform their doctor. In other respects patients should be assured of total confidentiality.

Part of reducing stress is ensuring that patients have optimal support on discharge and that they are aware of any state benefits that they are entitled to. Thus you may need to refer them to social and voluntary services. It is important, however, to ensure that increased social support is acceptable to the patient before organizing it.

A Hospital Anxiety and Depression (HAD) scale (Zigmond & Snaith 1983) can be used to aid diagnosis of anxiety and depression. It can identify patients who need further professional help, e.g. a clinical psychologist, and can also be used for monitoring levels of anxiety and depression over time. It may be useful to ask patients to complete a HAD scale prior to discharge, 4 weeks post discharge/event and 3 months after discharge/event. Continued high scores would demonstrate a need for professional psychological intervention.

The HAD scale has been validated for use within a cardiac population. To use the scale it is necessary to purchase a starter pack from NFER-NELSON (tel: 01753 858961; e-mail: information@nfer-nelson.co.uk).

Discharge planning

Return to work Employment issues that must be considered include stress at work, physical demands and restrictions operating in certain jobs such as driving heavy goods vehicles or public transport vehicles. In these circumstances the local driving authority guidelines, such as those of the DVLA in the UK, should be followed. However, it is important to discourage patients from making a decision about returning to work or other long-term plans too early in their recovery, for as patients progress their feelings may change drastically from how they feel very early on in their recovery. All patients should be encouraged to discuss their thoughts and feelings with their family, GP, hospital consultant and rehabilitation staff before coming to a final decision.

Driving (general) Driving can resume within 4 weeks of MI and 4–6 weeks of CABG. Patients should be advised that driving whilst they have chest pain or dizziness is dangerous and should be avoided. Patients who have had a heart attack should also inform their insurance company.

Resuming sexual relations Resumption of sexual activity may be discussed, recognizing that this is a very personal area and patients may not be ready to discuss it with you. Thus written advice can also be given. Simple advice can state that they wait for a period of about 2 weeks and that they generally be guided by how well they are feeling. If a patient can climb two flights of stairs without angina or extreme breathlessness, it is safe to have sexual intercourse. Other issues to consider include the following:

- Anal sex can sometimes induce vasovagal episodes.
- Viagra is a powerful vasodilator and guidance should be given if patients are using this drug.
- Blood pressure can rise rapidly during sex so consideration must be given to uncontrolled hypertension.

Drug therapy If patients are to comply with drug therapy it is important that they are given the information that they need to facilitate compliance. Patients may need to understand why they have been prescribed certain drugs and the likely effects and side-effects of the medications before they are willing to take them. Patients and their families should be encouraged to discuss fears and outline other personal difficulties that may affect compliance, e.g. poor memory and dementia, poor eyesight and financial constraints. Aids such as a dosette may be required or large print on bottles. The pharmacist must be involved to give specialist advice. A list of drugs and timings can be included on a patient-held record (see below). Patients should be encouraged to request a repeat prescription from their GP on discharge, as most acute trusts will only supply 5–7 days' worth of discharge medications.

Patient-held records Patient-held records have been used in areas such as obstetrics for many years. Patient-held records are also of use within cardiac rehabilitation as they are valuable tools for encouraging patients' ownership of their health and foster a sense of responsibility for lifestyle changes and compliance with treatment.

These records may include information on diagnosis, tests and treatments received, medications, risk factors and future plans and appointments. Patients are encouraged to take these record cards with them to all appointments with GP, consultant and practice nurse as well as to cardiac rehabilitation. Thus, they become a very useful aid for communication between primary and secondary care as well as a source of information for the patient.

Patient-held records should include the patient's goals and the patient's stage of change/readiness to change should also be documented at each consultation so that information can be directed to the patient appropriately. Many cardiac rehabilitation teams have developed their own patient-held record but a standardized format may be something to aim for once further audit and accreditation of cardiac rehabilitation has been carried out.

Phase two

In this early postdischarge period patients can feel isolated and anxious. Support can be provided at this time by keeping in contact with the patient and carer either by a home visit or by telephone contact (Fulmer et al 1999,

Gilliss et al 1993, Naylor & McCauley 1999, Roebuck 1999, Savage & Grap 1999, van Elderen-van Kemenade et al 1994). The plans, priorities and goals for rehabilitation set out in phase one should form the basis for the ongoing care plan taken into phase two. This should include cardiac risk assessment and interventions to address physical, psychological and social needs. The patient-held record should be kept up to date and progress with goals supported. Another important issue is to check the patient's progress with the home exercise plan and try to identify barriers or problems preventing the patient from following it. It could be that the patient is experiencing angina and needs to be 'fast tracked' for investigation plus or minus angiogram or that they are scared and just need reassurance that exercise is safe. Involvement of carers should be maintained and resuscitation training can be offered for family members, especially for those patients who may have had an out-of-hospital cardiac arrest.

A cardiac specialist nurse, health visitor or district nurse may visit patients at home or phone the patient. A home-visiting service is costly to provide but offers a useful insight into patients' lives, home and family circumstances and can facilitate appropriate educational and psychosocial interventions to reduce anxiety, improve physical and psychological functioning and support behaviour change (Lewin et al 1992).

Some services rely on the use of the *Heart manual* (Lewin et al 1992), a self-help programme for patients recovering from an MI that has proved an effective means of providing home-based, self-directed cardiac rehabilitation over a 6-week period. The manual includes information and advice about exercise, relaxation and stress management and is used in conjunction with audiotapes. The programme is supported by a trained nurse facilitator to guide and support primary care nurses in using the manual with CHD patients. Patients who have used the *Heart manual* have been shown to have lower hospital readmission rates and lower levels of anxiety and depression (Lewin et al 1992).

A home visit within 1 week of discharge will also allow the nurse to check that the patient has received the appropriate repeat prescriptions. Frequently prescriptions can be mixed up and the nurse can ensure (in most cases) that this does not happen.

Contact at this stage can be used to give the patient and carers more information about the outpatient cardiac rehabilitation programme and dispel any misconceptions, anxieties and fears that the patient may have about the outpatient programme.

Phase three

Traditionally this has taken the form of a structured exercise and health education programme that lasts for 4–12 weeks, starting about 2–4 weeks after discharge from hospital. Most programmes invite the patients to attend 1–3 times per week for sessions lasting from 1–2 hours. The recommendations in the SIGN guidelines (SIGN 2002) state that exercise sessions should be offered at least twice a week for a minimum of 8 weeks, educational and psychological interventions should be provided via a menu-based approach and that programmes target patients identified as either more distressed or in greater need of behavioural change, rather than deliver all aspects of the programme to every patient (Dusseldorp et al 1999, Linden et al 1996). The BACR (Coats et al 1995) and the Scottish Needs Assessment Programme (SNAP 2001) have also recommended this approach.

Psychological interventions could include:

- stress management
- relaxation techniques
- one-to-one or group counselling
- goal setting
- psychotherapy
- cognitive-behavioural approaches
- hypnotherapy.

Many of these interventions may need to be provided by professionals with highly developed skills in cognitive-behavioural therapy, health belief and illness representation models and motivational interviewing (DoH 2001, Lewin et al 1995, Miller & Rollnick 1991).

Educational interventions could include individual or group sessions on:

- process of CHD
- healthy eating
- cholesterol and lipids
- smoking cessation
- hypertension
- activity and exercise
- resuscitation training
- medication advice
- vocational advice.

A meta-analysis of 8988 patients reported that cardiac rehabilitation programmes that include psychological and educational interventions resulted in a 34% reduction in cardiac mortality and a 29% reduction in recurrent MI at 1–10-year follow-up (Dusseldorp et al 1999). Two other earlier meta-analyses reported similar cardiovascular outcomes (Linden et al 1996, Mullen et al 1992). Analysis of studies of health education in cardiac patients has found that the most important determinant of effectiveness is the quality of the intervention (Mullen et al 1997). The quality of the intervention was defined as adherence to the five principles of adult learning:

1. Relevance (tailored to patients' knowledge, beliefs, circumstances)
2. Individualization (tailored to personal needs)
3. Feedback (informed regarding progress with learning or change)
4. Reinforcement (rewarded for progress)
5. Facilitation (provided with means to take action and/or reduce barriers).

Any cardiac rehabilitation programme must take these principles into account when setting up its exercise, health education and psychological interventions.

Although cardiac rehabilitation has traditionally taken place in a hospital setting it is increasingly recognized that it can also be undertaken safely in a community setting, such as in a local sports centre or community centre (Bethell & Mullee 1990, Hamalainen et al 1991).

Exercise component of programme

The exercise component of cardiac rehabilitation has advanced a long way over the last 20 years or so. The formal exercise classes are an integral part of the overall therapeutic intervention of cardiac rehabilitation. Where possible, patients should be encouraged to attend the exercise component of cardiac rehabilitation, except of course if they have an unstable cardiac status or other limiting illness.

Before joining the classes patients must be risk stratified. For most patients it is sufficient to formulate risk based on history, examination and resting ECG combined with a functional capacity test such as a shuttle walk test or 6-minute walk test (Demers et al 2001, Tobin & Thow 1999). However, most patients will also have had a formal exercise tolerance test and echocardiography. These tests are particularly important in high-risk patients (poor LV systolic function, residual ischaemia, ventricular arrhythmias) or those who wish to participate in high-intensity exercise training.

Most cardiac rehabilitation programmes perform an initial assessment that includes a shuttle walk test or 6-minute walk test along with general assessment of symptoms, risk factors and psychological status. The assessment is usually multidisciplinary and is a very good way of continuing the care plan and goal setting carried out in phases one and two. Use of motivational interviewing techniques (Prochaska & Diclemente 1984) during these assessments can enhance work already started with the patient. These assessments can be carried out midway and at the end of the programme too.

Phase four

Phase four is traditionally where rehabilitation staff hand over care of CHD patients to primary care staff. It is important therefore that excellent communication is maintained and that the patient and primary care staff are aware of any outstanding issues or problems. A patient-held record is one tool that, if used properly, could ease the transition from phase three to phase four. In many areas practice nurses and other primary care staff are receiving further training to enable them to take on this role. The BACR is already providing training for health and fitness instructors to become accredited and provide phase four exercise classes in community settings. Patients completing phase three should be encouraged to attend this type of class.

WHO SHOULD ATTEND CARDIAC REHABILITATION?

Traditionally cardiac rehabilitation has been offered to patients who have sustained a myocardial infarction or coronary artery bypass surgery. These groups are known to benefit from comprehensive cardiac rehabilitation

(Carlsson 1998, Engblom et al 1997, Goble & Worcester 1999, Wosornu et al 1996). However, there is emerging evidence that other groups of patients may also benefit from a comprehensive cardiac rehabilitation programme, including those:

- post angioplasty (Hofman-Bang et al 1999)
- with stable angina (NHS CRD 1998, SHPIC 1998, Thompson & Bowman 1998, US DHHS 1995)
- with chronic heart failure (Berlardinelli et al 1999)
- post cardiac transplant (Hofman-Bang et al 1999).

AUDIT

As noted earlier, the NSF (DoH 2000), SIGN (2002) and the CHD Task Force (2001) state that multidisciplinary, menu-based rehabilitation should be provided across the nation. All these documents state the need to carry out audit as a way of improving and standardizing the service that is provided nationally. The BACR and British Heart Foundation have printed audit guidelines, as have SIGN, for cardiac rehabilitation. The Northern and Yorkshire Public Health Observatories (N & YPHO) have also produced a basic data set for cardiac rehabilitation as well as a package of valid, reliable and sensitive assessment and outcome measures appropriate to the aims of cardiac rehabilitation. This can be accessed through their website: www.cardiacrehabilitation.org.uk.

The cardiac rehabilitation guidelines and audit standards (Thompson et al 1996) state that data should be collected in four broad categories:

1. Clinical (e.g. heart rate, lipids)
2. Behavioural (e.g. smoking status, activity levels)
3. Health (mortality, health-related quality of life)
4. Psychological (anxiety, depression).

However, there are few validated and user-friendly tools available. Please access the N & YPHO article for more information.

NURSE-LED CLINICS

A literature is now emerging that demonstrates the effectiveness of nurse-led secondary prevention interventions for patients with CHD, particularly in primary care. This links in with the aims of phase four of cardiac rehabilitation, in terms of supporting the patients to maintain/encourage further changes in lifestyle (Campbell et al 1998). Nurse-led clinics could also be utilized at the start of phase three.

Clinics could be set up as a 'stand alone' or in conjunction with traditional cardiology clinics and could be used to assess patients' symptoms and risk stratification and also as a way of ensuring continuity and quality of care. This would of course include optimizing secondary prevention measures.

The nurse-led clinic could be linked into the patients' assessment before commencing rehabilitation. Thus a multidisciplinary approach could be useful, i.e. including physiotherapist, dietitian and pharmacist as well as nursing and medical staff. However, there needs to be more formal research into the effectiveness of such clinics.

■ **KEY POINTS**

- Comprehensive menu-based cardiac rehabilitation should be an integral part of care for patients with heart disease.
- Comprehensive menu-based cardiac rehabilitation reduces mortality and improves morbidity.
- Cardiac rehabilitation is an integral part of secondary prevention.
- A multidisciplinary team should provide cardiac rehabilitation.
- Cardiac rehabilitation interventions should be based on the principles of adult learning.
- Continued audit and research is required to improve standards of care.

■ **CASE STUDY 10.1**

Mrs B is admitted to a medical ward suffering an acute inferior myocardial infarction and with a history of hypertension. Her recovery is unremarkable and prior to discharge she is seen by the rehabilitation nurse and the physio-therapist. As she has stairs at home, she is supervised on a flight of stairs outside the ward by the physiotherapist and manages without any problems. Discussing her home circumstances with the rehabilitation nurse, she discloses that she never goes anywhere without her husband and that he does all of the shopping and all of the housework. Knowing that she was going home to full support, she was discharged and asked to return for exercise tolerance testing 1 week later.

The ECG technician was surprised to see Mrs B return for her exercise test in a wheelchair, which according to the husband was on the instructions of the GP. Mr B was very angry that Mrs B had been asked to undergo an exercise test so soon after her heart attack. Such was the situation that the doctor decided that he would postpone the exercise test until she had recuperated further.

How would the rehabilitation nurse resolve this problem?

Answer

Mrs B had been contacted on discharge and there had been no developments or complications since discharge. She had been mobilizing well around the ward and the only reason she had not been exercise-tested prior to discharge was that there was no appointment slot available. Mrs B and her husband were invited to come up to the hospital for a check on her blood pressure and to attend the series of talks available to patients after myocardial infarc-tion. Mrs B's blood pressure was within the normal parameters, she had no symptoms of angina and was complying with her medication. The nurse noticed how frequently Mr B answered questions asked of Mrs B and how involved in her care he was. He was completely responsible for her drug administration. The nurse praised Mr B for taking such good care of Mrs B but gently pointed out that all patients unless physically or mentally disabled must assume responsibility for their own care at some point.

A few weeks later the nurse managed to see Mrs B on her own and discussed her domestic relationship with her husband. Mrs B admitted that she would love to be allowed out on her own to visit friends or go shopping for an hour. It was agreed that the nurse would invite Mr and Mrs B for joint counselling to try to find options that would suit both of them. When they arrived for the counselling session, the nurse took great care to praise Mr B and asked him if it had been hard for him when his wife had been diagnosed as having had a heart attack. At this point Mr B started to weep. His mother had died when he was 18 years old as a result of 'heart disease'. He had had to shoulder the burden of responsibility for himself and his father and had never had the opportunity to grieve fully. Since his marriage, he had lived in fear of losing his wife and was terror-stricken when the diagnosis of heart attack was made. After hearing an explanation of how the care of the cardiac patient has progressed so dramatically, Mr B was able to understand the source of his fears and to acknowledge the restriction he was putting on his wife's recovery. Mrs B went on to have an exercise test and to participate in the exercise class. Her physical and psychological health improved immensely.

REFERENCES

Berlardinelli R, Georgiou D, Cianci G, Purcarno A 1999 Randomized, controlled trial of long-term moderate exercise training in chronic heart failure: effects on functional capacity, quality of life and clinical outcome. Circulation 99: 1173–1182

Bethell HJ, Mullee MA 1990 A controlled trial of community based coronary rehabilitation. British Heart Journal 64: 370–375

Campbell NC, Ritchie LD, Thain J, Deans HG, Rawles LD, Squair JL 1998 Secondary prevention in coronary heart disease: a randomised trial of nurse led clinics in primary care. Heart 80(5): 447–452

Carlsson R 1998 Serum cholesterol, lifestyle, working capacity and quality of life in patients with coronary artery disease. Experiences from a hospital-based secondary prevention programme. Scandinavian Cardiovascular Journal 50(suppl): 1–20

Clinical Standards Board for Scotland (CSBS) 2001 National overview, coronary heart disease, heart attack: secondary prevention. NHS Scotland, Edinburgh

Coats A, McGee H, Stokes H, Thompson D (eds) 1995 BACR guidelines for cardiac rehabilitation. Blackwell Science, Oxford

Coronary Heart Disease/Stroke Task Force 2001 Report for NHS Scotland. Stationery Office, Edinburgh

Demers C, McKelvie RS, Negassa A, Yusuf S 2001 Reliability, validity and responsiveness of the six-minute walk test in patients with heart failure. American Heart Journal 142: 698–703

Department of Health 2000 National Service Framework. Modern standards and service, coronary heart disease. Department of Health, London, Edinburgh

Department of Health 2001 Treatment choice in psychological therapies and counselling – an evidence based clinical practice guideline. Department of Health, London

Dusseldorp E, van Elderen T, Maes S, Meulman J, Kraaij V 1999 A meta-analysis of psycho educational programmes for coronary heart disease patients. Health Psychology 18: 506–519

Engblom E, Korpilhati K, Hamalainen H et al 1997 Quality of life and return to work five years after coronary artery bypass surgery. Long-term results of cardiac rehabilitation. Journal of Cardiopulmonary Rehabilitation 17: 29–36

Fulmer TT, Feldman PH, Kim TS et al 1999 An intervention study to enhance medication compliance in community-dwelling elderly individuals. Journal of Gerontology Nursing 25: 6–14

Gilliss CL, Gortner SR, Hauck WW, Shinn JA, Sparcino PA, Tompkins C 1993 A randomised clinical trial of nursing care for recovery from cardiac surgery. Heart and Lung 22: 125–133

Goble AJ, Worcester MU 1999 Best practice for cardiac rehabilitation and secondary prevention. Heart Research Centre, on behalf of Department of Human Services, Melbourne, Australia

Hamalainen H, Kallio V, Knuts LR et al 1991 Community approach in rehabilitation and secondary prevention after acute myocardial infarction: results of a randomised clinical trial. Journal of Cardiopulmonary Rehabilitation 11: 221–226

Hofman-Bang C, Lisspers J, Nordlander R et al 1999 Two-year results of a controlled study of residential rehabilitation for patients treated with percutaneous transluminal coronary angioplasty. A randomised study of a multifactorial programme. European Heart Journal 20: 1465–1474

Johnston M, Foulkes J, Johnston DW, Pollard B, Gudmundsdottir H 1999 Impact on patients and partners of extended cardiac counselling and rehabilitation: a controlled trial. Pyschosomatic Medicine 61: 225–233

Jolliffe JA, Rees K, Taylor RS, Thompson D, Oldridge N, Ebrahim S 2001 Exercise-based rehabilitation for coronary heart disease (Cochrane review). Issue 3. Cochrane Library, Oxford

Lewin B, Robertson IH, Cay EL et al 1992 Effects of self-help post myocardial infarction rehabilitation on psychological adjustment and use of health services. Lancet 339: 1036–1040

Lewin B, Cay EL, Todd I et al 1995 The angina management programme: a rehabilitation treatment. British Journal of Cardiology 2: 221–226

Linden W, Stossel C, Maurice J 1996 Psychosocial interventions for patients with coronary artery disease: a meta-analysis. Archives of Internal Medicine 156: 745–752

Miller W, Rollnick S 1991 Motivational interviewing: preparing people to change addictive behavior. Guilford Press, New York

Mullen PD, Mains DA, Velez R 1992 A meta analysis of controlled trials of cardiac patient education. Patient Education and Counselling 19: 143–162

Mullen PD, Simons-Morton DG, Ramirez G, Frankowski RF, Green LW, Mains DA 1997 A meta-analysis of trials evaluating patient education and counselling for three groups of preventative health behaviours. Patient Education and Counselling 32: 157–173

Naylor MD, McCauley KM 1999 The effects of a discharge planning and home follow up intervention on elders hospitalised with common medical and surgical cardiac conditions. Journal of Cardiovascular Nursing 14: 44–54

NHS Centre for Reviews and Dissemination 1988 Cardiac rehabilitation. Effective Health Care 1998 (4): 4

Pell J 1997 Cardiac rehabilitation: a review of its effectiveness. Coronary Health Care 1: 8–17

Prochaska JO, Diclemente CC 1984 The transtheoretical approach: crossing traditional foundations of change. Don Jones, Irwin, Homewood, IL

Roebuck A 1999 Telephone support in the early post discharge period following elective cardiac surgery: does it reduce anxiety and depression levels? Intensive and Critical Care Nursing 15: 142–146

Savage LS, Grap MJ 1999 Telephone monitoring after early discharge for cardiac surgery patients. American Journal of Critical Care 8: 154–159

Scottish Health Purchasing Information Centre (SHPIC) 1998 Cardiac rehabilitation. SHPIC, Southampton

Scottish Intercollegiate Guideline Network (SIGN) 2002 Cardiac rehabilitation: a national clinical guideline. SIGN, Edinburgh

Scottish Needs Assessment Programme (SNAP) 2001 Provision for cardiac rehabilitation services in Scotland – needs assessment and guidelines for decision makers. Public Health Institute of Scotland, Glasgow

Shepherd RJ, Franklin B 2001 Changes in life: a major goal in cardiac rehabilitation. Journal of Cardiopulmonary Rehabilitation 21(4): 189–200

Thompson DR 1989 A randomised controlled trial of in-hospital nursing support for first time myocardial infarction patients and their partners: effects on anxiety and depression. Journal of Advanced Nursing 14: 291–297

Thompson DR, Bowman GS 1998 Evidence for the effectiveness of cardiac rehabilitation. Intensive and Critical Care Nursing 14: 38–48

Thompson DR, Coldie CJ 1988 Support of wives of myocardial infarction patients. Journal of Advanced Nursing 13: 223–228

Thompson DR, Bowman R, Kitson Al, de Bono DP, Hopkins A 1996 Cardiac rehabilitation guidelines in the United Kingdom: guidelines and audit standards. Heart 75: 89–93

Thompson DR, Bowman GS, Kitson AL, de Bono DP, Hopkins A 1997 Cardiac rehabilitation services in England and Wales: a national survey. International Journal of Cardiology 59: 299–304

Tobin D, Thow MK 1999 The 10 m-shuttle walk test with Holter monitoring: an objective outcome measure for cardiac rehabilitation. Coronary Health Care 3: 3–17

US Department for Health and Human Services 1995 Cardiac rehabilitation. Clinical practice guideline no. 17. AHCPR publication No 96-0672. US Department for Health and Human Services, Rockville, MD

van Elderen-van Kemenade T, Maes S, van den Broek Y 1994 Effects of health education programme with telephone contact during cardiac rehabilitation. British Journal of Clinical Psychology 33: 367–378

Williams RB, Haney TL, McKinnis RA et al 1986 Psychosocial and physical predictors of anginal pain relief with medical management. Psychosomatic Medicine 48: 200–210

World Health Organization 1993 Cardiac rehabilitation and secondary prevention: long-term care for patients with ischaemic heart disease. WHO Regional Office for Europe, Copenhagen

Wosornu D, Bedford D, Ballantyne D 1996 A comparison of the effects of strength and aerobic exercise training on exercise capacity and lipids after coronary artery bypass surgery. European Heart Journal 17: 854–863

Zigmond AS, Snaith RP 1983 The Hospital Anxiety and Depression Scale. Acta Psychiatra Scandinavica 67: 36

FURTHER READING

Ware JE Jr, Snow KK, Kosinski AS, Gandek B 1993 SF-36: Health survey manual and interpretation guide. Nimrod Press, Boston, MA

Women and coronary heart disease

Elizabeth Farish   Grace Lindsay

INTRODUCTION

It is important to explain why we believe a chapter specifically devoted to coronary heart disease (CHD) in women should be included in this book. CHD has been well recognized as a major cause of mortality and disability in males but as a less important threat to the health of women. Yet, in all the developed countries CHD is the leading cause of death in women past the age of the menopause, accounting for more deaths than all the cancers combined. CHD death rates for women range from almost 1% of deaths (0.76%) in age group 40–44 years to 7.4% in age group 55–59 years to 42.5% in the 85–89 years age band (Tunstall-Pedoe 1998).

Most epidemiological studies and intervention trials conducted to investigate the cause of CHD involved only male subjects. The results from such studies have been used as a basis for CHD prevention practice for both men and women. This may or may not be appropriate. The natural course of CHD is different in males and females. Analysis of the limited data collected in women has been undertaken in an effort to improve our understanding of the nature of CHD risk in women.

This chapter aims to discuss the CHD risk factors that are particularly important or unique to women. It will include a discussion on the impact of the traditional CHD risk factors that may exert a more potent effect on women and aspects of life unique to females that may have a bearing on CHD risk, with particular reference to menopausal status and the use of postmenopausal hormone replacement therapy (HRT).

PROFILE OF CORONARY HEART DISEASE IN WOMEN

CHD risk in women

For the purpose of the clinical evaluation of CHD risk in women, it is important to understand the differences that occur among women and not only the differences between women and men. The traditional CHD risk factors that have been shown to be operative in men are also important in women (Manson et al 1992). These include smoking, hypercholesterolaemia and hypertension. However, their effect on CHD risk is different and they have been shown to be less predictive of subsequent CHD in women than in men (Wilhelmsen et al 1977). These CHD risk factors are discussed in more detail in Chapters 3, 4 and 5.

Age and the menopause

Since the early decades of the 20th century it has been noted that there is a marked gender difference in risk of CHD, with a significant age disparity in males and females who succumb to CHD (Glendy et al 1937). Although many disease patterns have changed since that early work, the natural course of CHD with increasing age still differs in males and females today. Premenopausal women appear to be protected from CHD when compared to men. However, with advancing age this gender difference in CHD risk changes and in the UK, CHD is the leading cause of death and disability in women past the age of the menopause (Fig. 11.1).

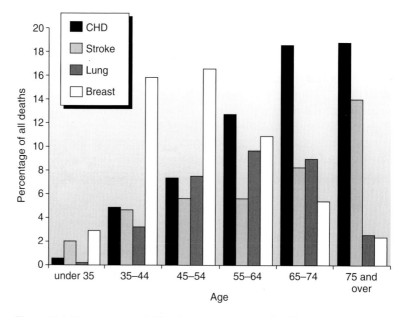

Figure 11.1 The percentage of all female deaths per year attributable to coronary heart disease, stroke, lung cancer and breast cancer across all age groups (data from BHFHPRG 2002).

It has long been widely believed that the increase in CHD risk with increasing age in females is linked with the menopause and its accompanying decline in ovarian hormones. This belief has arisen due to several observations. There is a delayed rise in coronary deaths in women compared with men, the incidence of CHD being very low in women of premenopausal age, while the ratio of male to female death rates from CHD decreases sharply at about the time of the natural menopause. In addition, it was noted that women who had an early sudden menopause as a result of bilateral oophorectomy and who did not receive oestrogen replacement therapy were at a significantly higher risk of CHD than premenopausal women of similar age (Colditz et al 1987). Furthermore, loss of ovarian function is associated with changes in lipid levels, principally an increase in LDL-cholesterol, resulting in a more atherogenic profile (Jensen 1991). Nevertheless, population data on CHD mortality indicates that CHD risk in women increases exponentially with age and it is not possible to discern any change in the rate of acceleration at the age of menopause (Fig. 11.2). It has been argued that this is because the natural menopause occurs at different ages in different individuals and marks an arbitrary time point in a variable and gradual decline in ovarian function. However, this explanation has been refuted (Barrett-Connor 1997), on the grounds that the menopause occurs almost universally within a fairly narrow age range (45–55 years) and within this age range it is easy to detect an abrupt change in the death rate from breast cancer, a disease which is almost certainly dependent on oestrogen levels. Moreover, the decline in the ratio of male to female deaths that occurs with age can be explained by a decrease in the acceleration of CHD rate in men. The absolute difference between male and female rates actually increases after the menopause, although the total number of female deaths finally outstrips that of men in old age (Table 11.1).

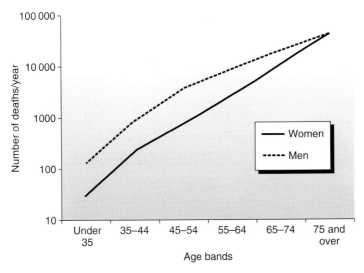

Figure 11.2 A comparison of mortality from coronary heart disease in men and women according to age, for 2001 (adapted from BHFHPRG 2002).

Table 11.1 The total numbers of male and female deaths in various age brackets that have been attributed to coronary heart disease and the associated death rate per million population (OPCS 1995)

Age group	Population (Thousands)		No. CHD deaths		CHD deaths per million	
	Male	Female	Male	Female	Male	Female
15–19	1665	1569	3	0	1.8	0.0
20–24	1606	1525	5	1	3.1	0.7
25–29	1895	1790	25	6	13.2	3.4
30–34	2164	2047	73	16	33.7	7.8
35–39	2193	2098	231	51	105.3	24.3
40–44	1857	1822	526	127	283.3	69.7
45–49	1674	1669	1043	237	623.1	142.0
50–54	1805	1813	2063	440	1143	242.7
55–59	1432	1453	3039	715	2122	492.1
60–64	1253	1298	4543	1443	3626	1112
65–69	1095	1189	6758	2746	6172	2310
70–74	941	1131	9677	5030	10284	4447
75–79	739	1043	11963	8701	16188	8342
80–84	406	710	9761	9763	24042	13751
85–89	206	477	7119	10550	34558	22117
90+	80	291	3279	8501	40988	29213

Thus it would appear that the natural menopause does not significantly impact on CHD event rates. The 'gender gap' in CHD mortality which is remarkably consistent worldwide remains unexplained and it is still unclear what role, if any, oestrogen has to play in it.

Socio-economic class

The detrimental effects of deprivation on the health of both sexes have been clearly documented (Black 1980), but it appears that in areas of high deprivation, women are particularly disadvantaged in terms of increased CHD risk when compared with their better-off counterparts.

A comparison of age-standardized mortality rates for CHD and stroke in relation to social class reveals a large gradient in mortality (British Heart Foundation 2002). Table 11.2 shows CHD mortality rates according to social class, with higher social class groups at the top. There is a higher incidence of CHD and stroke in the lower social class groups. However, for women, the relationship between CHD and stroke mortality according to social class is greater than that observed in males.

Smoking

The evidence for the role of cigarette smoking as a major risk factor for CHD exists for females as well as males. In a prospective study of 121 000 middle-aged female nurses, the risk of CHD was six times greater among the heaviest smokers compared to non-smokers (Willett et al 1987). Furthermore, the risk of sudden cardiac death in smokers was also increased between two- and fourfold (Nyboe et al 1991).

Table 11.2 Age-standardized mortality rates per 100 000 population from CHD and stroke between males and females in relation to social class 1986–1992 (men and women aged 35–64 years) (adapted from BHFHPRG 2002)

	Men	Women
Coronary Heart Disease		
I/II Professional/Intermediate	160	29
IIIN Skilled non-manual	162	39
IIIM Skilled manual	231	59
IV/V Partly skilled/unskilled	266	78
Ratio of lowest–highest social class	1.66	2.69
Stroke		
I/II Professional/Intermediate	29	14
IIIN Skilled non-manual	27	22
IIIM Skilled manual	33	18
IV/V Partly skilled/unskilled	40	34
Ratio of lowest–highest social class	1.38	2.43

However, the impact of smoking on CHD risk may have a more detrimental effect on women's cardiovascular health compared to age-matched males (Njoistad et al 1996, Prescott et al 1998). On average, first myocardial infarctions (MI) occur 7 years earlier in male smokers than in male non-smokers. Strikingly, in comparison, first MIs in women who smoke precede those in non-smokers by 19 years (Hansen et al 1993).

Smoking may have an additional effect on CHD risk in women. Women who smoke become menopausal on average 1–2 years earlier than non-smokers (USDHHS 1989). Studies have reported lower plasma oestrogen levels in women smokers when compared to age-matched non-smokers (Mattison & Thorgeirsson 1978). Recent work suggests that the polycyclic hydrocarbons in smoke induce premature egg cell death, resulting in early ovarian failure (Matikainen et al 2001). If oestrogen protects against CHD, it is clear that smoking, a well-documented major contributor to CHD risk in both sexes, has an additional adverse effect that is specific to women.

Hypertension

Isolated systolic hypertension and combined systolic and diastolic hypertension are documented risks for morbidity and development of CHD in both men and women (British Heart Foundation 2002). In young adults, systolic and diastolic blood pressures tend to be higher in men than women (Table 11.3). Throughout adulthood blood pressure gradually rises in both sexes (Whelton et al 1994). However, the gradient of increase is slightly steeper in women. The resultant effect is that by the fifth to sixth decade blood pressure levels are similar in males and females. With advancing years, mean levels of systolic blood pressure continue to rise in the population. Isolated systolic hypertension is more prevalent in elderly females than males, since women make up a larger proportion of the elderly population (Silagy & McNeil 1992), and is estimated to affect about one third of women

Table 11.3 Average blood pressure levels in young adults

	Females	Males
Systolic pressure (mmHg)	110–120	120–130
Diastolic pressure (mmHg)	70–75	75–80

over 65 years of age (BHFHPRG 2002). The risk is significant: each 10 mmHg increase in systolic blood pressure is associated with a 20–30% increase in risk of CHD and stroke (Bush 1990). Hypertension is associated with adverse changes in the structure and function of arterial walls and endothelium, reduction in compliance of small peripheral arteries, increased left ventricular wall mass and abnormal diastolic function (Rizzoni et al 1998). Left ventricular hypertrophy often co-exists with hypertension. The associated increases in wall tension and oxygen demand have been reported to be greater in women (Liao et al 1995).

Health-care practitioners should therefore be vigilant in identifying this common modifiable CHD risk factor in women. Recent well-conducted clinical trials of hypertension therapy that have included women suggest comparable responsiveness to therapy and benefits for women and men (Hansson et al 1998, SHEP Co-operative Research Group 1991, Staessen et al 1997).

Hypertension during pregnancy

Hypertension has been documented to occur in between 5% and 10% of pregnancies. Not all hypertensive states during pregnancy are the result of the same underlying process, which in turn has important implications for subsequent CHD risk. There are three broad classes of hypertension in pregnancy:

- co-existing hypertension
- 'pregnancy-induced' hypertension
- 'pre-eclampsia'.

Co-existing hypertension or essential hypertension is present prior to the pregnancy and continues throughout. The impact on future CHD risk is similar to that observed in the general population with similar blood pressure levels. This is discussed in more detail in Chapter 4.

Specific to pregnancy, there are two main classes of hypertension: 'pregnancy induced' and 'pre-eclampsia'. The former hypertensive state tends to arise in the third trimester and is characterized by moderate elevations in both systolic and diastolic blood pressure that may require treatment. Blood pressure returns to normal after delivery and is thought not to be linked to an increased likelihood of hypertension or risk of CHD in the future. The latter, 'pre-eclampsia', is a specific disorder of pregnancy that is dangerous and poorly understood. It is rare before the 20th week of gestation but can occur at any time beyond and is characterized by the presence of hypertension, proteinuria and oedema; earlier onset is associated with greater severity of the condition. Follow-up work has reported an association between pre-eclampsia and subsequent CHD (Croft & Hannaford 1989, Rosenberg et al 1983).

In practice, particularly when reviewing case records retrospectively, the potential for confusion regarding diagnosis of hypertensive states during pregnancy is significant and the ability to target appropriate individuals lost. However, during pregnancy may be the first time that a woman has a blood pressure check and any woman who has a record of hypertension during pregnancy warrants follow-up to ensure that blood pressure levels remain within the normotensive range post partum. Such women are therefore targets for early monitoring and prevention strategies.

Oral contraceptives

The use of the older high-dose contraceptive pill (known as first generation) increased risk of CHD, in particular risk of myocardial infarction. This was shown to be mediated through increasing levels of LDL-cholesterol, lowering HDL-cholesterol, raising blood pressure and promoting clotting mechanisms (Stadel 1981). Because younger women are at lower absolute risk of CHD, the additional risk was small particularly in women who were non-smokers. However, there was a greatly increased risk of myocardial infarction when the combination of high-dose oral contraceptives and cigarette smoking was present (Hennekens et al 1979), with the risk of MI and stroke increasing exponentially among those who smoked and were older than 35 years (Salonen et al 1982).

Second-generation contraceptive preparations evolved based on lower doses of oestrogen. These were shown to have a less deleterious effect on risk of CHD (Colditz 1994). In a meta-analysis of 13 studies of health outcome in past users it was shown that the deleterious effects of these and earlier preparations applied to current users and that duration of use did not affect risk (Stampfer et al 1990). The authors concluded that there was a rapid return to baseline CHD risk following discontinuation of therapy and that increased risk of thrombosis, a short-term mechanism, explained most, if not all, of the increased risk in current users.

By the early 1990s third-generation oral contraceptive preparations were introduced with similar levels of oestrogen as their second-generation counterparts but now with non-androgenic progestogens in the hope that the better lipid profile would reduce CHD risk. Evaluation of their impact on risk of MI revealed no increased risk in women who did not smoke cigarettes (Colditz 1994). However, there were reports that this new generation of contraceptive pills was associated with increased risk of venous thromboembolism (Lewis et al 1997). After much debate and reanalysis of the evidence, the conclusion reached was that although there was a small increase in risk of venous thromboembolism in users compared to non-users, this was not considered to be clinically important given the overall low absolute risk of venous thromboembolism in younger women (Kemmeren et al 2001).

Diabetes mellitus

Diabetes is an even stronger risk factor for CHD in women than in men (Howard et al 1998). Mortality rates for CHD in diabetic women are three- to sevenfold higher than in non-diabetic women. This is in comparison to a two- to fourfold increase in risk in male diabetics over male non-diabetics (Barrett-Connor & Wingard 1983, Howard et al 1998, Kannel & Wilson 1995, Manson et al 1991). The mechanism for this observation is not clear although it has been hypothesized that diabetes exacerbates the effects of other risk factors (Goldschmid et al 1994), impairs oestrogen binding (Ruderman & Haudenschild 1984) and attenuates the ability of oestrogen to stimulate nitric oxide production in endothelial cells (Cohen 1993), thus negating the protective effects that oestrogens confer on premenopausal women (Kannel & Wilson 1995).

In type 2 diabetes, there is increasing evidence that tight glycaemic control prevents or slows the progression of microvascular complications, although it is less clear if optimal control of diabetes decreases macrovascular problems. These areas are the subject of current research (UKPDS 1998a,b,c).

Gestational diabetes

Gestational diabetes, which occurs in 3% of pregnancies in the UK, may be a marker for increased CHD risk. Long-term follow-up studies reviewed by Rich-Edwards and colleagues (1995) have shown an increased incidence of hypertension, insulin resistance and adverse lipid profiles in women who had gestational diabetes compared to women who had normal pregnancies. More than one third of women who had gestational diabetes subsequently developed non-insulin dependent diabetes compared to a rate of 5% in women who had normal pregnancies (Mestman 1988). Postnatal follow-up usually involves an oral glucose tolerance test to exclude the presence of diabetes mellitus. Longer term follow-up could help to identify earlier those women who develop diabetes mellitus and would provide the opportunity for more comprehensive CHD risk factor assessment and intervention.

Lipid profile

The lipid profile of total cholesterol, triglyceride, LDL-cholesterol and HDL-cholesterol measurements is important in both genders in risk factor assessment. In the Framingham study (Castelli 1984), CHD risk factors and events were observed over a 6-year period. It was shown that at any cholesterol level the risk of CHD over that time period in women was only one third of that observed in men, irrespective of smoking and blood pressure status. The lack of predictive power of total cholesterol in CHD risk assessment in women has been documented by others (Isles 1993).

It has been suggested that in females, more emphasis should be placed on levels of the other lipid parameters, namely triglyceride, LDL-cholesterol and HDL-cholesterol, rather than relying on a total cholesterol measurement alone. Elevated triglyceride levels have been identified as posing a greater threat to women than men (Castelli 1986). The independent nature of their effect in women remains in debate with some studies (Castelli 1986), demonstrating an independent association with increased CHD risk (after adjusting for the effect of other key risk factors) while other work does not (Bush et al 1987). HDL-cholesterol levels in the population are higher in females than males and it has been suggested that this effect may account for at least some of the CHD protection observed in younger females (Kannel & Brand 1985). A low HDL-cholesterol is a particularly strong indicator of increased CHD risk (Jacobs et al 1990). Thus, both elevated triglyceride and lower HDL-cholesterol levels, themselves metabolically inversely linked, may have an important role in assessing risk of CHD in women.

After menopause, total cholesterol and LDL-cholesterol levels increase, reaching levels higher than those of age-matched men, and the highly atherogenic, small, dense LDL particles, enriched with apolipoprotein B_{100}, are also increased. Small decreases in HDL-cholesterol occur, accompanied by increases in triglyceride levels and Lp(a) concentrations, which further exacerbate the lipid risk profile (Jenner et al 1993).

Although some trials of CHD prevention which treated hyperlipidaemia contained no women (Shepherd et al 1995), those that included a significant proportion of women (Downs et al 1998, Miettinen et al 1997) demonstrated that lipid-lowering therapy appears to be at least as beneficial in women as men. There is evidence that women and men may respond differently to dietary modification (reduction in total fat to <30% and saturated fat to <7% of total calorie intake) (Walden et al 1997). Although similar reductions in total cholesterol and LDL-cholesterol were observed, in hypercholesterolaemic women reduced HDL levels occurred which were not evident in males.

Obesity

In the Nurses' Health Study, Manson et al (1990) studied over 120 000 females, aged between 30 and 55 years old. The risk of CHD was over three times higher in women with a body mass index (BMI) (calculated as weight in kilograms divided by the square of height in metres) of 29 and above compared to those women with a BMI of less than 21. A large proportion of the excess risk could be attributed to effects of obesity on blood pressure, glucose intolerance and lipid levels. However, after adjustment for these factors, an effect of obesity per se on CHD risk was still discernible.

Waist circumference reflects total and abdominal fat accumulation and has been shown to relate strongly to health risk, including the risk of CHD (Han & van Leer 1995, Lean et al 1995). In a cross-sectional study, a range of health outcomes were investigated according to waist circumference in 5887 men and 7018 women aged 20–59 years from the general population in The Netherlands (Lean et al 1998). Waist measurement was assessed in terms of action levels which were defined for both genders as (men (women)): less than action level 1, <94.0 (80.0) cm, action levels 1–2, 94.0–101.9 (80.0–87.9) cm and more than action level 2, ≥102.0 (88.0) cm. The group with waist measurement less than action level 1 was used as the comparative reference group. A 4.5-fold increase (95% CI, 2.5–3.7) in risk of non-insulin dependent diabetes mellitus was documented in men above waist action level 2 and 3.8-fold increase (95% CI, 1.9–7.3) in risk for women; a 4.2-fold increase (3.6–5.0) and 2.8-fold increase (2.4–3.2) respectively in the risk of having at least one other cardiovascular risk factor.

Localization of adipose tissue may be even more important for women than the degree of adiposity. Central obesity (android pattern) is associated with a number of metabolic derangements (glucose intolerance, hyperlipidaemia, hypertension) and an increased risk of CHD compared with a gynoid obesity pattern, with body fat concentrated in the hips and thigh (Kissebah & Krakower 1994). The risk of CHD rises steeply with increasing waist:hip ratios above 0.80 (Bjorntorp 1985).

Parity

Studies of CHD risk and its relationship to number of pregnancies have produced differing results; some studies show a positive correlation, some a negative and others no association at all. The subject is reviewed by Barrett-Connor & Bush (1991) who conclude that women with five or more pregnancies have a 1.8-fold increase of myocardial infarction compared to nulliparous women before taking into account smoking status and social class. Among parous women the relative risk estimate for five or more births relative to fewer births was 1.4. The greatest increase in risk was observed for women who had both an early age at first birth and five or more children (Palmer et al 1992). Most studies have failed to take into account the confounding variable of social class. Lower social class is associated with earlier first pregnancy which in turn is related to number of pregnancies. It is also postulated that it is the number of miscarriages, not the number of live births, that increases CHD risk. This suggests that it may not be the hormonal changes during and after pregnancy that increase risk but the possible presence of an adverse hormonal status that is also responsible for the poor reproductive history. Pregnancy, childbirth and parenthood obviously involve many fundamental changes with lasting consequences that further complicate the interpretation of any effect multiparity may impose on future risk of CHD.

HORMONE REPLACEMENT THERAPY

For almost 40 years hormone replacement therapy (HRT) has been used to treat women suffering from the distressing symptoms of the menopause, such as hot flushes and psychological disturbances, and long-term oestrogen use has been accepted since the 1970s as an effective prophylactic measure that reduces the incidence of osteoporotic fractures. More recently, attention has focused on its effects on the cardiovascular system.

Over the past 20 years a large body of observational data has been accumulated, all of which suggest that postmenopausal oestrogen use significantly reduces a woman's risk of CHD. Additionally, many trials have shown oestrogen to have beneficial effects on lipids and direct effects on blood vessels which would be expected to confer cardiovascular protection (Mosca 2000). However, data emerging recently from randomized controlled trials are challenging the belief that HRT confers cardiovascular benefits and its use for the prevention of CHD is currently being questioned.

Effects of HRT on cardiovascular risk markers
Effects on lipoproteins

The most commonly prescribed postmenopausal oestrogens in the UK are conjugated equine oestrogens and human oestrogens (17β-oestradiol, oestradiol valerate). Treatment with 0.625 mg/day conjugated equine oestrogens, which is the standard dose recommended for prevention of bone loss, results in a small increase in triglyceride levels, a reduction in LDL levels and an increase in HDL levels (Fig. 11.3). 17β-oestradiol or oestradiol valerate in the standard dose recommended for bone protection (2 mg/day) has also been shown to decrease LDL-cholesterol and increase HDL-cholesterol but to have little or no effect on triglycerides. Thus oestrogen has a beneficial effect on the main lipoprotein risk factors for CHD (Jensen 1991).

Lipoprotein changes are dose related and depend on the pretreatment lipid status of the patient. On average, in the normolipidaemic woman, the above-mentioned doses of oral postmenopausal oestrogen would effect a decrease in LDL-cholesterol of between 4% and 10% and an increase in HDL of around 10–15%. The rise in HDL is very consistent, being almost invariably seen, whereas there is sometimes no change in LDL, particularly in women with low pretreatment levels.

Although the traditional route of oestrogen administration is the oral one, in recent years there has been increasing interest in parenteral administration, mainly by means of oestradiol-releasing skin patches or subcutaneous implants. Replacement by these methods avoids 'first-pass' effects on the liver and is often well tolerated in women who experience gastrointestinal side-effects on oral therapy. The lipid changes exerted by these forms of therapy are much less marked than those induced by oral oestrogens. In particular, there is no rise in HDL-cholesterol.

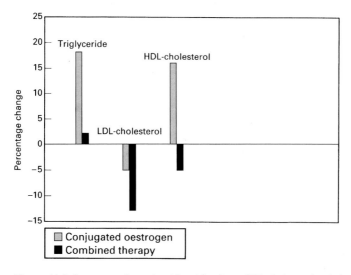

Figure 11.3 Percentage change in triglyceride, plasma LDL-cholesterol and plasma HDL-cholesterol on conjugated equine oestrogens alone and combined therapy of conjugated equine oestrogens and norgestrel (adapted from Farish et al 1991).

Unopposed (without a progestogen) oestrogen therapy has been associated with an increased risk of endometrial cancer. Therefore, for women who have not had a hysterectomy a progestogen is added to the regimen to prevent oestrogen-induced hyperplasia of the endometrium and eliminate the potential increased risk of carcinoma.

The progestogens used in combined HRT fall into two main categories, namely derivatives of 19-nortestosterone, such as norethisterone or norgestrel, and 17-hydroxyprogesterone derivatives, such as medroxyprogesterone acetate or dydrogesterone. Most of the combined therapies currently available in the UK contain progestogens of the 19-nortestosterone series. These progestogens have androgenic as well as progestogenic activity and tend to counteract the beneficial effects of oestrogen on lipid metabolism. Most importantly, they markedly reduce HDL-cholesterol levels. However, they also induce a small decrease in triglyceride levels and reduce levels of lipoprotein(a) (Farish et al 1991), elevated levels of which are associated with increased risk of CHD and stroke. Reports on the effects of these progestogens on LDL-cholesterol are inconsistent. Progesterone-related compounds are less androgenic and have much less marked effects on lipids (Jensen 1991). The effects of combined preparations vary according to the relative doses and potencies of the oestrogens and progestogens which they contain. In most oral preparations which employ norethisterone or norgestrel the balance is such that the oestrogen-induced rise in HDL is negated (Fig. 11.3). Triglyceride levels are unchanged or reduced and lipoprotein(a) levels are decreased. In regimens which include MPA the oestrogen-induced rise in HDL may be blunted, while those with dydrogesterone appear to affect lipids in a similar manner to oestrogen monotherapy.

Oestrogen as a treatment for hyperlipidaemia Hyperlipidaemic women are likely to experience much greater lipid changes than normolipidaemic women. In 1978 a Swedish group published a study in which oestrogen was used as a treatment for type II hyperlipoproteinaemia in postmenopausal women (Tikkanen et al 1978). The women had an average cholesterol of 8.7 mmol/l. After 6 months' treatment with 2 mg oestradiol valerate, LDL-cholesterol was reduced by 18%, HDL-cholesterol increased by 30% and triglyceride levels were unchanged. The magnitude of the decrease in LDL was positively correlated with the initial level. The authors suggested that hyperlipidaemia should be regarded as an additional indication for oestrogen therapy in postmenopausal women and in 1993 the Expert Panel on Detection, Evaluation and Treatment of High Blood Cholesterol in Adults recommended that oestrogen should be considered as a first-line treatment for hyperlipidaemic postmenopausal women.

Nowadays the most effective agents available for reduction of LDL levels are HMG co-enzyme A reductase inhibitors or statins (Gotto 1997). These drugs reduce LDL levels in hypercholesterolaemic women by 25–45% and also significantly reduce triglyceride levels. However, statins produce only modest rises (around 5%) in HDL levels, as opposed to greater than 20% increases routinely induced by oral oestrogens (Davidson et al 1997). The use of combination statin and HRT has been shown in several trials to have a more beneficial effect on lipid profile than either therapy alone, although there are no data on clinical endpoints as yet.

Non-lipid effects on cardiovascular risk

Oestrogen receptors are present in the vasculature and in addition to its beneficial effects on lipids, oestrogen has been shown to have potentially beneficial direct effects on blood vessels. It increases vasodilatation and inhibits the response of blood vessels to injury and the development and progression of atherosclerosis (Mendelsohn & Karas 1999).

Ongoing research suggests that oestrogen may have beneficial effects on carbohydrate metabolism and body fat distribution, both of which are associated with CHD risk.

The susceptibility of LDL to oxidative modification has been implicated in the pathogenesis of atherosclerosis. Oestrogen has been found to have antioxidant effects in vitro. However, studies to date on the effects of post-menopausal oestrogen therapy have produced conflicting results.

There is a large amount of data on the effects of HRT on markers of coagulation and fibrinolysis. The effects on haemostasis are complex. Oral oestrogen alone and with the addition of a progestogen has been shown to reduce fibrinogen, the antifibrinolytic protein, plasminogen activator inhibitor 1, and in some studies factor VII, which should favour fibrinolysis. However, oestrogen also decreases the anticoagulant proteins antithrombin III and protein S (Mendelsohn & Karas 1999). Transdermal oestrogen has a minimal effect on haemostatic parameters. As in the case of lipoproteins, the net effect of HRT on coagulation factors depends on the preparation, the route of administration and the duration of therapy.

Two biochemical markers for coronary artery disease in which there has recently been a great deal of interest are the amino acid homocysteine and C-reactive protein (CRP), increased plasma levels of which are associated with increased incidence of disease. Homocysteine has been shown to be an independent marker, and is thought to exert its influence via several mechanisms, including direct injury to the endothelium, increased platelet aggregation, increased auto-oxidation of LDL and causing abnormalities in clotting (Stein & McBride 1998). It would appear likely that reducing homocysteine should decrease cardiac disease, but there are no intervention studies as yet to confirm this. Homocysteine increases with age, males have higher levels than females and postmenopausal women higher levels than premenopausal women so it was expected that oestrogen might decrease it. There have been few studies published so far and results have been variable, some workers finding a reduction with oestrogen or oestrogen plus progestogen, others failing to detect any difference.

CRP has recently been shown to be one of the strongest predictors of CVD in women (Ridker et al 2000) and is one of the few biochemical risk markers adversely affected by HRT (Cushman et al 1999). However, it is not clear whether the increase in this inflammatory marker induced by oral oestrogen or oestrogen plus progestogen, but not by non-oral therapy, has any clinical relevance, although it has been hypothesized that increased

CRP is associated with decreased plaque stability and increased probability of thrombosis and that this effect may explain the early increase in CHD events seen in the first of the randomized placebo controlled HRT studies to report (Hulley et al 1998).

HRT and CHD events
Observational studies

Oestrogen-only HRT Results from a number of large studies carried out in the USA have indicated that postmenopausal oestrogen use is associated with a significant reduction in CHD risk. Meta-analyses of observational studies suggest a reduction in CHD risk of 30–50% in oral oestrogen users compared with non-users (Barrett-Connor & Grady 1998, Stampfer & Colditz 1991).

One of the most important earlier studies was the Lipid Research Clinic's follow-up study, which compared oestrogen users with non-users over an 8-year period and found that users had about one third of the risk of fatal CHD compared with non-users (Bush et al 1987). Both groups had a similar distribution of most risk factors (age, blood pressure, smoking, etc.) but users had higher triglyceride levels, lower LDL-cholesterol and higher HDL-cholesterol levels. Statistical analysis of the data suggested that about half of the protective effect could be accounted for by the lipid changes, particularly the increase in HDL-cholesterol. No correlation was found between triglyceride levels and CHD risk. The Nurses' Health Study, a large, very well-designed study involving over 70 000 postmenopausal women, has recently published 20-year follow-up data (Grodstein et al 2000) which is in line with their findings at 10 years, showing an incidence in CHD in oestrogen-treated women half of that observed in untreated women.

Observational studies have also indicated that oestrogen has a protective effect in women who already have CHD. One of the larger trials followed over 2000 women with established CHD for a 10-year period and found that oestrogen users had a significantly better overall survival than non-users (Sullivan et al 1990).

Combined therapy In most of the large epidemiological studies, oral unopposed oestrogen was used exclusively. There are no epidemiological data available for parenteral oestrogen and very little for oestrogen/progestogen therapy, although the little there is suggests that the effects of combined preparations are similar to oestrogen-only regimens (Barrett-Connor & Grady 1998). A Swedish study followed over 20 000 women who had been prescribed HRT, two thirds of which was oestrogen only and one third cyclical combined therapy, for 6 years (Falkeborn et al 1992). The group treated with combined therapy had approximately half the incidence of myocardial infarction of that expected from the incidence rates for the population of the region (relative risk = 0.53), while those treated with oestrogen alone had a relative risk of 0.69. This finding was somewhat unexpected since the most commonly used combined preparation was one containing a high-dose androgenic progestogen, which would be expected to reduce HDL-cholesterol levels.

An American group compared the use of HRT in over 500 postmenopausal women who had sustained a myocardial infarction with that of over 1000 age-matched controls. One third of those on HRT were taking oestrogen combined with the non-androgenic progestogen medroxyprogesterone acetate (MPA) while the rest had an oestrogen-only preparation. The relative risk of myocardial infarction for those on HRT compared with those not on treatment was 0.69 for those on oestrogen alone and 0.68 for those on combined therapy, indicating that the reduced risk associated with oestrogen use was not compromised by addition of MPA (Psaty et al 1994). More recently, the latest update from the Nurses' Study has indicated no difference in relative risk of CHD between users of oestrogen alone and users of combined oestrogen and MPA (Grodstein et al 2000). Additionally, 3-year data from the Postmenopausal Estrogen/Progestogen Interventions (PEPI) Trial, a large American multicentre randomized placebo-controlled study designed to assess the effects of unopposed oestrogen and three different oestrogen/ non-androgenic progestogen regimens on cardiovascular risk factors, indicated that all the regimens improved lipid profile and coagulation factors without adversely affecting blood pressure or insulin levels (Writing Group for the PEPI Trial 1995).

Randomized controlled trials

Observational studies have been criticized on the grounds of selection bias, since women taking HRT tend to be healthier, of higher socio-economic status and better educated than those who do not. Although the consistency and magnitude of the decrease in CHD risk observed in study after study made it extremely unlikely that all the apparent protection could be due to bias, it was generally agreed that evidence from randomized placebo-controlled trials was necessary for confirmation so the results from several large randomized controlled clinical trials being carried out to determine whether HRT does reduce the risk of heart disease in healthy women or the risk of new cardiovascular events in women who already have CHD were eagerly awaited.

The first two trials to publish were secondary prevention trials, the Heart and Estrogen/Progestin Replacement Study (HERS) (Hulley et al 1998) and the Estrogen Replacement and Atherosclerosis Trial (ERA) (Herrington et al 2000). The findings from both of these trials proved very disappointing. The HERS examined the effect of continuous combined oestrogen-progestogen therapy (conjugated equine oestrogens + MPA) in 2763 postmenopausal women (mean age 67 years) with established CHD. After 4 years there were no differences between the treatment and placebo groups for non-fatal MI or CHD death. However, there was a significant time trend, with more CHD events occurring in year 1 in the HRT group than in the placebo group, but fewer in subsequent years. More women in the hormone group experienced venous thromboembolic events and gall bladder disease. Based on these results, the authors concluded that HRT should not be started for the purpose of secondary prevention of CHD, but that it may be favourable for women already on treatment to continue.

The ERA Trial was a three-arm double-blind placebo-controlled trial set up to evaluate the effect of HRT on progression of coronary atherosclerosis in normocholesterolaemic women with angiographically verified coronary artery disease. There were 309 women enrolled, mean age 66 years. They were assigned to oral equine oestrogens with or without MPA or placebo and they were followed up for 3 years. No differences were found between the groups either in terms of changes in mean minimum coronary artery diameter or clinical cardiovascular event rates, although the two treatment arms showed a favourable effect on lipoproteins compared to the placebo arm. Unlike the HERS, there was no increase in events during the first year of treatment.

The unexpected results of these two trials have been discussed at length in the literature and limitations in each of them, such as age of subjects, type of HRT, trial duration, pointed out. Nevertheless, the consensus of expert opinion was that there is no longer any reason to start HRT in post-menopausal women with established CHD with the sole or main aim of producing a cardiovascular benefit.

A follow-up to the HERS (HERS II), undertaken to determine if the apparent decrease in CHD risk observed in the later years of the HERS persisted or became more marked, resulting in overall benefit, showed that after almost 7 years of HRT there was no evidence of benefit for any cardiovascular outcome (Grady et al 2002).

A third secondary prevention trial, Oestrogen in the Prevention of Reinfarction Trial (ESPRIT-UK) has just reported (ESPRIT Team 2002). This is a UK 2-year placebo-controlled trial of oestradiol valerate involving 1000 women who have already had a myocardial infarction. The results indicate that oestradiol valerate does not reduce the overall risk of further cardiac events in postmenopausal women who have survived a myocardial infarction. These findings lend additional support to the existing recommendation that HRT should not be used for secondary prevention of CHD.

However, the results of secondary prevention trials cannot be extrapolated to women without CHD and results from the Women's Health Initiative primary prevention trial were anxiously awaited. This trial was set up with a planned duration of 8.5 years. Between 1993 and 1998, 16 608 post-menopausal women were enrolled and randomly assigned to either continuous equine oestrogens + MPA or placebo. The trial was stopped early, after a mean follow-up of 5.2 years, on the grounds that interim analysis had showed that the health risks exceeded the benefit. The therapy did not protect against heart disease but actually increased heart attacks, stroke and blood clots in legs and lungs and the test statistic for invasive breast cancer exceeded the stopping boundary. There were decreases in colorectal cancers and osteoporotic fractures. There was no effect on all-cause mortality but the global index statistic supported risks exceeding benefits. The authors concluded that this regimen should not be initiated or continued for primary prevention of CHD (Writing Group for the Women's Health Initiative Investigators 2002). A separate WHI study, running in parallel, of oestrogen alone in women who have had a hysterectomy is continuing, because at this stage the balance of risks and benefits of oestrogen alone is uncertain.

The limitation common to all the above trials is that only oral oestrogen and one type of progestogen were tested. The results do not necessarily apply to lower dosages of these drugs or to other oral preparations or to HRT administered transdermally, which may give a different risk/benefit profile. Nevertheless, they are very disappointing, being so much at odds with those expected from observational trials and studies of surrogate markers. There are no further randomized trials ongoing at present. The Women's International Study of Long Duration Oestrogen after the Menopause (WISDOM), a multicentre UK, Australia and New Zealand trial set up recently, was to have recruited 22 000 healthy women and treat them with conjugated equine oestrogens with or without MPA and was planned to run for 10 years, due to end in 2012. However, it has just been halted, due to a number of factors, including the cost, slow recruitment, safety and the ethics of continuing in the light of recent information on HRT.

A lot of work is currently being conducted with low-dose formulations which show encouraging results for effects on lipids and arterial reactivity as well as efficacy in symptomatic control and prevention of bone loss. However, further randomized clinical trials would be necessary to clarify their effects on CHD and these are likely to be very difficult to carry out in view of recently published data.

A new development in the field of menopausal therapy is the advent of selective oestrogen modulators, known as SERMs. These drugs exert oestrogenic effects on bone and lipids, while behaving as oestrogen antagonists on breast and endometrial tissue. The hope is that they will have beneficial effects on heart and bone, while exhibiting no adverse effects on breast or endometrium. A randomized double-blind, placebo-controlled study of the SERM raloxifene, entitled Raloxifene Use for the Heart (RUTH) which involves approximately 10 000 patients, is under way at present.

CONCLUSION

In summary, most of the risk factors for CHD and the preventive strategies advocated in men are applicable to women. For several of these risk factors the magnitude of their effect on prevalence rate differs from that observed in males and warrants particular attention in women. These include diabetes mellitus, triglyceride and HDL-cholesterol levels, isolated systolic hypertension in the elderly and central obesity. They should be considered in association with the factors that are unique to women, namely menopausal status, oral contraceptive use, pre-eclampsia and gestational diabetes.

The data from a large number of observational studies of HRT use, both in healthy women and those with established CHD, have suggested that oral oestrogen replacement therapy significantly reduces the risk of cardiovascular mortality and its effects on surrogate risk markers, particularly lipoproteins, provide a biologically plausible explanation for these findings.

However, randomized controlled trials which have recently reported have failed to confirm expectations. Three secondary prevention trials have found no evidence of cardiovascular benefit from either oral oestrogen alone or with a progestogen. The only primary prevention trial to report so far has shown an increased risk of CHD with combined oestrogen/progestogen therapy. The role of oestrogen monotherapy in primary prevention is currently unclear.

■ KEY POINTS

- CHD is the leading cause of death in women.
- The traditional risk factors for CHD and the preventive strategies advocated in men are applicable to women.
- Diabetes mellitus, triglyceride and HDL-cholesterol levels, pre-eclampsia, isolated systolic hypertension in the elderly and central obesity warrant particular attention in women.
- The likelihood of a role for HRT in the prevention of CHD has become unconvincing in the light of recent evidence from randomized trials.

REFERENCES

Barrett-Connor E 1997 Sex differences in coronary heart disease. Circulation 95: 252–264
Barrett-Connor E, Bush TL 1991 Estrogen and coronary heart disease in women. Journal of the American Medical Association 265: 1861–1867
Barrett-Connor E, Grady D 1998 Hormone replacement therapy, heart disease and other considerations. Annual Review of Public Health 19: 55–72
Barrett-Connor E, Wingard DL 1983 Sex differential in ischaemic heart disease mortality in diabetics: a prospective population-based study. American Journal of Epidemiology 118: 489–496
Bjorntorp P 1985 Regional patterns of fat distribution. Annals of Internal Medicine 103: 994–995
Black D 1980 Inequalities in health: report of a Research Working Group chaired by Sir Douglas Black. DHSS, London
British Heart Foundation Health Promotion Research Group (BHFHPRG) 2002 Coronary Heart Disease Statistics. Department of Public Health, University of Oxford, Oxford
Bush TL 1990 The epidemiology of cardiovascular disease in post-menopausal women. Annals of the New York Academy of Science 592: 263–271
Bush TL, Barrett-Connor E, Cowan LD et al 1987 Cardiovascular mortality and non contraceptive use of estrogen in women: results from the Lipid Research Clinics Program Follow-up Study. Circulation 75: 1002–1009
Castelli WP 1984 Epidemiology of coronary heart disease: the Framingham Study. American Journal of Medicine 76(2A): 4–12
Castelli WP 1986 The triglyceride issue: a view from Framingham. American Heart Journal 112: 432–437
Cohen RA 1993 Dysfunction of vascular endothelium in diabetes mellitus. Circulation 87(suppl 5): V67–V76
Colditz GA 1994 Oral contraceptive use and mortality during 12 years of follow-up: the Nurses' Health Study. Annals of Internal Medicine 120: 821–826
Colditz GA, Willett WC, Stampfer MJ, Rosner B, Speizer FE, Hennekens CH 1987 Menopause and the risk of coronary heart disease in women. New England Journal of Medicine 316: 1105–1110
Croft P, Hannaford PC 1989 Risk factors for acute myocardial infarction in women: evidence from the Royal College of General Practitioners' Oral Contraception Study. British Medical Journal 298: 165–168

Cushman M, Legault C, Barrett-Connor E et al 1999 Effect of postmenopausal hormones on inflammation-sensitive proteins: the Postmenopausal Estrogen/Progestogen Interventions (PEPI) study. Circulation 100: 717–722

Davidson MH, Testolin LM, Maki KC, von Duvillard S, Drennan KB 1997 A comparison of estrogen replacement, pravastatin and combined treatment for the management of hypercholesterolaemia in postmenopausal women. Archives of Internal Medicine 157: 1186–1192

Downs JR, Clearfield M, Weis S et al 1998 Primary prevention of acute coronary events with lovastatin in men and women with average cholesterol levels: results of AFCAPS/TexCAPS. Journal of the American Medical Association 279: 1615–1622

ESPRIT Team 2002 Oestrogen therapy for prevention of reinfarction in post menopausal women: a randomized placebo-controlled trial. Lancet 360: 2001–2008

Falkeborn M, Persson I, Adami HI et al 1992 The risk of acute myocardial infarction after oestrogen and oestrogen–progestogen replacement. British Journal of Obstetrics and Gynaecology 99: 821–828

Farish E, Rolton HA, Barnes JF, Hart DM 1991 Lipoprotein(a) concentrations in postmenopausal women taking norethisterone. British Medical Journal 303: 694

Glendy RE, Levine SA, White SA, White PD 1937 Coronary disease in youth: comparison of 100 patients under 40 with 300 persons past 80. Journal of the American Medical Association 109: 1775–1778

Goldschmid MG, Barrett-Connor E, Edelstein SL, Wingard DL, Cohn BA, Herman WH 1994 Dyslipidemia and ischemic heart disease mortality among men and women with diabetes. Circulation 89: 991–997

Gotto AM 1997 Cholesterol management in theory and practice. Circulation 96: 4424–4430

Grady D, Herrington D, Bittner V et al 2002 Cardiovascular disease outcomes during 6.8 years of hormone therapy. Journal of the American Medical Association 288: 49–57

Grodstein F, Manson J, Colditz GA, Willett WC, Speizer FE, Stampfer MJ 2000 A prospective, observational study of postmenopausal hormone therapy and primary prevention of cardiovascular disease. Annals of Internal Medicine 133: 933–941

Han TS, van Leer EM 1995 Waist circumference action levels in the identification of cardiovascular risk factors: prevalence study in a random sample. British Medical Journal 311: 1041–1045

Hansen EF, Andersen LT, von Eyben FE 1993 Cigarette smoking and age at first acute myocardial infarction, and influence of gender and extent of smoking. American Journal of Cardiology 71: 1439–1442

Hansson L, Zanchetti A, Carruthers SG et al 1998 Effects of intensive blood-pressure lowering and low-dose aspirin in patients with hypertension: principal results of the Hypertension Optimal Treatment (HOT) randomised trial. Lancet 351: 1755–1762

Hennekens CH, Evans D, Peto R 1979 Oral contraceptive use, cigarette smoking and myocardial infarction. British Journal of Family Planning 5: 66–67

Herrington DM, Reboussin DM, Brosnihan KB et al 2000 Effects of estrogen replacement on the progression of coronary artery atherosclerosis. New England Journal of Medicine 343: 522–529

Howard BV, Cowan LD, Go O, Welty TK, Robbins DC, Lee ET 1998 Adverse effects of diabetes on multiple cardiovascular disease risk factors in women: the Strong Heart Study. Diabetes Care 21: 1258–1265

Hulley S, Grady D, Bush T, Furberg C, Herrington D, Riggs B, Vittinghoff E 1998 Randomised trial of estrogen plus progestin for secondary prevention of coronary heart disease in women. Journal of the American Medical Association 280: 605–613

Isles C 1993 Prevention of coronary disease in women. Scottish Medical Journal 38(4): 103–106

Jacobs DR, Meban IL, Bangdiwala SI, Criqui MH, Tyroler HA 1990 High density lipoprotein cholesterol as a predictor of cardiovascular disease mortality in men and women: the follow-up study of the Lipid Research Clinics Prevalence Study. American Journal of Epidemiology 131: 32–47

Jenner JL, Ordovas JM, Lamon-Fava S et al 1993 Effects of age, sex, and menopausal status on plasma lipoprotein(a) levels: the Framingham Offspring Study. Circulation 87: 1135–1141

Jensen J 1991 Effects of sex steroids on serum lipids and lipoproteins. Baillière's Clinical Obstetrics and Gynaecology 5: 867–887

Kannel WB, Brand FN 1985 Cardiovascular risk factors in the elderly. Fertility and Sterility 6(suppl 2): 176S–179S

Kannel WB, Wilson PW 1995 Risk factors that attenuate the female coronary disease advantage. Archives of Internal Medicine 155: 57–61

Kemmeren JM, Algra A, Grobbee DE 2001 Third generation oral contraceptives and risk of venous thrombosis: meta-analysis. British Medical Journal 323: 131–134

Kissebah AH, Krakower GR 1994 Regional adiposity and morbidity. Physiological Review 74: 761–811

Lean MEJ, Han TS, Morrison CE 1995 Waist circumference as a measure for indicating need for weight management. British Medical Journal 311: 158–161

Lean MEJ, Han TS, Seidell JC 1998 Impairment of health and quality of life in people with large waist circumference. Lancet 351: 853–856

Lewis MA, Spitzer WO, Heinemann LAJ, Macrae KD, Bruppacher R 1997 Lowered risk of dying of heart attack with third generation pill may offset risk of dying of thromboembolism. British Medical Journal 315: 679–680

Liao Y, Cooper RS, Mensah GA, McGee DL 1995 Left ventricular hypertrophy has a greater impact on survival in women than in men. Circulation 92: 805–810

Manson JE, Colditz GA, Stampfer MJ et al 1990 A prospective study of obesity and risk of coronary disease in women. New England Journal of Medicine 322: 882–889

Manson JE, Colditz GA, Stampfer MJ et al 1991 A prospective study of maturity-onset diabetes and risk of coronary heart disease and stroke in women. Archives of Internal Medicine 151: 1141–1147

Manson JE, Tosteson H, Ridker PM et al 1992 The primary prevention of myocardial infarction. New England Journal of Medicine 326: 1406–1416

Mattison DR, Thorgeirsson SS 1978 Smoking and industrial pollution, and their effects on menopause and ovarian cancer. Lancet i: 187–188

Mendelsohn ME, Karas RH 1999 The protective effects of oestrogen on the cardiovascular system. New England Journal of Medicine 340: 1801–1811

Mestman JH 1988 Follow-up studies in women with gestational diabetes mellitus: the experience at Los Angeles County/University of Southern California Medical Center. In: Weiss PAM, Coustan DR (eds) Gestational diabetes. Springer-Verlag, Vienna, pp 191–198

Miettinen TA, Pyorala K, Olsson AG et al 1997 Cholesterol-lowering therapy in women and elderly patients with myocardial infarction or angina pectoris: findings from the Scandinavian Simvastatin Survival Study (4S). Circulation 96: 4211–4218

Mosca L 2000 The role of hormone replacement therapy in the prevention of postmenopausal heart disease. Archives of Internal Medicine 160: 2263–2272

Njoistad I, Arnesen E, Lund-Larsen PG 1996 Smoking, serum lipids, blood pressure, and sex differences in myocardial infarction: a 12-year follow-up of the Finnmark Study. Circulation 93: 450–456

Nyboe J, Jensen G, Appleyard M, Schnohr P 1991 Smoking and the risk of first acute myocardial infarction. American Heart Journal 122: 438–447

Office of Population Censuses and Surveys (OPCS) 1995 Series OH2 No 20. HMSO, London

Palmer JR, Rosenberg L, Shapiro S 1992 Reproductive factors and risk of myocardial infarction. American Journal of Epidemiology 136(4): 408–416

Prescott E, Hippe M, Schnohr P, Hein HO, Vestbo J 1998 Smoking and risk of myocardial infarction in women and men: longitudinal population study. British Medical Journal 316: 1043–1047

Psaty BM, Heckbert SR, Atkins D et al 1994 The risk of myocardial infarction associated with the combined use of estrogens and progestogens in postmenopausal women. Archives of Internal Medicine 154: 1333–1339

Registrar General for Scotland 1994 Report of the Registrar General for Scotland. HMSO, Edinburgh

Rich-Edwards JW, Manson JE, Hennekens CH, Buring JE 1995 The primary prevention of coronary heart disease in women. New England Journal of Medicine 333: 1758–1766

Ridker PM, Hennekens CH, Buring JE, Rifai N 2000 C-reactive protein and other markers of inflammation in the prediction of cardiovascular disease in women. New England Journal of Medicine 342: 836–843

Rizzoni D, Muiesan ML, Porteri E et al 1998 Relations between cardiac and vascular structure in patients with primary and secondary hypertension. Journal of the American College of Cardiology 32: 985–992

Rosenberg L, Miller DR, Kaufman DW 1983 Myocardial infarction in women under 50 years of age. Journal of the American Medical Association 250: 2801–2806

Ruderman NB, Haudenschild C 1984 Diabetes as an atherogenic factor. Progress in Cardiovascular Diseases 26: 373–412

Salonen JT, Puska P, Tuomilehto J 1982 Physical activity and risk of myocardial infarction, cerebral stroke and death: a longitudinal study in eastern Finland. American Journal of Epidemiology 115: 526–537

SHEP Co-operative Research Group 1991 Prevention of stroke by antihypertensive drug treatment in older persons with isolated systolic hypertension: final results of the Systolic Hypertension in the Elderly Program (SHEP). Journal of the American Medical Association 265: 3255–3264

Shepherd J, Cobbe SM, Ford I et al West of Scotland Coronary Prevention Study Group 1995 Prevention of coronary heart disease with pravastatin in men with hypercholesterolemia. New England Journal of Medicine 333: 1301–1307

Silagy CA, McNeil JH 1992 Epidemiologic aspects of isolated systolic hypertension and implications for future research. American Journal of Cardiology 69: 213–218

Stadel BV 1981 Oral contraceptives and cardiovascular disease. New England Journal of Medicine 305: 672–677

Staessen JA, Fagard R, Thijs L et al Systolic Hypertension in Europe (Syst-Eur) Trial Investigators 1997 Randomised double-blind comparison of placebo and active treatment for older patients with isolated systolic hypertension. Lancet 350: 757–764

Stampfer MJ, Colditz GA 1991 Estrogen replacement therapy and coronary heart disease: a quantitative assessment of the epidemiological evidence. Preventive Medicine 20: 47–63

Stampfer MJ, Willett WC, Colditz GA, Speizer FE, Hennekens CH 1990 Past use of oral contraceptives and cardiovascular disease: a meta-analysis in the context of the Nurses' Health Study. American Journal of Obstetrics and Gynaecology 163: 285–291

Stein JH, McBride PE 1998 Hyperhomocysteinaemia and atherosclerotic vascular disease. Archives of Internal Medicine 158: 1301–1306

Sullivan JM, van der Swaag R, Hughes JP et al 1990 Estrogen replacement and coronary heart disease: effect on survival in post menopausal women. Archives of Internal Medicine 150: 2557–2562

Tikkanen MJ, Nikkila EA, Vartiainen E 1978 Natural oestrogen as an effective treatment for type II hyperlipoproteinaemia in post menopausal women. Lancet 2: 490–492

Tunstall-Pedoe H 1998 Myth and paradox of coronary risk and the menopause. Lancet 351: 1425–1427

UK Prospective Diabetes Study (UKPDS) Group 1998a Tight blood pressure control and risk of macrovascular and microvascular complications in type 2 diabetes: UKPDS 38. British Medical Journal 317: 703–713

UK Prospective Diabetes Study (UKPDS) Group 1998b Intensive blood glucose control with sulphonylureas or insulin compared with conventional treatment and risk of complications in patients with type 2 diabetes (UKPDS 33). Lancet 352: 837–853

UK Prospective Diabetes Study (UKPDS) Group 1998c Effect of intensive blood-glucose control with metformin on complications in overweight patients with type 2 diabetes (UKPDS 34). Lancet 352: 854–865

US Department of Health and Human Resources (US DHHS) 1989 Reducing the consequences of smoking: 25 years of progress: a report of the Surgeon General. US Department of Health and Human Services, Rockville, MD

Walden CE, Retzlaff BM, Buck BL, McCann BS, Knopp RH 1997 Lipoprotein lipid response to the National Cholesterol Education Program Step II diet by hypercholesterolemic and combined hyperlipidemic women and men. Arteriosclerosis, Thrombosis and Vascular Biology 17: 375–382

Whelton PK, He J, Klag MJ 1994 Blood pressure in westernized populations. In: Swales JD (ed) Textbook of hypertension. Blackwell Scientific Publications, Oxford

Wilhelmsen L, Bengtsson C, Elmfeldt D et al 1977 Multiple risk prediction of myocardial infarction in women as compared to men. British Heart Journal 39: 1179–1185

Willett WC, Green A, Stampfer MJ et al 1987 Relative and absolute excess risks of coronary heart disease among women who smoke cigarettes. New England Journal of Medicine 317: 1303–1309

Writing Group for the PEPI Trial 1995 Effects of estrogen and estrogen/progestin regimens on heart disease risk factors in postmenopausal women. Journal of the American Medical Association 273: 199–208

Writing Group for the Women's Health Initiative Investigators 2002 Risks and benefits of estrogen plus progestin in healthy postmenopausal women. Journal of the American Medical Association 288: 321–333

Type 2 diabetes and coronary heart disease

Parijat De   Marc Evans   Alan Rees

12

■ CONTENTS

INTRODUCTION

Diabetes mellitus is a major public health problem and is now assuming epidemic proportions. Type 2 diabetes mellitus (T2DM) increases the risk of all manifestations of vascular disease, including coronary heart disease (CHD), cerebrovascular disease and peripheral vascular disease, with CHD accounting for the majority of type 2 diabetes-related morbidity and mortality (Laakso & Lehto 1998). The risk of cardiovascular disease is increased 2–4-fold in T2DM (Wingard & Barrett-Connor 1995) and as many as 75% of deaths in people with T2DM will be from cardiovascular disease (King's Fund 1996). Furthermore, the prevalence of T2DM is at least 2–3-fold higher in people with established CHD than in the general population (Currie et al 1997). It is also known that patients with T2DM but with no history of cardiovascular disease have the same risk of subsequent myocardial infarction over 7 years as non-diabetic patients who survive their initial MI. This means that patients with T2DM have the same absolute risk of CHD as those who have survived their initial MI (Haffner et al 1998). The life expectancy of a person with T2DM is reduced by 8–10 years in the 40–70 year age group but improvements can be achieved by aggressive management of risk factors. Thus T2DM should be regarded as an aggressive vascular disease needing early diagnosis and multiple CHD risk factor interventions.

This chapter addresses cardiovascular risk in relation mainly to T2DM and focuses on the management of risk factors using currently available evidence.

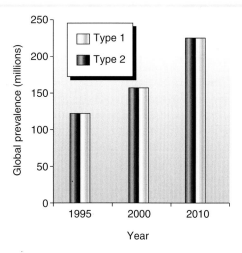

Figure 12.1 Projected increase in global prevalence of diabetes. (Reproduced with permission from Day C 2001. The rising tide of type 2 diabetes. British Journal of Diabetes and Vascular Disease 1(1): 37–43.)

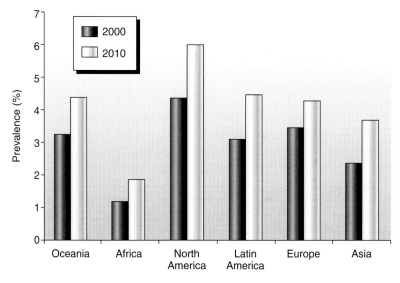

Figure 12.2 Estimated prevalence of T2DM as a percentage of the population in different areas of the world in 2000 and 2010. (Reproduced with permission from Day C 2001. The rising tide of type 2 diabetes. British Journal of Diabetes and Vascular Disease 1(1): 37–43.)

PREVALENCE

Globally, more than 150 million people (2% of the world's population) have diabetes. This is expected to exceed 220 million by 2010 and double by 2025 (Fig. 12.1). The prevalence of diabetes will more than double in Asia, Africa and Eastern Mediterranean countries (Fig. 12.2). In Europe, prevalence will increase from 3.5% to 4.7%, mainly in older adults (WHO 1997). In the UK alone it is estimated that there are over 2 million people (overall prevalence around 3–4%) with T2DM (Amos et al 1997) and for each diagnosed case, there is one undiagnosed case of diabetes.

The predominant clinical phenotype of diabetes is T2DM, accounting for around 90% of all cases. There is a wide variation in the prevalence of diabetes amongst different racial groups. The Afro-Caribbean and Indo-Asian population in the UK, for instance, have a 2–5-fold higher prevalence. The main reasons for the increase in prevalence are increasing obesity (both adult and childhood), decreasing levels of physical activity, increasing age, urbanization and increase in ethnic admixture.

COST IMPLICATIONS

In most of the developed countries of the world, diabetes exerts its influence on health by means of its long-term complications. Alongside incidence and prevalence, the direct health-care costs of diabetes prevention, treatment, care and rehabilitation are important indicators of the impact diabetes has on our society. According to the CODE-2 study (Costs of Diabetes in Europe, type 2) in the UK, the average cost of care for 1 year of a patient with T2DM is around £1500 or just over 4% of the annual NHS budget (Baxter et al 2000). Hospital admission is the single largest contributor to NHS costs and the presence of complications is the most important cost driver (Figs 12.3,12.4). For example, the presence of both microvascular and macrovascular complications increases personal and carer expenditure more than threefold. Thus, T2DM is costly not only for the patient, in terms of premature morbidity and mortality, but also financially for the National Health Service.

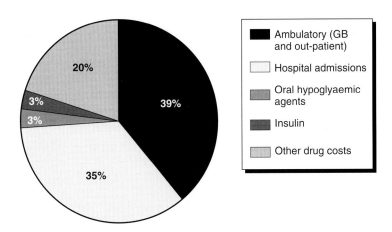

Figure 12.3 Direct health-care costs by category. (Reproduced from Williams with permission from the Medical Education Partnership.)

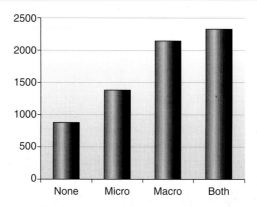

Figure 12.4 Direct health-care costs (£ per patient per annum) in relation to presence or absence of complications. (Reproduced from Williams with permission from the Medical Education Partnership.)

NEW DIAGNOSTIC CRITERIA FOR DIABETES

The diagnosis of diabetes is not in doubt when patients present with symptoms, glycosuria and elevated blood glucose over 11 mmol/l. There is no need for a confirmatory glucose tolerance test in such patients. In June 2000 the UK adopted the World Health Organization criteria for diabetes (British Diabetic Association 2000). In essence, the fasting glucose cut-off value is now 7 mmol/l instead of 7.8 mmol/l as this has been shown in epidemiological studies to have a closer relationship to the 2-hour value of 11.1 mmol/l and thus of developing complications of diabetes. Many patients will have fasting plasma glucose values between 6 and 7 mmol/l. In the new criteria, a fasting plasma value between 6.1 and 6.9 mmol/l is termed impaired fasting glycaemia (IFG), which is broadly analogous to the previous impaired glucose tolerance (IGT). This category of subjects is at increased risk of developing diabetes in the future together with an increased risk of ischaemic heart disease (but not of microvascular complications). Those who have a fasting blood sugar between 6.1 and 7 should have an oral glucose tolerance test to exclude or confirm diabetes. If the 2-hour value after an oral glucose tolerance test is >11.1 mmol/l, diabetes is diagnosed. If the result at 2 hours is >7.8 but <11.1 mmol/l, impaired glucose tolerance is diagnosed. It is important to remember that in subjects with no symptoms, diagnosis should not be based on a single glucose determination. At least one additional glucose test on another day with a value in the diabetic range is essential, either fasting, from a random sample, or from the 2-hour oral glucose tolerance test.

With increased awareness amongst susceptible individuals at risk of developing T2DM and with the help of these new diagnostic criteria, it is presumed that more patients will now be diagnosed as having T2DM than previously.

PATHOPHYSIOLOGY

Type 2 diabetes is characterized by chronic fasting and meal-time hyperglycaemia and this is probably a result of a complex interaction between a number of environmental factors and genetic susceptibility.

■ **BOX 12.1 Type 2 diabetes classification. Reproduced from Williams with permission from the Medical Education Partnership.**

A. **Common type 2 diabetes mellitus** (combination of insulin resistance and relative insulin deficiency)
B. **Specific forms of diabetes in adults**
- **Genetic defects associated with β-cell dysfunction**
  - a) Mitochondrial diabetes and deafness (MIDD)
  - b) Maturity-onset diabetes of the young (MODY) due to: HNF-4α, glucokinase, HNF-1α, IPF-1, HNF-1β gene mutations
  - c) Latent autoimmune diabetes in adults
  - d) Exocrine pancreatic disease
- **Genetic defects associated with insulin resistance**
  - a) Mutations in the insulin receptor gene
    Leprachuanism and Rabson–Mendenhall syndrome
    Some cases of type A insulin resistance
  - b) Defects in genes related to postreceptor signal transduction
    Polycystic ovary syndrome
    Lipoatrophic diabetes
    Some cases of type A insulin resistance
  - c) Genetic mutations affecting adipose tissue
    LMNA gene, PPAR-γ, leptin
- **Drug-induced diabetes**
  Glucocorticoids, thiazides, nicotinic acid, etc.
- **Endocrine diseases**
  Cushing's syndrome, acromegaly, phaeochromocytoma, glucagonoma, hyperthyroidism, etc.
- **Diabetes associated with other genetic syndromes**
  Obesity syndromes: Prader–Willi syndrome, Lawrence Moon–Biedl syndrome, etc. Others: Friedrich's ataxia, myotonic dystrophy, haemochromatosis, porphyria, thalassaemia, etc.

The basic pathophysiological abnormality is a combination of inadequate insulin secretion, i.e. β-cell dysfunction and the inability of insulin to promote glucose uptake by tissues such as muscle, liver and adipose tissue, i.e. insulin resistance (Kumar & Barnett 1997, Leslie 1993, Yki-Jarvinen 1994). Patients with T2DM have both these defects and there has been considerable debate as to which one comes first. However, it is well recognized that by the time hyperglycaemia is established, both insulin resistance and β-cell dysfunction are present. Whether a patient becomes diabetic or not is entirely dependent on β-cell deficiency, since insulin resistance is almost universal in T2DM and has also been shown to precede the onset of diabetes.

Insulin resistance is now known to be the major culprit in the conglomeration of cardiovascular risk factors collectively termed the 'metabolic syndrome'. It includes hyperinsulinaemia, insulin resistance, obesity, hypertension, hypertriglyceridaemia and reduced high-density lipoprotein (HDL) cholesterol concentration. In addition to the above risk factors, other thrombotic risk factors correlating with insulin resistance include elevated levels of plasminogen activator inhibitor I (PAI-I), factor VII and fibrinogen. Hyperinsulinaemia and insulin resistance thus help promote development of the atheromatous plaque (by promoting macrophage migration and proliferation and stimulating lipid synthesis) and, together with a pro-thrombotic antifibrinolytic state, promote cardiovascular disease. Various studies have shown that increased cardiovascular risk in T2DM is already established in the prediabetic, insulin-resistant state (Mansfield et al 1996, Zavaroni et al 1989).

Microvascular complications are associated with the development of clinical diabetes whereas macrovascular complications are initiated by hyperinsulinaemia in the prediabetic state (Haffner et al 1990). This explains why so many T2DM patients (at diagnosis) already have established macrovascular complications.

Insulin resistance is a known feature of obesity and central obesity is independently associated with features of metabolic syndrome and predicts T2DM. Metabolically active intra-abdominal fat is associated with high flux of non-esterified fatty acids (NEFA) into the liver, causing hypertriglyceridaemia and reduced hepatic extraction of insulin leading to peripheral insulinaemia. Again, high circulating NEFA levels also cause insulin resistance by interfering with uptake and utilization of glucose. Another area of major interest and research is endothelial dysfunction in T2DM wherein there is reduced bio-availability of nitric oxide resulting in impaired smooth muscle relaxation and vasodilatation.

Thus, it is clear that if insulin resistance is the key underlying factor in the pathogenesis of chronic cardiovascular risk factors such as hypertension and dyslipidaemia, modifying insulin sensitivity may have long-term benefits for the reduction of complications of T2DM, in particular the cardiovascular complications.

RISK FACTOR MANAGEMENT

Obesity

Scale of the problem

The WHO defines overweight when the BMI $<25\,\text{kg/m}^2$ and obesity when it is $>30\,\text{kg/m}^2$. The prevalence of obesity is increasing throughout the world and in the UK and many other developed societies, the prevalence rate amongst adults is 17–25% and up to 40% of the remaining adults are overweight according to the WHO definition (WHO 2000). More than 90% of T2DM is associated with overweight and obesity. Both the site and degree of obesity influence the level of associated health risk. Waist measurements of more than 102 cm and 88 cm for men and women respectively represent high risk of diabetes and CHD (Lean et al 1995). Obesity is a powerful risk factor for T2DM and the Nurses' Health Study has clearly defined the obesity–diabetes relationship throughout the entire spectrum of BMI as compared to lean women and men (BMI <22). Those women with a BMI more than 35 had a 93-fold increased risk of developing T2DM (Colditz et al 1990) and men with BMI more than 35 had an equivalent risk which

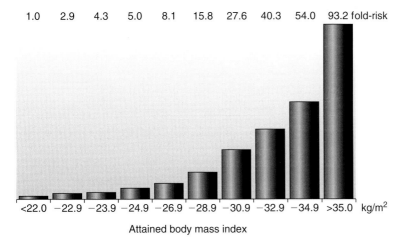

1.0   2.9   4.3   5.0   8.1   15.8   27.6   40.3   54.0   93.2 fold-risk

<22.0 −22.9 −23.9 −24.9 −26.9 −28.9 −30.9 −32.9 −34.9 >35.0 kg/m²

Attained body mass index

Figure 12.5 Obesity and the risk of type 2 diabetes (US women aged 30–55 years in 1876 followed for 14 years). (Reproduced with permission from Pinkney J 2001. Implications of obesity for diabetes and coronary heart disease in clinical practice. British Journal of Diabetes and Vascular Disease 1(2): 103–106.)

was increased by 40-fold (Chan et al 1994). From Figure 12.5 it will be clear that a small upward shift in the average BMI of the population can translate into a large shift in the prevalence of T2DM. Apart from obvious genetic causes, lifestyle changes, eating habits and physical activity have become important determinants of obesity.

Obesity is also a clear risk factor for CHD, though the absolute risks are less than those for T2DM, e.g. women with BMI >29, as compared to women with BMI <21, have a three-fold increased risk of CHD (Manson et al 1990). Obesity, interacting with the other risk factors, namely smoking, diabetes, hypertension and dyslipidaemia, has a major impact on CHD. Central obesity (excessive visceral intra-abdominal fat) rather than general obesity is the main risk factor for CHD in the population. Thus, measurement of the waist circumference will help identify individuals who are at a higher risk of developing diabetes and coronary heart disease.

Treatment modalities

The first step in the management of obese patients is to initiate a change in lifestyle by concentrating on eating habits, physical activity and behaviour modification. Low-fat diets and very low-calorie diets (VLCDs) have been shown to induce weight loss and facilitate weight maintenance. Fat intake should be reduced to less than 40 g per day and information and suggestions about healthy eating and alcohol intake should be given. Very low-calorie diets containing 400–800 calories (mainly as protein) have been shown to induce a weight loss in the order of 15–25 kg over 3 months. However, at the end of 12 months, the amount of weight loss was similar to that of a lifestyle programme (Richman et al 1992). The problem, however, with VLCDs is the predisposition to gain weight after stopping such a dietary regime. Physical activity in the form of walking or exercise programmes has been shown to be effective in aiding weight loss.

■ BOX 12.2 Benefits of 10 kg weight loss (Reproduced with permission from Pinkney J 2001. Implications of obesity for diabetes and coronary heart disease in clinical practice. British Journal of Diabetes and Vascular Disease 1(2): 103–106.)

Mortality	20–25% fall in total mortality
	30–40% fall in diabetes-related deaths
	40–50% fall in obesity-related cancer deaths
Blood pressure	10 mmHg fall in systolic blood pressure
	20 mmHg fall in diastolic blood pressure
Angina	91% reduction of symptoms
	33% increase in exercise tolerance
Lipids	10% fall in total cholesterol
	15% fall in LDL cholesterol
	30% fall in triglycerides
	8% increase in HDL cholesterol
Diabetes	>50% fall in risk of developing diabetes
	30–50% fall in fasting blood glucose
	15% fall in HbA_{TC}

The initial treatment targets in obese type 2 diabetic subjects should be modest weight loss of around 10 kg (5–10% body weight) and this has been shown to significantly improve glycaemic control (Jung 1997). Benefits of a 10 kg weight loss on various cardiovascular risk profiles and mortality are shown in Box 12.2.

Behavioural therapy has been shown to improve HbA1c concentrations by up to 3% (Henry et al 1986) and the addition of exercise to behavioural therapy has been shown to improve weight loss and weight maintenance in obese type 2 diabetic patients (Wing et al 1987).

In subjects with impaired glucose tolerance (who are at high risk of subsequent development of T2DM), it has been recently shown in a prospective study that combined lifestyle changes and weight loss averaging only 3–4 kg reduced the subsequent risk of developing T2DM by 58% over 4 years (Tuomilehto et al 2001). This study (Diabetes Prevention Programme) was a trial of over 3000 subjects with IGT involving 27 centres in the USA and was conducted over 4 years to assess the effect of different interventions on the progression to T2DM. Intensive lifestyle intervention with regular exercise and weight loss reduced the risk of progression to T2DM in 58% while treatment with metformin also reduced progression to T2DM by a lesser percentage of 31%. This finding is not new but provides further confirmation that diet, exercise and weight control can be used effectively to reduce progression of prediabetic states and impaired glucose tolerance to frank type 2 diabetes.

In terms of drug therapy, metformin remains the drug of choice in the obese (BMI more than 30) diabetic patients, because it causes less weight gain than sulphonylureas and insulin (UKPDS 1995a) and has also been shown to reduce mortality (UKPDS 1998b). All sulphonylureas, with the possible exception of glimepiride (Amaryl), promote weight gain and caution must be exercised prior to using such treatments in the obese type 2 diabetic patients. Thiazolidinediones (rosiglitazone and pioglitazone) have been shown to induce modest weight gain and their role remains to be established in the management of patients with T2DM (Werner & Travaglini 2001).

Antiobesity drugs such as orlistat (Xenical) and sibutramine (Reductil) have been shown to induce weight loss in obese type 2 diabetic subjects. Both of them have specific side-effects and contraindications and there are few long-term morbidity/mortality data to support their regular use in clinical practice. Moreover, they are not licensed for long-term use in the UK.

Gastric restriction surgery is an approach often utilized in morbidly obese type 2 diabetic patients. There is good evidence that substantial weight loss brought about by gastric bariatric surgery frequently leads to withdrawal of therapy, including insulin, and often remission of accompanying diabetes (Karlsson et al 1998). This should only be undertaken in selected patients with full explanation, by a multidisciplinary team with a good follow-up programme.

The presence of obesity substantially magnifies any cardiovascular risk factor and its prevention, together with treatment in appropriate circumstances, would greatly reduce the development of T2DM and diminish the problems of CHD. A structured multidisciplinary programme of exercise, diet and drug therapy can achieve weight loss in both primary and secondary care settings. This requires time, trained individuals, resources and patient commitment.

Glycaemic control

It is now well established that optimally, blood glucose should be maintained as near to physiological levels as possible in subjects with T2DM. The association between diabetes and premature cardiovascular disease suggests that improving glycaemia would be of long-term vascular benefit to all patients with diabetes.

UKPDS

The landmark United Kingdom Prospective Diabetes Study (UKPDS) was reported in 1998. It involved 5000 newly diagnosed type 2 diabetic patients who were studied over 20 years. Patients were randomized to receive either a 'conventional' or an 'intensive' treatment regimen. In the former group patients were treated with diet alone, although additional drugs were allowed if glycaemic control deteriorated. The intensively treated subjects were managed on oral hypoglycaemic agents or insulin. In the latter group, there was nearly a 1% difference in HbA1c in favour of the intensively treated group (7.0% vs 7.9%) and this was associated with significant benefits from the risk of microvascular endpoints and reduction in any diabetes-related complications. The incidence of macrovascular disease, i.e. myocardial infarction, was reduced but did not reach statistical significance (UKPDS 1998a). Epidemiological extrapolation of the UKPDS data, however, did suggest that improvement in glycaemic control would be associated with reduced cardiovascular risk (Table 12.1). It did not matter whether the intensively treated

Table 12.1 Relative risks of complications in intensive versus conventional blood glucose control and tight versus less tight blood pressure control studies. (Reproduced with permission from Levy JC 2001. UKPDS Odyssey – 2001. British Journal of Diabetes and Vascular Disease 1(1): 114–121.)

	Glucose control study		Blood pressure control study	
	Relative risk on intensive policy	Log-rank p	Relative risk on tight control	Log-rank p
Any diabetes-related endpoint	0.88 (0.79 to 0.99)	0.029	0.76 (0.62 to 0.92)	0.0046
Deaths related to diabetes	0.90 (0.73 to 1.10)	0.34	0.68 (0.49 to 0.94)	0.019
All-cause mortality	0.94 (0.80 to 1.10)	0.44	0.82 (0.63 to 1.08)	0.17
Myocardial infarction	0.84 (0.71 to 1.00)	0.052	0.79 (0.59 to 1.07)	0.13
Stroke	1.11 (0.81 to 1.51)	0.52	0.56 (0.35 to 0.89)	0.013
Peripheral vascular disease	0.65 (0.36 to 1.18)	0.15	0.51 (0.19 to 1.37)	0.17
Microvascular disease	0.75 (0.60 to 0.93)	0.0099	0.63 (0.44 to 0.89)	0.0092

Table 12.2 Risk reductions and NNT values for recent large trials in diabetes care. (Reproduced with permission from Patel V et al 2001. The HOPE Study and The MICRO HOPE Substudy. British Journal of Diabetes and Vascular Disease 1(1): 44–51.)

Endpoint	UKPDS glycaemic control trial		UKPDS metformin subtrial		UKPDS hypertension trial		HOPE MICRO-HOPE	
	RR	nnt/yr	RR	nnt/yr	RR	nnt/yr	RR	nnt/yr
Any diabetes endpoint	5.1%	196	13.5%	74	16.5%	61	–	–
Death from diabetes	–	–	5.2%	192	6.6%	152	–	–
Death from all causes	–	–	7.1%	141	–	–	24%	141
Myocardial infarction	2.7%	370	7%	143	–	–	22%	167
Stroke	–	–	–	–	5.1%	196	33%	237
Microvascular complications	2.8%	357	–	–	7.2%	138	15%*	180*

*Overt nephropathy, laser therapy or dialysis; RR = risk reduction; nnt = number needed to treat.

group used sulphonylurea or insulin as the net benefit was the same. In the UKPDS subgroup, obese type 2 diabetics who were randomized to intensive treatment with metformin had a significantly reduced risk of any diabetes-related deaths (by 42%) and myocardial infarction (by 39%) compared to the conventionally treated group (UKPDS 1998b). This was also significant when compared to the sulphonylurea and insulin-treated group (Table 12.2). This effect of metformin on reduction of cardiovascular risk may be related to its capacity to modify insulin resistance.

The UKPDS also helped outline the nature and progression of T2DM and has now incontrovertibly established that glycaemic control deteriorates progressively with time and this appears to be linear and not affected by any of the therapies used (UKPDS 1995b). It also showed that in over 80% of patients diet and lifestyle measures failed to achieve good sustained glycaemic control and that by 3 years, approximately 50% of patients needed combination therapy (UKPDS 1999). Thus, there is now a clear rationale for introducing combination therapy early to help minimize the risk of complications. There is now ample evidence that one should strive to achieve as near normal glycaemic control as possible in type 2 diabetic patients. This may not be easy and to achieve optimum care we need to identify high-risk patients and implement risk factor reduction using robust management protocols in a co-ordinated manner between the primary care and secondary care interface.

Insulin resistance

Type 2 diabetes is regarded as a condition of premature vascular disease with clustering of major cardiovascular risk factors such as hypertension, dyslipidaemia, hyperinsulinaemia, atherosclerosis and a procoagulant state in the individual patient. It is now well recognized that the common underlying abnormality is insulin resistance (impaired effectiveness of insulin) and new therapies are constantly being developed to target this specifically. Insulin resistance predates the onset of T2DM and is also well established as a cause of complications, particularly in T2DM.

The role of insulin resistance in the pathogenesis of diabetic complications is further substantiated by the UKPDS which clearly showed that there was no significant reduction of macrovascular complications of T2DM, despite the use of sulphonylurea and insulin, suggesting that factors such as insulin resistance (apart from glycaemic control) may have an important role in the pathogenesis of complications. A precedent for targeting insulin resistance has already been established with the use of metformin as shown in the UKPDS.

Role of thiazolidinediones

Although glycaemic control remains a priority in the management of T2DM, new management strategies for combating insulin resistance and its metabolic sequelae are being developed. The class of drugs called thiazolidinediones (TZDs) are new oral antidiabetic agents acting on nuclear peroxisome proliferator-activated receptor γ (PPAR-γ) and help mediate their anti-hyperglycaemic effect by their insulin-sensitizing activity. In addition, they help decrease circulating insulin levels, free fatty acids and triglycerides whilst LDL and HDL-cholesterol concentrations are either unchanged or slightly increased, with little alteration in their ratio. These agents enhance insulin action without stimulating insulin secretion and are currently licensed for use in obese patients in combination with metformin or a sulphonylurea where metformin is contraindicated once monotherapy has failed (Day 1999, Schoonjans & Auwerx 2000). They have a slowly generated antihyperglycaemic effect which may take up to 2–3 months to achieve maximal efficacy. Some patients show little or no response to thiazolidinediones.

Common contraindications currently employed in the UK are impaired liver function and cardiac failure. These drugs have been associated with an early weight increase but this has been claimed to be in part due to redistribution of fat. As yet, in the UK, they are not licensed as monotherapy or for triple therapy. Thus, although thiazolidinediones are important new therapeutic agents specifically tackling insulin resistance, there are limited outcome data to clarify their role. There are many outcome studies currently in progress to assess their long-term clinical impact in the treatment of T2DM and cardiovascular disease.

Microalbuminuria

Microalbuminuria in a diabetic patient is not just a marker of worsening renal function but also a marker for increased cardiovascular risk. Microalbuminuria occurs within the first 10 years of diabetes and clinical proteinuria in a further 5–10 years. Its development in T2DM patients imparts a 2–5-fold increase in mortality, predominantly from cardiovascular causes (Alzaid 1996).

The presence of microalbuminuria in T2DM indicates that the patient is at risk of a vascular event in the next 5–10 years and aggressive management of all risk factors of the 'metabolic syndrome' is advised. The prevalence of microalbuminuria in the type 2 diabetic patient is around 20–25% although there is a reported variability in various cross-sectional studies. This probably reflects the general heterogeneity of T2DM, particularly in relation to the presence of hypertension, deterioration of hyperglycaemia before diagnosis and perhaps ethnic background. Mortality is as high as 70–80% in microalbuminuric patients, compared to 20% of those with normal urinary albumin excretion. Patients with microalbuminuria show some features of the 'metabolic syndrome' with central obesity, insulin resistance and dyslipidaemia. They also show evidence of endothelial dysfunction. Those microalbuminuric type 2 diabetic patients who progress to overt nephropathy have characteristically raised glycated haemoglobin levels, increased blood pressure, particularly systolic, high initial urinary albumin excretion, hyperlipidaemia and are smokers (Klein et al 1995).

Evidence-based treatment strategies

Tight blood glucose and blood pressure control have been shown to prevent the development and progression of microalbuminuria. The use of angiotensin-converting enzyme (ACE) inhibitors, other antihypertensive agents and angiotensin II receptor antagonists has also been explored.

In the UKPDS, the majority of type 2 diabetic patients had normal albumin excretion at baseline. The relative risk of developing microalbuminuria was 33% lower in the intensively controlled group (glycated haemoglobin <7%) at 12 years compared to the conventionally treated group (glycated haemoglobin 7.9%).

Normotensive type 2 diabetic patients with microalbuminuria when treated with ACE inhibitors show a reduction in the progression to overt nephropathy and reduction of cardiovascular endpoints. This was shown in relatively young microalbuminuric type 2 diabetic patients whose blood pressure was <140/90 mmHg. The ACE inhibitor enalapril reduced the 5-year risk of progression to overt nephropathy by 60% compared to placebo (Ravid et al 1996).

The Hypertension in Diabetes Study (part of the UKPDS) has demonstrated a reduction in the development of microalbuminuria in a group of hypertensive type 2 diabetic patients after 4.5 years of tight blood pressure control. The relative risk of developing microalbuminuria was reduced by 29% in the tightly controlled group (achieving a blood pressure of 144/82 mmHg). There was no difference in the incidence of proteinuria in those allocated to atenolol or captopril, though this study was not powered to detect relatively small differences. However, to achieve tight blood glucose control, up to three antihypertensive agents had to be used in more than 30% of patients (UKPDS 1998c). Both ACE inhibitors (HOPE Study 2000, Ravid et al 1998) and angiotensin II receptor antagonists (Parving et al 2001) show clear renoprotective effects in terms of reducing microalbuminuria and decline in creatinine clearance in patients with T2DM with or without hypertension.

Thus, there is no doubt that early detection and treatment of microalbuminuria by strict control of glycaemia and blood pressure are very important in the management of patients with T2DM. The judicious use of ACE inhibitors will delay the development of end-stage renal disease and time to renal replacement therapy, but will also have a significant effect on the incidence of cardiovascular events in such patients. To date, angiotensin II receptor antagonists have also been shown to delay progression to nephropathy but have not been shown to influence CHD morbidity/mortality.

MANAGEMENT OF HYPERTENSION IN DIABETES

Hypertension and diabetes mellitus are independent risk factors for CHD and frequently co-exist in the same patient. Hypertension exacerbates both macrovascular and microvascular complications of diabetes. Hypertension is twice as prevalent in patients with diabetes compared to the general population. The prevalence of hypertension in T2DM varies between 30% and 80% and it is possibly the single most important factor in the initiation and progression of diabetic nephropathy.

Aetiology

Factors which contribute to the high prevalence of hypertension in diabetic subjects include sodium retention, vascular hyperreactivity and diabetic nephropathy. Additional factors contributing to increased cardiovascular complications are reduction in vascular compliance, loss of nocturnal blood pressure dips, increased prevalence of left ventricular hypertrophy and clustering of other cardiovascular risk factors (Feher 2001).

Blood pressure and plasma glucose levels are positively correlated (Kelleher et al 1998). It has been shown that tight blood glucose control decreases blood pressure in diabetes, despite increases in plasma volume and exchangeable sodium (Ferriss et al 1985). The combined result of glucose and insulin has major independent but perhaps additive effects that contribute to abnormal blood pressure regulation in patients with T2DM. Circulating plasma renin activity levels are low in T2DM but it is thought that tissue rather than circulating levels may have a more important role in vascular autoregulation and this perhaps is a key factor in the aetiology of hypertension in T2DM (Stern & Tuck 1996).

Important trials

Evidence for management of hypertension in diabetes is derived from several prospective antihypertensive outcome trials. However, many of the trials are limited in that data were derived from either post hoc subgroup analysis of diabetic patients (SHEP, CAPP, SYST-EUR and HOT trials) or secondary endpoints in trial protocol (ABCD and FACET trials).

The three important hypertension trials that we will focus on are the UKPDS Hypertension Substudy, Hypertension Optimal Treatment (HOT; Hansson et al 1998) and the Heart Outcomes Prevention Evaluation (HOPE) Study.

The UKPDS Hypertension in Diabetes Study subgroup compared relatively tight blood pressure control versus less tight blood pressure control. Over 1100 of the original 5000 patients were hypertensive and investigators achieved a 10 mmHg difference in systolic blood pressure (154 versus 144 mmHg) and a 5 mmHg difference in diastolic blood pressure (87 versus 82 mmHg) in favour of the tightly controlled group. Table 12.2 summarizes the important findings of the study. Intensive blood pressure treatment was associated with a 24% reduction in diabetes-related endpoints ($p = 0.005$), 32% for diabetes-related deaths ($p = 0.02$), 44% reduction in fatal and non-fatal stroke ($p = 0.013$), 56% for congestive cardiac failure and 37% for microvascular complications ($p = 0.01$). The tight control arm part of the study was further randomly allocated to either a β-blocker (atenolol) or an ACE inhibitor (captopril). Atenolol and captopril were both equally effective in reducing the incidence of diabetic complications but the study was not sufficiently powered to determine which antihypertensive agent was superior. This suggests that blood pressure reduction itself may be more important than the actual treatment used (UKPDS 1998d). The important point for the clinician, therefore, relating to hypertension is that single drug therapy resulted in tight blood pressure control in less than 50% of patients and that in more than 30% of patients, three or more agents had to be used. Moreover, after 9 years of treatment, only 56% of the tight controlled group had attained a target blood pressure of <150/85 mmHg. The practical implications of these observations are self-evident.

In the HOT study a cohort of nearly 1500 patients from the main subgroup were identified as having diabetes mellitus. These patients were randomized to a target diastolic blood pressure of <80 mmHg. The risk of immediate cardiovascular events was halved in comparison with the group randomized to achieving a diastolic blood pressure of <90 mmHg. The study also showed the particular benefits of using low-dose aspirin in reducing vascular morbidity and mortality, but the greatest benefit was seen in terms of reduction in myocardial infarction.

A lot of debate has revolved around the use of ACE inhibitors and whether they have a specific vascular protective effect over and above their blood pressure-lowering effects. The HOPE study has not only strengthened the view that ACE inhibitors have specific renoprotective effects (reduction of intraglomerular pressures) but also a specific cardiovascular protective effect. In this study, all the 9500 patients who had high cardiovascular risks were randomized to receive either the ACE inhibitor ramipril or placebo. Patients were 55 years and over and had a history of coronary artery disease, stroke, peripheral vascular disease or diabetes mellitus plus one other cardiovascular risk factor such as hypertension, elevated total cholesterol, low HDL-cholesterol, documented microalbuminuria or history of smoking. This study was terminated early as results were dramatically in favour of ACE inhibition, particularly in the diabetic subgroup of 6500 patients. In the whole group, ACE inhibition was associated with a 22% reduction in risk. Total mortality was also reduced by 22% in the general population and by 24% in the diabetic population (Table 12.2). The cardiovascular benefit appeared greater than that attributable to the small difference in blood pressure and it is likely that the benefits of the ACE inhibitor ramipril were over and above its blood pressure-lowering effect. Of major interest in this study was the reduction in the diagnosis of new diabetes (105 versus 154; relative risk 0.068, $p = 0.002$) in the ramipril arm. Thus there is encouraging evidence for the use of ACE inhibitors as first-line therapy in CHD prevention in patients with a high cardiovascular risk such as those with diabetes mellitus.

Treatment

Most antihypertensive drugs have been assessed in patients with diabetes with regard to surrogate endpoints. There is good evidence for various regimens based on diuretics (SHEP trial; Curb et al 1996), β-blockers (UKPDS), ACE inhibitors (UKPDS) and calcium channel blockers (HOT, SYST-EUR trial; Tuomilehto et al 1999) used either as monotherapy and/or in combination. Therapy should be tailored to the individual diabetic patient, taking into account other potential diabetes-related problems including peripheral vascular disease, renal artery stenosis, autonomic neuropathy, erectile dysfunction, alterations in glucose homeostasis and lipid metabolism. Although any class of drugs in any combination can be used to treat hypertension in patients with T2DM, the side-effect profile of these drugs must be remembered.

The initiation of antihypertensive therapy must be based on the estimation of absolute risks for the development of cardiovascular disease.

The British Cardiac Society, the British Hyperlipidaemia Association and the British Hypertensive Society have co-operated in preparing national recommendations which have been endorsed by Diabetes UK (Wood et al 1998). All these current guidelines emphasize the importance of risk assessment in order to identify patients who will benefit from treatment. A formal estimation of 10-year CHD risk should be performed using the chart of the Joint British Recommendations on Prevention of CHD (see Chapter 2).

In patients with T2DM, the threshold for starting antihypertensive treatment is a blood pressure $\geqslant 140/90$ mmHg and the target blood pressure should be $< 140/80$ mmHg ($\leqslant 130/75$ mmHg if there is evidence of proteinuria or nephropathy). If the systolic blood pressure (SBP) is > 160 mmHg (for any level of diastolic blood pressure), patients should be treated. If the SBP is between 140 and 159 mmHg and diastolic < 90 mmHg, they should be treated only if there is evidence of target organ damage, complications or if the overall 10-year CHD risk is greater than 15% (Wood et al 1998). An ACE inhibitor titrated to the maximum recommended and tolerable dose is preferable as first-line therapy. Clinical trial evidence suggests that patients with diabetes may require combinations of several antihypertensive agents to adequately control their blood pressure. ACE inhibitors, low-dose diuretics, calcium channel blockers and both α- and β-blockers are all suitable agents.

DIABETIC DYSLIPIDAEMIA

Lipid abnormalities are common in patients with T2DM and are present both at the time of diagnosis and in the prediabetic state. Diabetic dyslipidaemia is affected by various lifestyle characteristics and by genetic factors and is said to persist despite usual hypoglycaemic therapy. Dyslipidaemia (high LDL and triglyceride and low HDL levels) is an established risk factor for CHD in both the diabetic and non-diabetic population (Box 12.3).

Aetiology

In patients with T2DM there are diverse alterations in lipid and lipoprotein metabolism, including both quantitative and qualitative changes in lipoprotein concentration and composition (Syvanne & Tasiken 1997, Syvanne et al 1994, Tasiken 1995). The hallmark of diabetic dyslipidaemia is hypertriglyceridaemia with reduced HDL levels, seen in up to one third of type 2 diabetic patients even with good glycaemic control (Betteridge 1996). The total and LDL-cholesterol levels are similar to those in subjects without diabetes as was found in the Multiple Risk Factor Intervention (MRFIT) study (Stamler et al 1993). It has also been shown that the typical dyslipidaemia of

---

■ **BOX 12.3 Typical lipid profile of patients with T2DM**

↑ Plasma concentrations of VLDL, LDL and apolipoprotein A
↓ Plasma concentrations of HDL cholesterol
↑ Plasma concentration of triglycerides

T2DM is more severe in women than in men, consistent with a reported excess CHD risk in diabetic women (Kannel & McGee 1979, Malmstorm et al 1997).

The aetiology of diabetic dyslipidaemia is complex and involves a variety of factors including insulin resistance (Reaven & Greenfield 1981), hyper-insulinaemia, hyperglycaemia (Howard 1987) and disturbed fatty acid meta-bolism (Lewis et al 1995). Type 2 diabetes with insulin resistance results in increased fatty acid release from adipose tissue to the liver and overpro-duction of triglyceride-rich VLDL particles (TG-VLDL). This, together with the defective inhibitory control of insulin on hepatic synthesis of VLDL, results in increased hepatic production of large TG-VLDL particles and thus of elevated plasma triglyceride levels. This is further aggravated by the fail-ure of insulin to maintain a regulatory balance between the intestinally derived triglyceride-containing lipoprotein (chylomicrons) and the VLDL of hepatic origin. Again, in T2DM there is an impaired catabolism of trig-lyceride-rich lipoproteins due to the defective function of enzyme lipo-protein lipase (LPL) and this is most striking in those diabetic patients with CHD.

Hypertriglyceridaemia is associated with accelerated atherogenesis in patients with T2DM by a number of different mechanisms. Firstly, remnant particles which are also cholesterol rich and contain apoproteins B and C-II accumulate in T2DM and are directly proatherogenic. Secondly, fasting hypertriglyceridaemia is associated with abnormal postprandial lipaemia, which is again believed to be atherogenic (Foger & Patsch 2000). This post-prandial lipaemia is associated with changes in lipoprotein metabolism, namely reduction in HDL-cholesterol and formation of small dense LDL particles. Furthermore, hypertriglyceridaemia is associated with increased levels of PAI-1 which is associated with increased thrombosis and coagula-tion (Hamsten & Karpe 1996).

HDL-cholesterol is decreased in T2DM largely due to reduced concen-trations of lipid-rich HDL particles largely mediated by hypertriglyceri-daemia.

Although, as previously mentioned, there is little difference between total LDL-cholesterol concentrations in T2DM, LDL-cholesterol is a very impor-tant risk factor for coronary artery disease. There are both quantitative and qualitative changes in LDL-cholesterol resulting in increased atherogenicity. The LDL-cholesterol particles in T2DM are smaller and denser and are more prone to oxidation and glycation, thus increasing their atherogenicity (Betteridge 1997, Steinberg 1997). Indeed, there is a strong association between the small dense LDL particles and CHD risk (Austin et al 1996). In the UKPDS study, LDL-cholesterol was found to be the major determinant of coronary heart disease (Turner et al 1998). In addition, there are a wide variety of qualitative changes in lipoprotein composition and structure resulting in increased viscosity, glycation and overall atherogenicity.

There has been much debate over the association of triglycerides in relation to CHD. There are some studies that have found triglycerides to be a better predictor of CHD risk than LDL-cholesterol. The Diabetes Intervention Study followed over 1000 newly diagnosed type 2 diabetic subjects for an average of 12 years. Multivariate analysis showed that triglycerides, together with hypertension and blood glucose, were significant predictors of both myocardial infarction ($p = 0.05$) and death ($p = <0.01$) (Hanefeld et al 1996). In both the PROCAM population (Assman & Schulte 1992) and the Helsinki Heart Study (Manninen et al 1992), hypertriglyceridaemia was associated with the highest CHD risk in individuals with LDL:HDL-cholesterol ratio >5. Recently, the concept of hyperinsulinaemia cluster (positive correlation for BMI, triglycerides, insulin and a negative correlation for HDL-cholesterol) was found to be predictive of CHD-related death in T2DM (Lehto et al 2000). Again, a meta-analysis from six studies involving more than 4500 patients followed for between 7 and 13 years has shown an association between hypertriglyceridaemia and coronary events in patients with T2DM (Tasiken 1999).

Postprandial hyperlipaemia, oxidative stress and endothelial dysfunction

There is now convincing evidence that exaggerated postprandial lipaemia is associated with atherosclerotic disease severity and progression in both diabetic and non-diabetic subjects (Karpe et al 1993, 1994). Recent evidence suggests that potential mechanisms accounting for the strong association between postprandial lipaemia and the production of triglyceride-rich lipoproteins and atherosclerosis, in both diabetic and non-diabetic subjects, may involve enhanced oxidative stress and endothelial dysfunction (Evans et al 2000, Plotnick et al 1997). Available evidence suggests that the extent of endothelial dysfunction may reflect the degree of oxidative stress imposed on the endothelium, more so because antioxidants have been shown to improve endothelial dysfunction in both diabetic and non-diabetic subjects.

Thus, it is clear that disturbed postprandial lipaemia in T2DM with excess production of triglyceride-rich lipoproteins appears to be an important factor in the atherogenesis in such patients, by mechanisms which involve enhanced oxidative stress and endothelial dysfunction. Furthermore, there is good evidence that attenuating postprandial lipidaemia in T2DM may provide therapeutic benefit of reducing cardiovascular risk in such patients.

Important trials

Lifestyle modification, including physical activity and a low-calorie diet aiming to maintain normal body weight, should be the first priority in the treatment of diabetic dyslipidaemia. A number of studies have shown that such changes improve insulin sensitivity, increase HDL and decrease triglyceride concentrations in patients with T2DM. Glycaemic control also improves diabetic dyslipidaemia, particularly the reduction of plasma triglyceride levels, although many studies do not confirm the latter. If dyslipidaemia persists despite lifestyle modification, lipid-lowering therapy should be considered after estimation of the 10-year CHD risk, using the Joint British Guidelines for the Prevention of CHD.

Unfortunately many clinical trials of lipid intervention and CHD prevention have been conducted in study populations that have specifically excluded patients with diabetes. A few trials have conducted post-hoc analysis of subgroups of patients with T2DM. The Helsinki Heart Study was one such primary prevention study with gemfibrozil. Although there was a reduction in cardiovascular events by 60%, this did not achieve statistical significance as the study design was underpowered to reveal such benefit.

The Scandinavian Simvastatin Survival Study (4S; 1994) and the Cholesterol and Recurrent Events (CARE) study (Pyorala et al 1997) are secondary prevention trials using simvastatin and pravastatin respectively. These two trials present the most compelling evidence in support of lipid reduction in secondary prevention of CHD but the data on patients with diabetes represent a post-hoc subgroup analysis and some caution must be exercised in extrapolation of this evidence to clinical practice. In the 4S study, overall mortality was reduced by 43% in patients with diabetes, although this effect was not statistically significant due to the small number of patients. The incidence of major CHD and atherosclerotic events was reduced by 55% and 37% respectively in patients with diabetes compared with 32% and 36% respectively in non-diabetic patients.

In the CARE study, the relative risk of coronary events was reduced by 25% in patients with diabetes compared to 23% for non-diabetic patients. However, due to the higher initial risk of CHD in patients with diabetes, the absolute reductions achieved were greater (8.1% versus 5.2% respectively).

Two studies, SENDCAP and DAIS, have investigated the effect of lipid-lowering therapy with fibrates on surrogate endpoints (Elkeles et al 1998, Steiner et al 2001). In the St Mary's, Ealing, Northwick Park Diabetes Cardiovascular Disease Prevention (SENDCAP) study, patients with T2DM and no history of cardiovascular disease were randomized to receive bezafibrate or placebo in addition to their existing conventional treatment and followed up for 3 years. There was a significant reduction in events, mainly documented MI and ischaemic changes on resting ECG. Patients treated with bezafibrate had significantly greater reductions in serum triglycerides, total cholesterol, total:HDL-cholesterol ratio and a significantly greater increase in HDL-cholesterol.

In the Diabetes Atherosclerosis Intervention Study (DAIS; Steiner et al 2001), 418 men and women with T2DM received fenofibrate or placebo for at least 3 years. Patients had at least one visible coronary lesion on angiography and half of them had a history of CAD. Patients had good glycaemic control and had total cholesterol:HDL ratio >4 plus either triglyceride concentration 1.7–5.2 mmol/l and LDL-cholesterol 4.5 mmol/l or less. Fenofibrate therapy was associated with significantly less increase in the percentage diameter of angiographically visible stenoses. This trial was not powered for clinical endpoints but there were fewer events, albeit not statistically significant, in the fenofibrate group (38 versus 50).

Several ongoing studies will provide further insights into the potential benefits of lipid-lowering therapy in the diabetic population using fibrates, statins or a combination. The MRC/BHF Heart Protection Study, a large and well-designed randomized study, included 6000 men and women aged 40–80 years (90% with T2DM) who were followed up for over 6 years (Heart Protection Study 2002). Baseline total cholesterol was 3.5 mmol/l or greater and patients included were considered to be at increased risk of

CHD. Simvastatin 40 mg as compared to placebo reduced heart attacks, strokes and other vascular events in 70 out of every 1000 patients treated (overall 33% reduction in MI and ischaemic strokes and a 12% reduction in all-cause mortality). These benefits were irrespective of patient's presenting cholesterol levels and in addition to other effective treatments like aspirin and antihypertensive medications. Clear benefits, perhaps for the first time, were seen in several subgroups of patients who were poorly represented in previous trials. These subgroups include women, those over 75 years of age, individuals with diabetes and no vascular events and those with known cerebrovascular and peripheral arterial disease and patients with LDL-cholesterol below 2.5 mmol/l. This landmark study will perhaps change the way we approach lipid-lowering therapy and perhaps steer us away from waiting for cholesterol levels prior to treatment if the absolute cardiovascular risk is considered high, particularly in patients with T2DM with even 'low' and 'normal' lipid values.

Treatment

There should be a multi-risk factor approach to ameliorating CHD risk in patients with diabetes. There should be particular focus on good control of blood pressure, statin therapy, optimal glycaemic control and stopping smoking. Both primary and secondary prevention strategies to reduce cardiovascular outcomes in patients with diabetes are summarized in Box 12.4.

■ **BOX 12.4   Strategies to reduce cardiovascular mortality in T2DM. (Reproduced with permission from Patel V et al 2001. The HOPE Study and The MICRO HOPE Substudy. British Journal of Diabetes and Vascular Disease 1(1): 44–51.)**

Primary prevention by treatment of cardiovascular risk factors
- Exercise, healthy diet, obesity management, smoking cessation
- Control of hypertension (BP = 140/80)
- Glycaemic control (HbA$_{IC}$ = 7%)
- Cholesterol reduction with statins (T. chol = 5.0, LDL = 3.0, HDL = 0.9)

Secondary prevention of cardiovascular disease
- Aspirin 75 mg od
- Beta blockers
- ACE inhibitors
- Intensive insulin therapy (Digami protocol)
- Cholesterol reduction with statins

Other preventive measures
- Ramlpril 10 od (HOPE study)
- Aspirin 75 mg od

Surgical treatment of coronary heart disease
- Interventional cardiology
- Surgical

Fasting plasma lipid profile needs to be included in the annual assessment of all T2DM subjects. Guidelines and recommendations for cut-off levels of triglycerides and total/LDL-cholesterols have been proposed by both European and American authorities. For example, the European guidelines propose the use of statins if the LDL-cholesterol is $\geqslant 3$ mmol/l with the equivalent threshold in the US being $\geqslant 2.6$ mmol/l. Similarly, in the European guidelines fibrate therapy is advised if total triglycerides $\geqslant 2.2$ mmol/l with LDL-cholesterol $\leqslant 3$ mmol/l. It is expected that clinicians will continue to use absolute CHD risk criteria from charts for the individual patients. Joint British guidelines recommend that the total cholesterol be <5 mmol/l and LDL-cholesterol <3 mmol/l in patients with diabetes with a 10-year CHD risk of $\leqslant 15\%$. The evidence base at present supports statin therapy as first-line intervention for the treatment of diabetic dyslipidaemia.

In some high-risk patients combination therapy with statins and fibrates will be required with regular monitoring of muscle enzymes and hepatic function. It is of paramount importance that patients with diabetes receive high-quality evidence-based care to reduce the risk of macrovascular disease. The high risk of CHD in patients with T2DM, the acceptance of T2DM as a CHD equivalent in the recent guidelines (NCEP 2001), suggests that all patients with T2DM may qualify for statin therapy based on a threshold of 10-year CHD risk of $\geqslant 15\%$.

It is important to remember that hyperinsulinaemia and insulin resistance are independent risk factors for CHD and are closely associated with dyslipidaemia in the metabolic syndrome and treatments must be geared to improving insulin sensitivity. Therapy should also be targeted towards prevention as there is encouraging evidence that T2DM can be prevented by lifestyle measures as shown in the Finnish Diabetes Prevention Study (Lindstrom et al 2003).

CONCLUSION

Type 2 diabetes mellitus is a vascular disease and patients often have clustering of cardiovascular risk factors. According to the third report of the National Cholesterol Education Programme (NCEP) Expert Panel on Detection, Evaluation and Treatment of High Blood Cholesterol in Adults (Adult Treatment Panel III), diabetes is now considered a CHD risk equivalent as most patients with T2DM have multiple risk factors (NCEP 2001). Since CHD in patients with diabetes may be clinically covert or silent, the prevention of CHD is an important goal and must not be postponed until clinically overt CHD is present. Patients with diabetes benefit more in absolute terms from risk factor modification, as their initial risk is higher. Thus, there needs to be a low threshold for intervention in such patients. Apart from glycaemic control and treatments targeting insulin resistance, aggressive management of risk factors, including treatment of blood pressure and dyslipidaemia, is advocated. The widespread use of aspirin is to be encouraged and cessation of smoking is a top priority. Recognition that T2DM is a major risk factor for CHD and an aggressive multiple risk factor approach to managing the patients with diabetes should improve the prognosis in this high-risk group of patients.

■ KEY POINTS

- The global prevalence of T2DM is projected to rise alarmingly in the near future.
- Diabetes and its complications contribute significantly to health-care costs in the United Kingdom.
- T2DM is a major risk factor for cardiovascular disease with a 2–4-fold increased risk compared to non-diabetic individuals.
- Patients with T2DM often have clustering of cardiovascular risk factors.
- The UKPDS has clearly shown the progressive nature of T2DM and the substantial benefits of metformin when used as a first-line treatment in obese patients with T2DM.
- New and stringent targets for blood pressure control have now emerged for patients with T2DM, often requiring multiple antihypertensive agents.
- Targeting insulin resistance is an important consideration in T2DM and new therapeutic options are now available.
- Dyslipidaemia associated with T2DM is characterized by increased levels of dense LDL, elevated levels of triglycerides and low HDL-cholesterol levels.
- CHD risk factors need to be aggressively managed in patients with T2DM.
- There is good evidence that lifestyle intervention, with regular exercise and weight loss, reduces the risk of progression and development of diabetes mellitus.

REFERENCES

Alzaid AA 1996 Microalbuminuria in non-insulin dependent diabetes. Diabetes Care 19: 79–89

Amos AF, McCarty DJ, Zimmet P 1997 The rising global burden of diabetes and estimates and projection to the year 2010. Diabetic Medicine 14 (suppl 5): S7–85

Assman G, Schulte H 1992 Relation of high density lipoprotein cholesterol and triglycerides to incidence of atherosclerotic coronary artery disease (the PROCAM experience). American Journal of Cardiology 70: 733–737

Austin A, Braslow J, Hennekens C et al 1996 Low density lipoprotein subclass patterns and risk of myocardial infarction. Journal of the American Medical Association 276: 875–881

Baxter H, Bottomley J, Burns E et al 2000 CODE-2 UK: the current costs of type 2 diabetes in the UK. Diabetic Medicine 17 (suppl 1): 13

Betteridge DJ 1996 Diabetic dyslipidemia – implications for vascular risk. In: Betteridge DJ (ed) Lipids: current perspectives. Martin Dunitz, London

Betteridge DJ 1997 LDL heterogeneity: implications for atherogenicity in insulin resistance and NIDDM. Diabetologia 40: S149–S151

British Diabetic Association 2000 New diagnostic criteria for diabetes. BDA, London

Chan JM, Rimm EB, Colditz GA, Stampfer MJ, Willett WC 1994 Obesity, fat distribution, and weight gain as risk factors for clinical diabetes in men. Diabetes Care 17: 961–969

Colditz GA, Willet WC, Stampfer MJ et al 1990 Weight as a risk factor for clinical diabetes in women. American Journal of Epidemiology 132: 501–513

Curb JD, Pressel SL, Cutler JA et al 1996 Effects of diuretic-based anti-hypertensive treatment on cardiovascular disease risk in older diabetic patients with isolated systolic hypertension. Systolic Hypertension in the Elderly Cooperative Research Group. Journal of the American Medical Association 276: 1886–1892

Currie CJ, Morgan CLI, Peters JR 1997 Patterns and costs of hospital care for coronary heart disease related and not related to diabetes. Heart 78 (6): 544–549

Day C 1999 Thiazolidinediones: a new class of antidiabetic drugs. Diabetic Medicine 16: 179–192

Day C 2001 The rising tide of type 2 diabetes. British Journal of Diabetes and Vascular Disease 1(1): 37, 38

Elkeles RS, Diamond JR, Poulter C et al 1998 Cardiovascular outcomes in type 2 diabetes. A double-blind, placebo-controlled study of bezafibrate: the St Mary's, Ealing, Northwick Park Diabetes Cardiovascular Disease Prevention (SENDCAP) Study. Diabetes Care 21: 641–648

Evans M, Anderson RA, Graham J et al 2000 Ciprofibrate therapy improves endothelial function and reduces post-prandial lipaemia and oxidative stress in type 2 diabetes. Circulation 101: 1773–1779

Feher MD 2001 Hypertension in diabetes. Practical Diabetes International 18 (6): 197–200

Ferriss JB, O'Hare JA, Kelleher CC et al 1985 Diabetic control and the renin-angiotensin system, catecholamines and blood pressure. Hypertension 7(suppl 2): 58–63

Foger B, Patsch JR 2000 Postprandial lipaemia. In: Betteridge DJ (ed) Lipids and vascular disease: current issues. Martin Dunitz, London

Haffner SM, Stern MP, Hazuda HP et al 1990 Cardiovascular risk factors in confirmed pre-diabetic individuals. Does the clock for coronary artery disease start ticking before the onset of clinical diabetes? Journal of the American Medical Association 263: 2893–2898

Haffner SM, Lehto S, Ronnemaa T, Pyorala K, Laasko M 1998 Mortality from coronary heart disease in subjects with type 2 diabetes and in non-diabetic subjects with and without prior myocardial infarction. New England Journal of Medicine 339: 229–234

Hamsten A, Karpe F 1996 Triglycerides and coronary heart disease – has epidemiology given us the right answer? In Betteridge DJ (ed) Lipids: current perspectives. Martin Dunitz, London

Hanefeld M, Fischer S, Julius U et al 1996 Risk factors for myocardial infarction and death in newly detected NIDDM: the Diabetes Intervention Study, 11-year follow-up. Diabetologia 39: 1577–1583

Hansson L, Zanchetti A, Carruthers SG et al 1998 Effects of intensive blood pressure lowering and low dose aspirin in patients with hypertension: principal results of the Hypertension Optimal Treatment (HOT) randomized trial. Lancet 351: 1755–1762

Heart Outcomes Prevention Evaluation (HOPE) Study Investigators 2000 Effects of ramipril on cardiovascular and microvascular outcomes in people with diabetes mellitus. Results of the HOPE study. Lancet 355: 253–259

Heart Protection Study Collaborative Group 2002 Study of cholesterol lowering with Simvastatin in 20,536 high-risk individuals: a randomized placebo-controlled trial. Lancet 360: 7–22

Henry RR, Wallace P, Olefsky JM 1986 Effects of weight loss on mechanisms of hyperglycemia in obese non-insulin-dependent diabetes mellitus. Diabetes 35: 990–998

Howard BV 1987 Lipoprotein metabolism in diabetes mellitus. Journal of Lipid Research 28: 613–628

Jung RT 1997 Obesity as a disease. British Medical Bulletin 53: 307–321

Kannel WB, McGee DI 1979 Diabetes and glucose intolerance as risk factors of cardiovascular disease: the Framingham Study. Diabetes Care 2: 120–126

Karlsson J, Sjostrom L, Sullivan M 1998 Swedish obese subjects (SOS) – an intervention study of obesity. Two-year follow-up of health related quality of life (HRQL) and eating behaviour after gastric surgery for severe obesity. International Journal of Obesity 22: 113–126

Karpe F, Bard JM, Steiner G, Carlson LA, Fruchart JC, Hamsten A 1993 HDL and alimentary lipaemia. Studies in men with myocardial infarction at young age. Atherosclerosis and Thrombosis 13: 11–22

Karpe F, Steiner G, Uffelman K, Olivecrona T, Hamsten A 1994 Postprandial lipoproteins and progression of coronary atherosclerosis. Atherosclerosis 106: 83–97

Kelleher C, Kingston SM, Barry DG et al 1998 Hypertension in diabetic clinic patients and their siblings. Diabetologia 31: 76–81

King's Fund Policy Institute 1996 Counting the cost: the real impact of non insulin dependent diabetes. A King's Fund Report commissioned by the British Diabetic Association. King's Fund, London

Klein R, Klein BEK, Moss SE, Cruickshank J 1995 Ten year incidence of gross proteinuria in people with diabetes. Diabetes 44: 916–923

Kumar S, Barnett AH 1997 Causes of non-insulin dependent diabetes mellitus. Medicine 7: 6–9

Laakso M, Lehto S 1998 Epidemiology of risk factors for cardiovascular disease in diabetes and impaired glucose tolerance. Atherosclerosis 137 (suppl): S65–73

Lean ME, Han TS, Morrison CE 1995 Waist circumference as a measure for indicating need for weight measurement. British Medical Journal 12: 1284–1290

Lehto S, Ronnemaa T, Pyorala K, Laakso M 2000 Cardiovascular risk factors clustering with endogenous hyperinsulinaemia predict death from coronary heart disease in patients with type 2 diabetes. Diabetologia 43: 148–155

Leslie RDG (ed) 1993 Causes of diabetes: genetic and environmental factors. Wiley, Chichester

Levy JC 2001 UKPDS Odyssey – 2001. British Journal of Diabetes and Vascular Disease 1(1): 16

Lewis GF, Uffelman KD, Szeto LW, Wellar B, Steiner G 1995 Interaction between free fatty acids and insulin in the acute control of very low density lipoprotein production in humans. Journal of Clinical Investigation 95: 158–166

Lindstrom J, Eriksson JG, Valle TT 2003 Prevention of diabetes mellitus in subjects with impaired glucose tolerance in the Finnish Diabetes Prevention Study: Results from a Randomized Clinical Trial. American Society of Nephrology 14(7 Suppl 2): S108–113

Malmstorm R, Packard CJ, Caslake M, Bedford D, Stewart P, Yehi-Jaronian H 1997 Defective regulation of triglyceride metabolism by insulin in the liver in non-insulin dependent diabetes mellitus. Diabetologia 40: 454–462

Manninen V, Tenkanen H, Koskinen P et al 1992 Joint effects of triglycerides and LDL cholesterol and HDL cholesterol concentrations on coronary heart disease risk in the Helsinki Heart Study. Implications for treatment. Circulation 85: 37–45

Mansfield MW, Haywood DM, Gran PJ 1996 Circulating levels of factor VII, fibrinogen and von Willibrand factor and features of insulin resistance in first-degree relatives of patients with NIDDM. Circulation 94: 2171–2176

Manson JE, Colditz GA, Stampfer MJ et al 1990 A prospective study of obesity and risk of coronary heart disease in women. New England Journal of Medicine 322: 882–889

Miles Fisher B 2000 Results of the Heart Outcome Prevention Evaluation (HOPE) study: implications for the care of people with diabetes. Modern Diabetes Management 1: 2–5

National Cholesterol Education Programme (NCEP) Expert Panel on Detection, Evaluation and Treatment of High Blood Cholesterol in Adults (Adult Treatment Panel III) 2001 Executive summary of the Third Report. Journal of the American Medical Association 285(19): 2486–2497

Parving HH et al, for the Irbesartan in Patients with Type 2 Diabetes and Microalbuminuria Study Group 2001 The effect of irbesartan on the development of diabetic nephropathy in patients with type 2 diabetes. New England Journal of Medicine 345: 870–878

Patel V et al 2001 The Hope study and the Micro Hope study. British Journal of Diabetes and Vascular Disease 1(1): 48, 50

Pinkney J 2001 Implications of obesity for diabetes and coronary heart disease in clinical practice. British Journal of Diabetes and Vascular Disease 1(2): 104, 105

Plotnick GD, Correti MC, Vogel RA 1997 Effect of antioxidant vitamins on the transient impairment of endothelium dependent brachial artery vasoactivity following a single high fat meal. Journal of the American Medical Association 278: 1682–1686

Pyorala K, Pedersen TR, Kjeksus J, Faergerman O, Olsson AG, Thorgeirsson G 1997 Cholesterol lowering with simvastatin improves prognosis of diabetic patients with coronary heart disease: a subgroup analysis of the Scandinavian Simvastatin Survival Study (4S). Diabetes Care 20: 614–620

Ravid M, Lang R, Rachmani R, Lishner M 1996 Longterm renoprotective effect of angiotensin converting enzyme inhibition in non-insulin dependent diabetes mellitus. A 7 year follow-up study. Archives of Internal Medicine 156: 286–289

Ravid M, Brosch D, Levi Z et al 1998 Use of enalapril to attenuate decline in renal function in normotensive, normoalbuminuric patients with type 2 diabetes. A randomised, controlled trial. Annals of Internal Medicine 128: 982–988

Reaven GM, Greenfield HS 1981 Diabetic hypertriglyceridaemia. Evidence for three clinical syndromes. Diabetes 31(suppl 2): 66–75

Richman RM, Steinbeck KS, Caterson ID 1992 Severe obesity: the use of very low energy diets or standard kilojoule restriction. Medical Journal of Australia 156: 768–770

Scandinavian Simvastatin Survival Study Group 1994 Randomized trial of cholesterol lowering in 4444 patients with coronary heart disease. Scandinavian Simvastatin Survival Study. Lancet 344: 1383–1389

Schoonjans K, Auwerx J 2000 Thiazolidinediones: an update. Lancet 355: 1008–1010

Stamler J, Vaccaro O, Neaton JD, Wentworth D, for the Multiple Risk Factor Intervention Trial Research Group 1993 Diabetes, other risk factors and 12-year cardiovascular mortality for men screened in the Multiple Risk Factor Intervention Trial. Diabetes Care 16: 434–444

Steinberg D 1997 Oxidative modification of LDL and atherogenesis. Circulation 95: 1062–1071

Steiner G and the DAIS Investigators 2001 Diabetes Atherosclerosis Intervention Study. Lancet 357: 9010

Stern N, Tuck ML 1996 Diabetes and hypertension. In: LeRoith D, Olefsky JM, Taylor S (eds) Diabetes mellitus: a fundamental and clinical test. Lippincott-Raven, New York

Syvanne M, Tasiken M-R 1997 Lipids and lipoproteins as coronary risk factors in non-insulin dependent diabetes mellitus. Lancet 350(suppl 1): 20–23

Syvanne M, Hilden H, Tasiken M-R 1994 Abnormal metabolism of post-prandial lipoproteins in patients with non-insulin dependent diabetes is not related to coronary artery disease. Journal of Lipids Research 35: 15–26

Tasiken M-R 1995 Dyslipidemia in non-insulin dependent diabetes. Cardiovascular Risk Factors 5: 22–29

Tasiken M-R 1999 Strategies for the management of diabetic dyslipidaemia. Drugs 58 (suppl 1): 47–51

Tuomilehto J, Rastenyte D, Birkenhager WH et al 1999 Effects of calcium-channel blockage in older patients with diabetes and systolic hypertension. New England Journal of Medicine 340: 677–684

Tuomilehto J, Lindstrom J, Eriksson JG et al 2001 Prevention of type 2 diabetes mellitus by changes in lifestyle among subjects with impaired glucose tolerance. New England Journal of Medicine 344: 1343–1350

Turner RC, Mills H, Neil HAW et al for the United Kingdom Prospective Diabetes Study (UKPDS) 1998 Risk factors for coronary artery disease in non-insulin-dependent diabetes mellitus: United Kingdom Prospective Diabetes Study (UKPDS 23). British Medical Journal 316: 823–828

UK Prospective Diabetes Study (UKPDS) 1995a Relative efficacy of randomly allocated diet, sulphonylureas, insulin, or metformin in patients with newly diagnosed non-insulin-dependent diabetes mellitus followed for three years (UKPDS 13). British Medical Journal 310: 83–88

UK Prospective Diabetes Study (UKPDS) 1995b Overview of 6 years' therapy of type 2 diabetes: a progressive disease (UKPDS 16). Diabetes 44: 1249–1258

UK Prospective Diabetes Study (UKPDS) 1998a Intensive blood glucose control with sulphonylureas or insulin compared with conventional treatment and risk of complications in patients with type 2 diabetes (UKPDS 33). Lancet 353: 837–853

UK Prospective Diabetes Study (UKPDS) 1998b Effect of intensive blood glucose control with metformin on complications in overweight patients with type 2 diabetes (UKPDS 34). Lancet 352: 854–865

UK Prospective Diabetes Study (UKPDS) 1998c Tight blood pressure control and risk of macrovascular and microvascular complications in type 2 diabetes (UKPDS 38). British Medical Journal 317: 703–713

UK Prospective Diabetes Study (UKPDS) 1998d Efficacy of atenolol and captopril in reducing risk of macrovascular and microvascular complications in type 2 diabetes (UKPDS 39). British Medical Journal 317: 713–720

UK Prospective Diabetes Study (UKPDS) 1999 Glycemic control with diet, sulphonylureas, metformin and insulin therapy in patients with type 2 diabetes: progressive requirement for multiple therapies. Journal of the American Medical Association 281: 2005–2012

Werner AL, Travaglini MT 2001 A review of rosiglitazone in type 2 diabetes mellitus. Pharmacotherapy 21: 1082–1099

Williams R The scale of problem of type 2 diabetes. In: Barnett AH (ed) The essence of type 2 diabetes. Medical Education Partnership, p 7

Wing RR, Epstein LH, Nowalk MP, Gooding W, Becker DL 1987 Long term effects of modest weight loss in type 2 diabetic patients. Archives of Internal Medicine 147: 1749–1753

Wingard DL, Barrett-Connor E 1995 Heart disease and diabetes. In: Harris MI (ed) Diabetes in America, 2nd edn. NIH publication 95-1468. National Institutes of Health, National Institutes of Diabetes and Digestive and Kidney Disease, Bethesda, MD

Wood D, Durrington P, McInnes G, Pulter N, Rees A, Wray A 1998 Joint British recommendations on prevention of coronary heart disease in clinical practice. Heart 80(suppl 2): S1–9

World Health Organization 1997 World Health Report. World Health Organization, Geneva

World Health Organization 2000 The Asia-Pacific perspective. Redefining obesity and its treatment. International Obesity Taskforce, International Association for the Study of Obesity, Hong Kong

Yki-Jarvinen H 1994 Pathogenesis of non-insulin-dependent diabetes mellitus. Lancet 343: 91–95

Zavaroni I, Bonora E, Pagliara M et al 1989 Risk factors for coronary artery disease in healthy persons with hyperinsulinemia and normal glucose tolerance. New England Journal of Medicine 320: 702–706

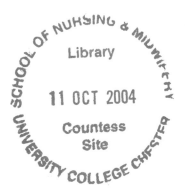

Index

Numbers in bold refer to boxes, figures and tables